# Pediatric Emergency Medicine
## BOARD REVIEW

Second Edition

William G. Gossman
Peter Emblad
Scott H. Plantz

**McGraw-Hill**
Medical Publishing Division

New York  Chicago  San Francisco  Lisbon  London
Madrid  Mexico City  Milan  New Delhi
San Juan  Seoul  Singapore
Sydney  Toronto

The McGraw·Hill Companies

**Pediatric Emergency Medicine Board Review, Second Edition**

Copyright © 2006 by The McGraw-Hill Companies, Inc. All rights reserved. Printed in the United States of America. Except as permitted under the United States Copyright Act of 1976, no part of this publication may be reproduced or distributed in any form or by any means, or stored in a data base or retrieval system, without the prior written permission of the publisher.

1 2 3 4 5 6 7 8 9 0    CUS/CUS    0 9 8 7 6 5

ISBN 0-07-146443-3

---

**Notice**

Medicine is an ever-changing science. As new research and clinical experience broaden our knowledge, changes in treatment and drug therapy are required. The authors and the publisher of this work have checked with sources believed to be reliable in their efforts to provide information that is complete and generally in accord with the standards accepted at the time of publication. However, in view of the possibility of human error or changes in medical sciences, neither the authors nor the publisher nor any other party who has been involved in the preparation or publication of this work warrants that the information contained herein is in every respect accurate or complete, and they disclaim all responsibility for any errors or omissions or for the results obtained from use of the information contained in this work. Readers are encouraged to confirm the information contained herein with other sources. For example and in particular, readers are advised to check the product information sheet included in the package of each drug they plan to administer to be certain that the information contained in this work is accurate and that changes have not been made in the recommended dose or in the contraindications for administration. This recommendation is of particular importance in connection with new or infrequently used drugs.

---

The editors were Catherine A. Johnson and Marsha Loeb.
The production supervisor was Phil Galea.
The cover designer was Handel Low.
Von Hoffmann Graphics was printer and binder.

This book is printed on acid-free paper.

**Cataloging-in-Publication data for this title is on file at the Library of Congress.**

# DEDICATION

*To my wife Sherry*

William Gossman

*To my daughter Annika, a source of endless amusement and amazement.
I look forward to watching you grow into the extraordinary woman
you are destined to become*

Peter Emblad

*To my wife Cynna*

Scott Plantz

**EDITORS:**

William Gossman M.D.
Assistant Professor
Department of Emergency Medicine
Chicago Medical School
North Chicago, IL

Peter Emblad, M.D.
Department of Emergency Medicine
San Franscisco Kaiser Hospital
San Francisco, CA

Scott H. Plantz, M.D.
Associate Professor
Department of Emergency Medicine
Chicago Medical School
Mt. Sinai Medical Center
Chicago, IL

**CONTRIBUTING AUTHORS:**

Bobby Abrams, M.D.
Attending Physician
Macomb Hospital
Macomb, MI

Jonathan Adler, M.D.
Instructor
Harvard Medical School
Boston, MA

Raymond C. Baker, M.D.
Professor of Clinical Pediatrics
University of Cincinnati College of Medicine
Associate Director
Division of General & Community Pediatrics
Children's Hospital
Cincinnati, OH

Kristen Bechtel, M.D., MCP
Assistant Professor of Emergency Medicine
Allegheny University of Health Sciences
Attending Physician
Department of Pediatric Emergency
St. Christopher's Hospital for Children
Philadelphia, PA

Michelle L. Bez, D.O.
Newcomb Medical Center
Vineland, NJ

Frank M. Biro, M.D.
Professor of Clinical Pediatrics
University of Cincinnati College of Medicine
Associate Director
Division of Adolescent Medicine
Children's Hospital
Cincinnati, OH

David F.M. Brown, M.D.
Instructor in Medicine
Harvard Medical School
Massachusetts General Hospital
Boston, MA

Sharona D. Bryant, M.D.
Assistant Professor of Emergency Medicine
Toxicology Fellow
Department of Emergency Medicine
MCP Hahnemann University
Attending Physician
Mercy Catholic Medical Center
Philadelphia, PA

Eduardo Castro, M.D.
Instructor in Medicine
Harvard Medical School
Massachusetts General Hospital
Boston, MA

Deandra Clark, M.D.
Department of Pediatrics
University of South Florida
Tampa, FL

David Cone, M.D.
Assistant Professor of Eme
Chief, Division of Emerger
Department of Emergency Medicine
Allegheny University of Health Sciences
Philadelphia, PA

Cheryl A. Coyle, RN, BSN, CCRN, CFRN, CEN, EMT
Life Flight Medical Crew Chief
University of Massachusetts Memorial Health Care
Worcester, MA

Carl W. Decker, M.D.
Madigan Army Medical Center
Fort Lewis, WA

Phillip G. Fairweather, M.D.
Clinical Assistant Professor
Mt. Sinai School of Medicine
New York, NY
Department of Emergency Medicine
Elmhurst Hospital Center
Elmhurst, NY

Craig Feied, M.D.
Associate Professor
Washington Hospital Center
George Washington University
Washington, D.C.

David Neal Franz, M.D.
Associate Professor of Pediatrics and Neurology
University of Cincinnati College of Medicine
Director
Tuberous Sclerosis Clinic
Children's Hospital
Cincinnati, OH

Anne Freter, RN, BSN
Intensive Care Unit
Hope Children's Hospital
Oak Lawn, IL

Lynn Garfunkel, M.D.
Assistant Professor of Pediatrics
Associate Director
Pediatrics Residency Training Program
Director
Combined Internal Medicine and Pediatric
Residency Training Program
University of Rochester School of Medicine and Dentistry
Rochester, NY

Marianne Gausche-Hill, MD, FACEP, FAAP
Associate Professor of Medicine,
UCLA School of Medicine
Director, Emergency Medical Services,
Harbor-UCLA Medical Center
Torrance, CA

Jay Gold, M.D.
MediStar
Madison, WI

Mitchell J. Goldman, DO, FAAEM, FAAP
Director, Pediatric Emergency Medicine
St. Vincent Emergency Physicians, Inc.
Indianapolis, IN

Javier A. Gonzalez del Rey, M.D.
Associate Professor
University of Cincinnati College of Medicine
Associate Director
Division of Emergency Medicine and
Pediatrics Residency Training Program
Director
Pediatrics Emergency Medicine Fellowship Program
Children's Hospital
Cinncinnati, OH

John Graneto, D.O.
Director, Pediatric Emergency Medicine
Lutheran General Children's Hospital
Park Ridge, IL

Michael I. Greenberg, M.D., MPH
Professor of Emergency Medicine
Professor of Public Health
Department of Emergency Medicine
Division of Toxicology
MCP Hahnemann University
Attending Physician
Mercy Catholic Medical Center
Philadelphia, PA

Guy H. Haskell, Ph.D., NREMT-P
Emergency Medical Services Instructor,
Educational Services
Emergency Paramedic, Ambulance Service
Bloomington Hospital and Healthcare System
Bloomington, IN

Ned Hayes, M.D.
Chief, Epidemiology Section
Bacterial Zoonoses Branch
Division of Vector-Borne Infectious Diseases
Centers for Disease Control and Prevention
Fort Collins, CO

Robert G. Hendrickson, M.D.
Instructor in Emergency Medicine
Toxicology Fellow
Department of Emergency Medicine
MCP Hahnemann University
Attending Physician
Mercy Catholic Medical Center
Philadelphia, PA

Melanie S. Heniff, MD, FAAEM, FAAP
Assistant Clinical Professor
Emergency Medicine and Pediatrics
Indiana University/Methodist Hospital
Indianapolis, IN

Rita Herrington-Mikels, BSN, RN, EMT-P
Emergency Medical Services Instructor
Bloomington Hospital and Healthcare System
Bloomington, IN

James F. Holmes, M.D.
University of California, Davis
School of Medicine
Sacramento, CA

Eddie Hooker, M.D.
Assistant Professor
University of Louisville
Louisville, KY

Ira Horowitz, M.D.
Director, Intermediate Intensive Care Unit
Department of Pediatrics
Division of Critical Care Medicine
Hope Children's Hospital
Christ Hospital and Medical Center
Oak Lawn, IL

Matt Kopp, M.D.
Department of Emergency Medicine
Rhode Island Hospital
Brown University School of Medicine
Providence, RI

Lieutenant Robert C. Krause, EMT-P
Toledo Fire & Rescue Department
Toledo, OH

Lance W. Kreplick, M.D.
Assistant Professor
University of Illinois
Christ Hospital
Oak Lawn, IL

Deborah A. Lee, M.D., Ph.D.
Assistant Professor
Department of Psychiatry
Clinical Assistant Professor
Department of Pediatrics
Director
Child Neurology TP
Tulane University
New Orleans, LA

Robert M. Levin, M.D.
Health Officer
Ventura County Public Health
Ventura, CA

Gillian Lewke Emblad, PA, CMA
Physician Assistant
San Mateo County Hospital
San Mateo, CA
St. Francis Hospital
San Francisco, CA
Summit Alta Bates
Oakland, CA

Bernard Lopez, M.D.
Assistant Professor
Thomas Jefferson Medical College
Thomas Jefferson University Hospital
Philadelphia, PA

Mary Nan S. Mallory, M.D.
Instructor
University of Louisville
Louisville, KY

Mariann M. Manno, M.D., FAAP
Assistant Professor of Pediatrics
Director, Division of Pediatric Emergency Medicine
University Of Massachusetts Medical School
Worcester, MA

Bridget A. Martell, M.D.
Yale New Haven Hospital
Huguenot, NY

David Morgan, M.D.
Jules Stein Eye Institute
Los Angeles, CA

Anthony Morocco, M.D.
Instructor in Emergency Medicine
Toxicology Fellow
Department of Emergency Medicine
MCP Hahnemann University
Attending Physician
Mercy Catholic Medical Center
Philadelphia, PA

James J. Nordlund, M.D.
Professor
Department of Dermatology
University of Cincinnati College of Medicine
Children's Hospital
Cincinnati, OH

Peter Noronha, M.D.
Associate Professor of Clinical Pediatrics
Associate Program Director of Pediatrics
University of Illinois College of Medicine
Chicago, IL

Scott E. Olitsky, M.D.
Assistant Professor
Residency Program Director
Department of Ophthalmology
State University of New York at Buffalo and the
Children's Hospital of Buffalo
Buffalo, NY

Robert L. Palmer, PA-C, REMT-P
Boston Medflight
Boston, MA

Geraldo Reyes, M.D.
Director
Critical Care Training
Hope Children's Hospital
Oak Lawn, IL

Luis R. Rodriquez, M.D., FAAP
Assistant Professor
Department of Pediatrics
Mt. Sinai School of Medicine
New York, NY
Elmhurst Hospital Center
Elmhurst, NY

Carlo Rosen, M.D.
Instructor
Harvard Medical School
Massachusetts General Hospital
Boston, MA

Bruce K. Rubin, M.D.
Professor of Pediatrics, Physiology and Pharmacology
Brenner Children's Hospital
Winston-Salem, NC

Howard M. Saal, M.D.
Professor of Clinical Pediatrics
University of Cincinnati College of Medicine
Head, Clinical Genetics
Director, Medical Genetics Residency Program
Children's Hospital
Cincinnati, OH

Alan Schooley, M.D.
Children's Hospital
Boston, MA

Girish D. Sharma, M.D., FCCP
Assistant Professor
Section of Pediatric Pulmonology
The University of Chicago Children's Hospital
Chicago, IL

Rejesh Shenoy, M.D.
Department of Pediatrics
University of Illinois College of Medicine
Chicago, IL

Mahesh Shrestha, M.D.
Assistant Professor of Emergency Medicine
Toxicology Fellow
Department of Emergency Medicine
MCP Hahnemann University
Attending Physician
Mercy Catholic Medical Center
Philadelphia, PA

Clifford S. Spanierman, M.D., FAAP
Pediatric Emergency Physician
Department of Emergency Medicine
Lutheran General Children's Hospital
Park Ridge, IL

Dana Stearns, M.D.
Instructor
Harvard Medical School
Massachusetts General Hospital
Boston, MA

Jack Stump, M.D.
Attending Physician
Rogue Valley Medical Center
Medford, OR

Loice Swischer, M.D.
Medical College of Pennsylvania
Philadelphia, PA

Nicholas Tapas, M.D.
General Pediatrician
Lutheran General Children's Hospital
Park Ridge, IL

Hector Trujillo, M.D.
General Pediatrician
Miami Children's Hospital
Miami, FL

William T. Zempsky, M.D.
Associate Director, Assistant Professor
Division of Pediatric Emergency Medicine,
University of Connecticut
Connecticut Children's Medical Center
Hartford, CT

Michael Zevitz, M.D.
Assistant Professor
Chicago Medical School
Chicago, IL

Huiquan Zhao, M.D., Ph.D.  
Divison of Human Genetics  
Department of Pediatrics  
Children's Hospital  
Cincinnati, OH

Stan Zuba M.D.  
Assistant Professor of Pediatrics  
RUSH/The Chicago Medical School  
Chicago, IL

# INTRODUCTION

Congratulations! *Pediatric Emergency Medicine Board Review: Pearls of Wisdom*, will help you learn some medicine. Originally designed as a study aid to improve performance on the Emergency Pediatric Written Board exams or Emergency Pediatric In-service exam, This book is full of useful information. A few words are appropriate discussing intent, format, limitations, and use.

Since *Pediatric Emergency Medicine Board Review* is primarily intended as a study aid, the text is written in rapid-fire question/answer format. This way, readers receive immediate gratification. Moreover, misleading or confusing "foils" are not provided. This eliminates the risk of erroneously assimilating an incorrect piece of information that makes a big impression. Questions themselves often contain a "pearl" intended to reinforce the answer. Additional "hooks" may be attached to the answer in various forms, including mnemonics, visual imagery, repetition, and humor. Additional information not requested in the question may be included in the answer. Emphasis has been placed on distilling trivia and key facts that are easily overlooked, that are quickly forgotten, and that somehow seem to be needed on board examinations.

Many questions have answers without explanations. This enhances ease of reading and rate of learning. Explanations often occur in a later question/answer. Upon reading an answer, the reader may think, "Hm, why is that?" or, "Are you sure?" If this happens to you, go check! Truly assimilating these disparate facts into a framework of knowledge absolutely requires further reading of the surrounding concepts. Information learned in response to seeking an answer to a particular question is retained much better than information that is passively observed. Take advantage of this! Use this book with your preferred source texts handy and open.

*Pediatric Emergency Medicine Board Review* has limitations. We have found many conflicts between sources of information. We have tried to verify in several references the most accurate information. Some texts have internal discrepancies further confounding clarification.

*Pediatric Emergency Medicine Board Review* risks accuracy by aggressively pruning complex concepts down to the simplest kernel—the dynamic knowledge base and clinical practice of medicine is not like that! Furthermore, new research and practice occasionally deviates from that which likely represents the right answer for test purposes. This text is designed to maximize your score on a test. Refer to your most current sources of information and mentors for direction.

*Pediatric Emergency Medicine Board Review* is designed to be used, not just read. It is an *interactive* text. Use a 3 x 5 card and cover the answers; attempt all questions. A study method we recommend is oral, group study, preferably over an extended meal or pitchers. The mechanics of this method are simple and no one ever appears stupid. One person holds the book, with answers covered, and reads the question. Each person, including the reader, says "Check!" when he or she has an answer in mind. After everyone has "checked" in, someone states his/her answer. If this answer is correct, on to the next one; if not, another person says their answer or the answer can be read. Usually the person who "checks" in first receives the first shot at stating the answer. If this person is being a smarty-pants answer-hog, then others can take turns. Try it, it's almost fun!

*Pediatric Emergency Medicine Board Review* is also designed to be re-used several times to allow, dare we use the word, memorization. A hollow bullet is provided for any scheme of keeping track of questions answered correctly or incorrectly.

We welcome your comments, suggestions and criticism. Great effort has been made to verify these questions and answers. Some answers may not be the answer you would prefer. Most often this is attributable to variance between original sources. Please make us aware of any errors you find. We hope to make continuous improvements and would greatly appreciate any input with regard to format, organization, content, presentation, or about specific questions. We also are interested in recruiting new contributing authors and publishing new textbooks. We look forward to hearing from you!

Study hard and good luck!

W.G., P.E., & S.P.

# TABLE OF CONTENTS

| | |
|---|---|
| EMERGENCY MEDICAL SERVICES | 13 |
| PEDIATRIC LIFE SUPPORT | 17 |
| INFECTIOUS DISEASES | 67 |
| CARDIOVASCULAR | 93 |
| SEDATION AND ANALGESIA | 125 |
| PULMONARY | 131 |
| GASTROINTESTINAL | 147 |
| TOXICOLOGY AND ENVIRONMENTAL | 163 |
| METABOLIC, ENDOCRINE AND NUTRITION | 231 |
| SUDDEN INFANT DEATH SYNDROME AND APPARENT LIFE-THREATENING EVENT | 243 |
| NEUROLOGY | 245 |
| RHEUMATOLOGY, IMMUNOLOGY AND ALLERGY | 257 |
| GENITOURINARY AND RENAL | 263 |
| HEMATOLOGY AND ONCOLOGY | 271 |
| DERMATOLOGY | 277 |
| SURGICAL EMERGENCIES | 283 |
| TRAUMA | 289 |
| ORTHOPEDIC EMERGENCIES | 301 |
| EYES, EARS, NOSE, THROAT & NECK | 309 |
| PSYCHOSOCIAL AND CHILD ABUSE | 317 |
| OBSTETRICS AND GYNECOLOGY | 325 |
| IMAGING PEARLS | 337 |
| STATISTICS AND PREVENTIVE | 347 |
| LEGAL PEARLS | 349 |
| RANDOM PEARLS | 357 |
| BIBLIOGRAPHY | 375 |

# EMERGENCY MEDICAL SERVICES

○ **At which three levels of government should EMS-C be integrated into EMS?**

It must be integrated at the state, regional and local levels.

○ **Which two agencies provide funding for education, training and research needed by EMS systems to treat pediatric patients?**

1. U.S. Dept. of Health and Human Services, Health Services and Resources Administration, Maternal and Child Health Branch.
2. The National Highway Traffic Safety Administration.

○ **Identify the four links in pediatric Chain of Survival.**

Injury prevention, early CPR, early access to EMS, and early advanced life support.

○ **List the two components of the first link (injury prevention) in the Chain of Survival for pediatric emergencies.**

Identification of problems and early intervention.

○ **When does entry into the EMS system occur?**

Entry into the EMS system occurs when the rescuer or bystander calls local EMS and speaks with a dispatcher.

○ **EMS dispatchers often provide a caller with pre-arrival directions. Who dictates what information is given to the caller?**

The information given callers varies widely and is controlled by local jurisdiction.

○ **Explain the advantages of using established dispatcher protocols when providing a caller with pre-arrival instructions.**

Use of dispatcher protocols will reduce the variability of information provided by dispatchers and ensure that succinct, accurate emergency information is provided to every caller in need of emergency assistance.

○ **In the broad scope, "who" is actually the first link in the Chain of Survival?**

The first link in the Chain of Survival is the general public.

○ **Who is included in this "first link" as it applies to children?**

Parents, caretakers, older siblings, and school personnel, who must be educated about the proper use of the EMS system.

○ **Approximately what percentage of EMS contacts in both rural and urban areas are children under 14 years of age?**

10%.

○ **For children younger than five years of age, is the EMS system most frequently activated for trauma or medical illness?**

Medical illness.

○ **Serious illness, including cardiopulmonary arrest, is most common in children of what age?**

2 years of age.

○ **A child-size ventilation bag used for resuscitation should have a reservoir of at least _____ ml but no more than _____ ml.**

450ml; 750ml.

○ **The use of a rigid cervical collar is often difficult in a small pediatric patient. Describe an alternative to this device.**

Cervical immobilization of small infants may be better achieved by the use of towels and tape rather than a rigid collar, which may not fit properly.

○ **Using a conservative estimate, how many persons aged 0 to 19 years have permanent disabilities from traumatic brain injuries annually?**

Approximately 29,000.

○ **How can a child acquire status of an "emancipated minor"?**

Marriage, judicial decree, military service, parental consent, failure of parents to meet legal responsibilities, living apart from and being financially independent of parents, motherhood.

○ **An EMT responds to a call where there is a question as to the authenticity of documents stating the victim's intent to refuse CPR. The victim is in cardiac arrest. What should the EMT do?**

The practice of initiating resuscitative efforts is generally accepted. CPR may be discontinued with further authentication of the patient's wishes or with a MD order.

○ **T/F: The Good Samaritan law protects the EMT from acts of negligence.**

False. The traditional legal concept holds the EMT to a "reasonable care" standard. The circumstances surrounding the incident are evaluated and the skill level of the rescuer is taken into consideration.

○ **Should the first responder attempt to assess resuscitatability of the cardiac arrest patient and then determine whether or not to initiate CPR?**

No. First responders are encouraged to initiate CPR in the cardiac arrest victim. Currently there are no accepted criteria for immediate determination of death by first responders. There are few exceptions to this rule.

○ **When does the legal duty to meet a "reasonable standard" of care commence for the healthcare provider?**

Once he or she performs an act that may be construed as rendering care.

○ **What are "mature minor" rules?**

Statutory rules that uphold the validity of consent given by minors if the treatment is appropriate and the minor is considered capable of comprehending the clinical circumstances and therapeutic options.

○ **T/F: Medical malpractice cases concerning CPR have been limited to in-hospital cases in which the risk of cardiac arrest could be anticipated.**

True. Successful action against laypersons that attempt out-of-hospital CPR seems unlikely.

○ **Once you have initiated CPR, do you incur a legal liability to continue?**

Once steps are initiated and termination would place the victim in a worse position or compromise the likelihood of assistance from others, the potential rescuer incurs a legal duty to perform appropriately.

○ **Do statutes cover events that take place during transport to a medical facility?**

Rescue settings vary by statute. In some states only actions at the site of the emergency are covered; other states include events during transport to a medical facility.

○ **Why should first responders not fear litigation from making reasonable attempts at CPR?**

Because CPR attempts in emergencies are likely to be viewed as reasonable, even when provided by an inadequately trained rescuer, as long as there is a good-faith belief that the possible benefits of the attempt outweigh the risk from the rescuer's incompetence.

○ **On what does the paramedic's scope of practice rely?**

Standing order protocols and offline medical direction (indirect medical control).

○ **Must pre-hospital personnel honor hospital DNR orders?**

Many state laws still make it illegal for pre-hospital personnel to honor a hospital DNR order.

○ **May an EMT disregard or countermand an order given by a physician?**

Not as a rule. However, most EMS systems have specific policies dealing with this issue. The procedure used varies widely from system to system.

○ **At what age can an automated external defibrillator (AED) be used in children?**

Eight or older.

○ **Why is hypothermia a particular concern in the field treatment of small children?**

Children have poorly developed heat regulation mechanisms (e.g. poor shivering), and a relatively larger surface area to volume ratio than adults. Accordingly, infants and small children are more likely to become hypothermic if exposed to the cold for prolonged periods, as may occur during extrication from a motor vehicle crash.

# PEDIATRIC LIFE SUPPORT

○ **T/F: Primary cardiac arrest is the most common cause of death in young children.**

False. It is uncommon in children. Respiratory arrest usually precedes cardiac arrest.

○ **What percent of children present with ventricular fibrillation as a cause of pulseless arrest outside of the hospital?**

10-15%. Most are in asystole.

○ **Ventricular fibrillation is more likely in which patients?**

Children > 10, submersion victims, those with congenital heart disease and in-hospital arrest.

○ **What is the common primary cause of pulseless cardiac arrest?**

Injury or disease leading to respiratory or circulatory failure.

○ **Cardiopulmonary arrest occurs predominately in which two pediatric age groups?**

Infants < 1year, and adolescents.

○ **What is the most common cause of death in children >1 year of age?**

Injury.

○ **Motor vehicle trauma accounts for what percent of all pediatric injuries and deaths?**

Almost 50%.

○ **What is the most important device to prevent pediatric motor vehicle injuries and deaths?**

A properly installed child restraint device.

○ **What percent of head injuries could bike helmets eliminate?**

85% of head injuries and 88% of brain injuries.

○ **What percent of fire-related deaths result from house fires?**

80%.

○ **T/F: Firearms are a leading cause of accidental death and injury in children.**

True.

○ **T/F: The presence of a gun in the home is linked to adolescent suicide.**

True.

○ **T/F: An awake child with respiratory distress should be laid on the ground or on a stretcher.**

False. Children with partial airway obstruction will find the most comfortable position on their own.

○ **If the child is conscious, when should EMS be activated?**

Immediately.

○ **If the child is unconscious, how long should the rescuer provide BLS before activating EMS?**

1 minute. Most pediatric arrests are respiratory in origin, so one minute may be enough to restore ventilation and oxygenation or prevent respiratory arrest from progressing to cardiac arrest.

○ **In an unconscious child, when should EMS be immediately activated?**

When two rescuers are present.

○ **What should be done if trauma is suspected?**

Complete immobilization of the spine.

○ **How can the airway be opened in an unconscious, apneic victim?**

Head tilt chin-lift, and jaw thrust.

○ **How can the airway be opened in an unconscious, apneic victim if neck trauma is suspected?**

Jaw thrust with neck immobilized.

○ **How is the head tilt-chin lift performed?**

One hand is used to tilt head and gently extend the neck. The index finger of the opposite hand lifts the chin outward.

○ **After the airway is established, how does the rescuer assess breathing?**

Looks for rise and fall of the chest, listens for exhaled air, feels for exhaled airflow at the mouth.

○ **What is the recovery position used for?**

When the victim is unconscious but has no evidence of trauma and is breathing effectively.

○ **How is the victim moved into the recovery position?**

The head, torso, and shoulders are moved simultaneously so that the victim is on his or her side.

○ **T/F: Rescue breathing is provided for all victims.**

False. Only those victims who have no spontaneous breathing.

○ **In infants, how should rescue breaths be provided?**

By placing your mouth over the victim's nose and mouth.

○ **How many breaths are supplied in rescue breathing?**

Two slow breaths, 1-1.5 seconds each separated by a pause to take a breath.

○ **What is the purpose of the pause between rescue breaths?**

To maximize oxygen content.

○ **How does the rescuer know if ventilation is not effective?**

The child's chest does not rise.

○ **Why should breaths be delivered slowly?**

To minimize the pressure required for ventilation, and prevent gastric distension.

○ **What is the most common cause of an airway obstruction?**

Laxity in the tongue causing it to fall back on the pharynx.

○ **What should the rescuer do if ventilation is unsuccessful?**

Reposition the head in the midline, place a towel under the shoulders and consider progressively extending the neck, provided trauma is not suspected.

○ **How may a second rescuer prevent gastric distension?**

Provide cricoid pressure.

○ **What happens when cricoid pressure is administered?**

The trachea is displaced posteriorly compressing the esophagus against the vertebral column.

○ **In a patient with a tracheostomy, how is air leakage prevented during rescue breathing?**

The victim's mouth and nose are sealed by the rescuer's hand or a tight fitting mask.

○ **When should the rescuer determine the need for chest compressions?**

After the airway is opened and two rescue breaths provided.

○ **T/F: If the child is not breathing, chest compressions are usually required.**

True. Heart rate and stroke volume are probably not adequate if the child is not breathing.

○ **What complications are common in children who receive CPR?**

None. Rib fractures in children are usually attributable to preceding trauma.

○ **How long should the layperson spend looking for a pulse in a non-breathing child?**

No time. Laypersons often have difficulty recognizing pulses and should begin chest compressions immediately if the patient is not breathing or moving.

○ **Where should the pulse be checked by health care professionals in infants?**

Brachial artery.

○ **Where should the pulse be checked by health care professionals in children?**

The carotid artery should be used in children greater than 1 year of age.

○ **If a pulse is present, how often should breaths be given?**

At a rate of 20 per minute.

○ **If a pulse is present, when should EMS be activated?**

After 20 breaths or one minute.

○ **What is the purpose of chest compressions?**

To circulate oxygen-containing blood to the vital organs.

○ **What are the two theories for the mechanism of blood flow during chest compressions?**

Thoracic pump theory and cardiac pump theory.

○ **To achieve optimal compressions, how should the child be positioned?**

Supine on a hard, flat surface.

○ **Where should you perform chest compressions on infants?**

Lower half of the sternum.

○ **How far should the infant's sternum be depressed during compressions?**

1/3 to 1/2 the depth of the chest.

○ **What should the rate of compressions be during infant CPR?**

At least 100 times per minute.

○ **What should the compression to ventilation ratio be?**

5:1.

○ **Children fall into what age-range for the purposes of BLS?**

Ages 1 year to 8 years.

○ **T/F: Compressions in children should be performed with the fingers.**

False. Compressions should be performed with the heel of the hand.

○ **What should the compression rate in children be?**

100 times per minute.

○ **What should the compression to ventilation ratio in children be?**

5:1.

○ **How often should the infant and child be reassessed?**

After 20 cycles of compressions and ventilation and every few minutes thereafter.

○ **How is airway patency maintained during compressions?**

The hand not doing compressions is used to maintain the head tilt.

○ **T/F: The majority of deaths from foreign body aspiration occur in children less than five years of age.**

True.

○ **When should attempts to clear the airway be considered?**

When foreign-body aspiration is witnessed or strongly suspected and when the airway remains obstructed during rescue breathing attempts.

○ **T/F: Relief of airway obstruction should be attempted for all patients with foreign body aspiration.**

False. Only if signs of complete obstruction are observed.

○ **For infants, what is the method by which complete foreign body obstruction is relieved?**

A combination of back blows and chest thrusts.

○ **Why should the Heimlich maneuver not be performed on infants?**

There is a potential for liver injuries in these patients.

○ **Why should blind finger sweeps be avoided?**

The foreign body may be pushed back into the airway.

○ **How should back blows be delivered in an infant?**

Hold the infant face down, resting on forearm. The head should be lower than the trunk. Deliver back blows between scapulae with heel of hand.

○ **T/F: Chest thrusts in a choking infant are delivered in the same manner as chest compressions.**

True.

○ **How many back blows should be given?**

Five.

○ **How long should the rescuer continue the series of back blows and chest thrusts?**

Until the object is expelled or the infant becomes unresponsive.

O    **How are foreign bodies expelled in the conscious child?**

Abdominal thrusts while standing behind victim.

O    **What method should be used to open the airway in the trauma victim?**

Jaw-thrust ensuring that spinal stabilization has been achieved.

O    **Why is it difficult to maintain neutral c-spine position in infants and young children?**

Prominent occiput predisposes the neck to slight flexion when the child is placed on a flat surface; this is why it is recommended to place a small towel under the shoulders to maintain the neck in neutral position.

O    **What is the dosing regimen for Lidocaine in RSI?**

1-2mg/kg IV.

O    **What is the dosing regimen for ketamine is RSI?**

1-4mg/kg IV/IM.

O    **What are the main negative side effects of ketamine?**

Hallucinations, emergence reaction, increasing intracranial pressure, laryngospasm, and increased intraocular pressure.

O    **What is the purpose of administering Lidocaine in RSI?**

To reduce ICP.

O    **What are the three main neuromuscular blocking agents used in RSI?**

Succinylcholine, vecuronium, rocuronium.

O    **Of the above medications, which is depolarizing?**

Succinylcholine.

O    **What is the dosing regimen for succinylcholine?**

1mg/kg in children, 2mg/kg in infants, IV/IM (IM dose double the IV dose).

O    **What is the duration of succinylcholine?**

3-5 minutes.

O    **What is the onset of action of succinylcholine?**

Very rapid.

O    **What is the dosing regimen for vecuronium?**

0.1-0.2mg/kg IV/IM.

○ **What is the duration of vecuronium?**

30-60 minutes.

○ **What is the onset of action of vecuronium?**

2-3 minutes.

○ **What is the dosing regimen of rocuronium?**

0.6-1.2mg/kg.

○ **What is the duration of rocuronium?**

30-45 minutes.

○ **What is the onset of action of rocuronium?**

Rapid.

○ **During mechanical ventilation the effectiveness of ventilation and oxygenation must be verified using what laboratory test?**

Arterial blood gas analysis.

○ **Your patient has been placed on a mechanical ventilator in preparation for transport. How long after the initial ventilatory settings have been made should an arterial blood gas analysis be completed?**

After ten to fifteen minutes.

○ **When using a volume-cycled ventilator, what is the recommended tidal volume that should be delivered to the patient?**

8 – 10 ml/kg.

○ **When discussing mechanical ventilators, what does the acronym PEEP stand for?**

Positive End-Expiratory Pressure.

○ **How often should the blood pressure of a hemodynamically unstable child be assessed?**

Blood pressure should be assessed every 5 minutes until stable and every 15 minutes thereafter. Attention to the patient's heart rate must also be closely monitored.

○ **Explain the advantage of inserting a nasogastric tube.**

The tube prevents gastric distention caused by air and is particularly useful during positive-pressure ventilation.

○ **You are caring for an infant that weighs 8 kg. What is the proper volume and rate of IV fluid administration for a patient smaller than 10kg?**

The proper fluid requirement in a patient smaller than 10kg is 4ml/kg per hour (e.g., the maintenance rate for an 8 kg baby is 4 ml x 8 kg = 32 ml/hour).

O  You have been asked to set the initial mechanical ventilator settings for a patient who is intubated. After assessing the patient's airway you determine the tube is properly placed and the patient has normal lung compliance. What is the recommended peak inspiratory pressure and inspiratory time for this patient with normal lung compliance?

Effective ventilation may be achieved at peak inspiratory pressures of 20 to 30 cm water and an inspiratory time of 0.5 to 1.0 second.

O  When mechanical ventilatory support is provided for the patient with normal lungs, a respiratory rate of _____ to _____ breaths per minute is typically required for infants and a rate of _____ to _____ breaths per minute for children.

Infants: 20 to 30 breaths per minute.
Children: 16 to 20 breaths per minute.

O  Explain the advantage of using neuromuscular blocking agents during mechanical ventilation of a child with air trapping?

The use of neuromuscular blocking agents is advisable during mechanical ventilation of the child with air trapping because the child's spontaneous respiratory effort often contributes to further airway obstruction.

O  Intubation bypasses glottic function and eliminates the physiologic positive end-expiratory pressure (PEEP) created during normal coughing, talking and crying. What should the PEEP setting be on the ventilator to maintain adequate functional residual capacity of the lungs?

To maintain adequate functional residual capacity, a PEEP of 2 to 4 cm water should be provided when mechanical ventilation is initiated.

O  List two primary advantages of using noninvasive monitoring devices such as pulse oximeters, transcutaneous oxygen and carbon dioxide monitors, and exhaled carbon dioxide monitors.

These tools are very useful because they allow continuous assessment of oxygenation, ventilation, or both.

O  Noninvasive monitoring devices such as those referenced in the above question may provide inaccurate data as a result of what types of medical conditions or equipment problems?

Hypothermia, poor peripheral perfusion, or endotracheal tube obstruction or displacement.

O  You are the attending physician in the ER. While evaluating a six year-old male (GCS 6), you observe the child has significant central nervous system depression following a fall from the front porch of his home. In addition to BLS care, what procedure should be initiated until intracranial pressure can be evaluated more thoroughly?

Intubate and hyperventilate with the $PaCO_2$ maintained at 30-35mm Hg until intracranial pressure can be evaluated more thoroughly. Also elevate the HOB to 30-35 degrees.

O  T/F: Hypotension is a late sign of shock and requires rapid intervention.

True.

O  If central venous access has been established, continuous or intermittent measurement of what type of pressure may help guide fluid administration and titration of vasoactive support?

Right heart filling.

○ **When should an orogastric or nasogastric tube be inserted into a patient, and what is its purpose?**

If bowel sounds are absent, abdominal distention is present, or the patient requires mechanical ventilation, an orogastric or nasogastric tube should be inserted to prevent or treat gastric distention.

○ **Why is blind nasogastric tube placement contraindicated in the patient with serious facial trauma?**

Intracranial tube placement may result.

○ **Congratulations! After months of work you have been selected to head the committee that is developing a pediatric transport system. Ideally, which institution should provide central control?**

The tertiary care facility.

○ **What minimum qualifications should the director of the transport service have?**

Training in pediatric emergency medicine or critical care.

○ **What is the lowest level of care that should be considered acceptable in a transport team?**

The transport team should be capable of providing pediatric ALS at the referring hospital and maintaining that level of care during transport.

○ **Which two agencies should be responsible for the establishment of well-defined protocols for specific clinical situations that arise during transport of an ill or injured child?**

The referring facility and the tertiary care unit.

○ **Once started, how long must a physician continue to administer CPR?**

As necessary until the victim is transferred to the care of other properly trained personnel or until cardiac death (as defined by cardiovascular unresponsiveness to acceptable resuscitative techniques) is determined.

○ **What is the most frequently used site for central venous cannulation and why?**

The femoral vein is the most frequently used central vein because it is large, anatomically reliable and can be cannulated without interrupting resuscitation.

○ **T/F: If a central line will soon be available, delay administering medications and fluids until it is established.**

False, establishment of a central line should not delay the administration of resuscitation medications and fluids.

○ **What equipment is important for the safe administration of fluids and medications in infants and young children?**

Infusion pumps or volume limiting devices such as minidrip chambers (if pumps are not available) should be used to safely administer fluid boluses and medication infusions in infants and young children.

❍ **During CPR in young children what strategy should be followed for establishing vascular access?**

In general, intraosseous access should be established following three attempts at peripheral vascular access (approximately 90 seconds).

❍ **Is intraosseous access appropriate for children older than 6 years of age?**

Yes. The PALS 2000 guidelines have removed the upper age limit for intraosseous access. However, keep in mind that intraosseous access becomes progressively more difficult in older children. If intraosseous access must be attempted in older patients, needles with threaded tips and alternative sites (iliac crest) should be considered to ensure success.

❍ **Does a particular site insure more rapid delivery of medications to the central circulation during CPR?**

There is no significant difference between peripheral, intraosseous or central access with respect to onset of drug action or peak drug levels.

❍ **What should always be done immediately following a bolus infusion?**

It is important to follow medication delivery with a 5 cc fluid bolus to flush the drug to the central circulation.

❍ **What is the most important factor in determining route of intravenous access?**

Rapid access should be sought using the technique with which the medical personnel are most familiar.

❍ **What is the indication for ETT medication administration?**

If IV/IO access cannot be established within 3-5 minutes, the ETT is an important route for administration of medications.

❍ **What resuscitation medications can be infused through the ETT?**

Lidocaine, epinephrine, atropine, naloxone (L.E.A.N.).

❍ **What veins should be attempted for peripheral access during resuscitation?**

Greater saphenous (medial surface of the ankle) and the median cubital (antecubital fossa of elbow).

❍ **When should scalp veins be used?**

Scalp veins are of value when nonemergent fluids and medications are needed or in postresuscitation treatment as a temporizing measure until definitive access is achieved.

❍ **What are the most common causes of sclerosis and skin sloughing following IV cannulation?**

Sclerosis and skin sloughing are most often related to necrotizing medications such as calcium and dextrose.

❍ **What are complications of intraosseous cannulation?**

Tibial fracture, compartment syndrome, osteomyelitis and skin cellulitis.

❍ **What site is generally recommended for the placement of an intraosseous needle?**

The anteromedial tibial surface 2-3 cm. below the tibial tuberosity is the preferred site for intraosseous needle placement in children.

❍ **What are signs that intraosseous insertion is successful?**

The subjective sense of a decrease in resistance as the needle passes through the cortex and into the marrow, the needle is stable in the bone and remains upright without support, marrow can be aspirated through the needle into a syringe and infusion through the needle does not show evidence of infiltration of the soft tissue.

❍ **What should you do if you are unsuccessful on your first attempt at intraosseous cannulation?**

This same site cannot be used again. The procedure should be attempted on the other leg.

❍ **What are two advantages of central venous access in resuscitation?**

Central venous access allows rapid delivery of drugs to the central circulation and also allows monitoring of central venous pressures.

❍ **Are central venous lines, peripheral lines, or intraosseous lines more subject to complications?**

Central lines are clearly associated with more serious complications then peripheral or intraosseous lines. The specific complications are a function of the site of the central line.

❍ **What complications are associated with all central lines?**

Local and systemic infection, bleeding, phlebitis, thrombosis, catheter fragment and embolism.

❍ **What complications are associated with central lines in the neck?**

Pneumothorax, hydrothorax, and hemothorax.

❍ **What general techniques have been employed in achieving central venous access in children?**

Both through the needle and over the needle catheter placement has been used to establish central venous access in children.

❍ **Are complications more common in central lines in children or adults?**

They are more common in younger patients.

❍ **What are the hazards of through the needle catheter placement?**

The catheter can be sheared off by the sharp needle during placement of a through the needle catheter.

❍ **When does catheter shear usually occur when placing a through-the-needle catheter?**

This usually occurs when resistance is encountered as the catheter is advanced and the catheter has been withdrawn through the needle.

❍ **What can be done to reduce the possibility of catheter shear?**

The catheter should never be withdrawn through the needle. The entire catheter and needle apparatus should be withdrawn as a unit to prevent the complications of catheter shearing.

○ **What is the most commonly used technique for central venous access in children?**

The Seldinger technique, which uses a guide wire to establish catheter placement.

○ **What is the most frequently used site for central venous access and why?**

The femoral vein is most frequently used because of its lower incidence of complications than central access in the neck, as well as the ease of starting a line far from the head and neck, which would interfere with CPR and airway management.

○ **What are the advantages of cannulating the external jugular vein?**

The external jugular vein is a superficial vessel that is easily visible. When cannulated there is a large IV that allows rapid infusion of drugs and medication. An external jugular line on occasion can be converted to a central line, but this is at times impossible because of the acute angle of the external jugular into the subclavian vein.

○ **Where is the saphenous vein most easily palpated?**

Anterior to the medial malleolus.

○ **What two methods are used for cannulating the saphenous vein?**

Blind stick or through a cut-down.

○ **What are complications of arterial catheters?**

Infection, embolus, arterial thrombus, ischemia or damage to the effective limb.

○ **What is the most common complication of radial artery catheterization in children?**

Radial artery occlusion.

○ **What are acceptable sites for arterial catheterization?**

Radial, brachial, axillary, femoral, dorsalis pedis, and posterior tibial arteries.

○ **Which two of the these are preferred?**

Radial and femoral artery.

○ **What is the most significant physiological change undergone by the neonate?**

The transition from fetal to neonatal circulation.

○ **What system must become instantly functional in this transition?**

The respiratory system, essentially nonfunctional in utero, must suddenly initiate and maintain oxygenation and ventilation.

○ **What is required to assist the majority of term newborns in making this transition?**

Maintenance of temperature, suctioning of the airway, and mild stimulation.

○ **Of the small number of newborns that require further intervention, most respond to what?**

Administration of a high concentration of inspired oxygen and ventilation with a bag and mask.

○ **What measure may be necessary if oxygen and bagging don't work?**

Chest compressions.

○ **What is the least commonly required intervention in newborn resuscitation?**

Resuscitative medications.

○ **What does the "inverted pyramid" illustrate?**

The relative frequencies and priorities of neonatal resuscitation.

○ **What must follow each step in the pyramid to prevent unnecessary intervention and potential complications?**

Reassessment.

○ **If there is a history of particulate meconium in the amniotic fluid, what should the resuscitation team be prepared to do?**

Suction the mouth and nose and consider suctioning of the trachea under direct visualization.

○ **Which critical metabolic derangement can be exacerbated by hypothermia in the newborn?**

Acidosis.

○ **How should the newborn be positioned?**

On his or her back or side with the neck in a neutral position.

○ **Why should hyperextension of the neck be avoided?**

It may produce airway obstruction.

○ **When placing the infant on his or her back, what can you do to insure neutral position?**

A rolled blanket or towel may be placed under the back and shoulders, thus elevating the torso 3/4 or 1 inch off the mattress to extend the neck slightly.

○ **How should the infant be positioned if copious secretions are present?**

On his or her side with the neck slightly extended to allow secretions to collect in the mouth rather than in the posterior pharynx.

○ **When should the trachea be suctioned if meconium staining is observed?**

Before other resuscitative steps are taken.

❍ **If meconium is absent but suctioning is required to ensure a patent airway, should the mouth or the nose be suctioned first?**

The mouth.

❍ **If mechanical suction is used, what negative pressure should not be exceeded?**

-100mm Hg (-136 cm $H_2O$).

❍ **What negative response can be produced by deep suctioning of the oropharynx?**

A vagal response that can cause bradycardia and/or apnea.

❍ **How long should you perform suctioning?**

No longer than 3-5 seconds per attempt.

❍ **What should you monitor during suctioning?**

The infant's heart rate.

❍ **What should you do between suctioning attempts?**

Time should be allowed between suction attempts for spontaneous ventilation or assisted ventilation with 100% oxygen.

❍ **What three forms of mild stimulation will be effective in stimulating breathing in most newborns?**

Drying, warming and suctioning.

❍ **What are two additional safe methods of stimulation?**

Slapping or flicking the soles of the feet and rubbing the infant's back.

❍ **What should you do if spontaneous and effective respirations are not established after a brief period (5 to 10 seconds) of stimulation?**

Positive-pressure ventilation.

❍ **If respirations are deemed adequate on assessment, what should you check next?**

Heart rate.

❍ **If respirations are inadequate or gasping is present, what should you do?**

Begin positive-pressure ventilation immediately.

❍ **If respirations are shallow or slow, what should you do?**

A brief period of stimulation may be attempted while 100% oxygen is administered. The rate and depth of respirations should increase after a few seconds of stimulation and administration of oxygen.

❍ **"The mere presence of respirations does not guarantee adequate ventilation." Explain.**

Shallow respirations may primarily ventilate airway dead space and thus provide inadequate alveolar ventilation, resulting in hypoxemia, hypercarbia, and slowing of the heart rate.

O **What vital sign is considered a reliable indicator of the newborn's degree of distress?**

Heart rate.

O **What three methods are used in evaluating heart rate?**

1. Palpation of the pulse at the base of the umbilical cord.
2. Palpation of the brachial or femoral pulse.
3. Auscultation of the apical heart sound with a stethoscope.

O **What should you do if the heart rate is less than 100 beats per minute?**

Positive-pressure ventilation with 100% oxygen should be initiated immediately.

O **What should you do if the heart rate is less than 60 bpm and not increasing rapidly despite effective ventilation with 100% oxygen?**

Chest compressions should be initiated.

O **T/F: An infant may be cyanotic despite adequate ventilation and a heart rate greater than 100 bpm.**

True.

O **What should you do if central cyanosis is present in a newborn with spontaneous respirations and an adequate heart rate?**

100% oxygen should be administered until the cause of the cyanosis can be determined.

O **What is acrocyanosis?**

Peripheral cyanosis.

O **Should you administer oxygen to an infant with peripheral cyanosis?**

No, it is a common condition in the first few minutes of life and is not indicative of hypoxemia.

O **What is the purpose of the Apgar scoring system?**

It enables rapid evaluation of a newborn's condition at specific intervals after birth.

O **What are the five objective signs measured by the Apgar?**

**A**ppearance (color)
**P**ulse (heart rate)
**G**rimace (reflex irritability)
**A**ctivity (muscle tone)
**R**espirations

O **At what intervals should the Apgar be measured?**

One and five minutes of age.

○ **When should you take additional scores?**

If the five-minute Apgar score is less than 7, additional scores are obtained every five minutes for a total of twenty minutes.

○ **Can the Apgar score be used to determine the need for resuscitation?**

No. If resuscitative efforts are required, they should be initiated promptly and should not be delayed while the Apgar score is obtained.

○ **How does prematurity affect the Apgar score?**

In preterm infants the Apgar score is more likely to be affected by gestational age than asphyxia.

○ **When should you be concerned about administering 100% oxygen in newborn resuscitation?**

Never. If oxygen is needed during the resuscitation of a newborn, 100% should be used without concern for its potential hazards.

○ **T/F: Only warmed and humidified oxygen should be administered.**

False. Ideally, oxygen should be warmed and humidified, but this may not be possible in an emergency situation.

○ **What methods can be used to administer oxygen to a newborn?**

A head hood, facemask attached to a non-self-inflating ("anesthesia") bag, or by a simple mask held firmly to the infant's face with at least 5 Lpm oxygen flow.

○ **What are three indications for positive-pressure ventilation?**

1. Apnea or gasping respirations. 2. Heart rate less than 100 bpm. 3. Persistent central cyanosis despite administration of 100% oxygen

○ **How can you determine the appropriate tidal volume for bagging a neonate?**

Begin bag-valve-mask ventilations carefully and determine visually the volume and force required to produce adequate chest expansion.

○ **For most newborns, what is the initial pressure required for lung inflation?**

30-40 cm $H_2O$. Less pressure (20 cm $H_2O$) is usually required for subsequent breaths.

○ **What should you do if adequate chest expansion is not achieved with initial assisted ventilation?**

The head and the facemask should be repositioned.

○ **What should you do if repositioning the head and facemask fail to produce effective chest expansion?**

Suction further and increase inflation pressure.

○ **What should you do if you still cannot achieve effective chest expansion and improvement in color and heart rate?**

Intubate immediately.

○ **When should you insert an orogastric tube?**

If BVM positive-pressure ventilation is required for more than approximately two minutes or if gastric distention develops.

○ **What size orogastric tube should be used?**

8F or 10F.

○ **Many self-inflating ventilation bags have a pop-off valve. At what pressure is this valve usually preset?**

30-45 cm $H_2O$.

○ **What is the problem with the pop-off valve in neonatal resuscitation?**

The initial inflation of a newborn's lungs may require higher inspiratory pressures, and the valve may prevent effective inflation unless it is occluded. Such bags should therefore have a pop-off valve that is easily bypassed.

○ **What is the ideal sized ventilation bag for neonatal resuscitation?**

450 – 750 ml.

○ **What is the range of neonatal tidal volume?**

6-8 ml/kg.

○ **Why are facemasks with cushioned rims recommended?**

They facilitate creation of an effective seal between face and mask.

○ **Should tapered tubes be used for neonates?**

No, only tubes with a uniform internal diameter.

○ **What is the preferred technique for performing chest compressions in the neonate and small infant?**

Two thumbs placed on the middle third of the sternum, with the fingers encircling the chest and supporting the back. The thumbs should be positioned side by side on the sternum just below the nipple line.

○ **What anatomical feature is important to avoid when performing chest compressions, and why?**

The xiphoid portion of the sternum. May cause liver damage.

○ **What is the depth of neonatal compression?**

One third the anterior-(posterior) diameter of the chest or to a depth that generates a palpable pulse.

○   **What is the rate of neonatal compressions?**

120 times per minute.

○   **T/F: The relaxation phase should be longer than the compression phase.**

False, they should both be smooth and equal.

○   **T/F: The compressing thumbs or fingers should not be lifted off the sternum during the relaxation phase.**

True.

○   **When should you cease compressions?**

When the heart rate reaches 60 or more bpm.

○   **What is the most common cause of bradycardia and shock in the neonatal period?**

Profound hypoxemia.

○   **When should medications be administered in cases of bradycardia and shock?**

If, despite adequate ventilation with 100% oxygen and chest compressions, the heart rate remains less than 60 bpm.

○   **What is the preferred site for vascular access during neonatal resuscitation?**

The umbilical vein, because it is easily located and cannulated.

○   **What preparation is required prior to umbilical catheterization?**

Skin prep, draped appropriately and the cord trimmed with a scalpel blade 1 cm above the skin attachment and held firmly with a ligature to prevent bleeding.

○   **How do you identify the umbilical vein?**

It is a thin walled single vessel. In contrast, the umbilical arteries are paired, have thicker walls, and are often constricted. The lumen of the vein is larger than that of the arteries; thus the vessel that continues to bleed after the cord is cut is usually the vein.

○   **What size catheter should be used?**

A 3.5F or a 5F umbilical catheter.

○   **How is the catheter prepared for insertion?**

It is flushed with heparinized saline (0.5 to 1 U/ml) and attached to a three-way stopcock.

○   **How far should the catheter be inserted?**

So that the tip is just below the skin and blood can be readily aspirated and any air bubbles evacuated. The umbilical venous catheter is inserted only until a good blood return is obtained. This should correspond to a depth of insertion of 1 to 4 cm.

○ **What complication can result from inserting the catheter too far?**

Advancement of the catheter tip into the portal vein or hepatic circulation. Neonatal liver injury (including hemorrhage) has been linked with the administration of hypertonic and alkaline solution (e.g., THAM or sodium bicarbonate into the portal vein, so this position of the catheter tip is avoided).

○ **What should be suspected if free blood return is absent?**

A wedged hepatic position.

○ **What should you do if you suspect such wedging?**

You should withdraw the catheter to a position where blood can be freely aspirated.

○ **How long can the umbilical catheter remain in place?**

It should be withdrawn as soon as possible after resuscitation to minimize the danger of infection or portal vein thrombosis.

○ **What is the advantage of cannulating the umbilical artery?**

It enables monitoring of blood pressure and blood sampling for blood gas analysis and evaluation of acid-base balance.

○ **What is the disadvantage of cannulating the umbilical artery?**

It is time-consuming and more difficult than venous cannulation.

○ **What other sites of cannulation can be used?**

Peripheral veins in the extremities and scalp.

○ **If fluid and medications are required but umbilical venous or arterial access cannot be obtained, what should you do?**

Attempt intraosseous cannula placement.

○ **Where is the intraosseous cannula inserted?**

In the medial aspect of the tibia, just inferior and medial to the tibial tuberosity on the flat surface of the proximal tibia.

○ **What route of medication administration should be used when vascular access cannot be achieved?**

Endotracheal.

○ **What two drugs can be administered to the neonate by this route?**

Epinephrine and naloxone.

○ **What epinephrine dosing regimen should be used for the endotracheal route in neonates?**

The dose is 0.01 to 0.03 mg/kg (1:10,000) or 0.1 to 0.3 ml/kg IV every 3 to 5 minutes. The drug should be diluted to a volume of 3-5 ml of normal saline (use smallest volume for smallest babies), followed by several positive-pressure ventilations.

O   **What are the indications for epinephrine in neonatal resuscitation?**

Asystole or spontaneous heart rate less than 60 bpm despite adequate ventilation with 100% oxygen and chest compressions.

O   **What is the dose?**

0.01 to 0.03 mg/kg (0.1 to 0.3 ml/kg of the 1:10,000 solution). May be repeated every 3 to 5 minutes if required.

O   **When is high dose epinephrine appropriate?**

Many randomized controlled studies failed to show improved outcomes routinely. However, may be considered for special circumstances suggesting catecholamine resistant condition eq. anaphylaxis. Known alpha or beta blocker overdose, severe sepsis already treated with high dose pressors.

O   **Does the current data support the use of high dose epinephrine in neonatal resuscitation?**

Data is inadequate at present to evaluate the efficacy of high doses of epinephrine in newborns, and the safety of these doses has not been established.

O   **What is the primary complication of high dose epinephrine in newborns?**

Prolonged hypertension, which may in turn lead to complications such as intracranial hemorrhage in preterm infants.

O   **What are the three primary volume expanders for neonates?**

1. O-negative blood crossmatched with mother's blood.  2. 5% albumin/saline solution or other plasma substitute.  3. Normal saline or Ringers lactate.

O   **What is the dosage for volume expanders in neonatal resuscitation?**

10 ml/kg. Reassess and administer additional boluses as needed.

O   **What are the routes of administration for naloxone?**

Intravenous, intraosseous, via the endotracheal tube, subcutaneous, or intramuscular (if perfusion is adequate).

O   **What is the dosing of naloxone?**

0.1 mg/kg. The initial does may be repeated every 2 to 3 minutes as needed.

O   **In addition to epinephrine and naloxone, what other drugs are useful in neonatal resuscitation?**

None. There is no evidence that atropine, calcium, or sodium bicarbonate is beneficial in the acute phase of neonatal resuscitation at delivery.

◯ **What percentage of all deliveries are complicated by the presence of meconium in the amniotic fluid?**

Approximately 12%.

◯ **What is the consistency of amniotic fluid containing meconium?**

Thin and watery or thick and particulate, resembling pea soup.

◯ **Meconium is found in the trachea of what percent of newborns with meconium staining despite suctioning?**

20-30%.

◯ **T/F: Suction should be applied directly to the endotracheal tube.**

True.

◯ **How is this accomplished?**

With a meconium aspirator.

◯ **What should you do if there is a significant amount of meconium?**

Repeat intubation and suction while withdrawing the ET tube, until the aspirated material is clear or until the heart rate indicates that resuscitation should proceed without delay.

◯ **What should you do if the patient's condition rapidly deteriorates before all meconium is removed?**

When an infant's condition is unstable, it may not be possible to clear the trachea of all meconium before positive-pressure ventilation must be initiated.

◯ **Why should an orogastric tube be placed in these infants?**

To empty the stomach, since it may contain meconium that could later be regurgitated and aspirated.

◯ **Why are preterm infants more subject to intracranial bleeds?**

Because the brain of the preterm infant has a fragile subependymal germinal matrix that is vulnerable to bleeding when injured by hypoxemia, rapid changes in blood pressure, or wide fluctuations in serum osmolality.

◯ **Why are preterm infants more likely to become hypothermic?**

Because their ratio of body surface area to volume is higher than that of full-term neonates.

◯ **Because of this increased risk of intracranial bleeding, what should be avoided in these patients?**

Administration of hyperosmolar solutions or large boluses of volume expanders.

◯ **What are the three most common complications in the postresuscitation period?**

1. Endotracheal tube migration (including dislodgment)

2. Tube occlusion by mucus or meconium
3. Pneumothorax

○ **Why is a pneumothorax difficult to diagnose by auscultation?**

Because breath sounds in the newborn are transmitted from all areas of the lung through the thin chest wall.

○ **When should you suspect pneumothorax?**

If a newborn deteriorates after an initial good response to ventilation or fails to respond to resuscitative efforts. Additional signs of pneumothorax include unilateral decrease in chest expansion, altered intensity or pitch of breath sounds, and increased resistance to hand ventilation.

○ **Some children may require sedation and administration of muscle relaxants to minimize the risk of endotracheal tube displacement during transport. Name three medications that are frequently used.**

Diazepam (0.1 to 0.2 mg/kg IV) and morphine sulfate (0.1mg/kg IV), Midazolam (0.1-0.2mg/kg IV/IM).

○ **What is the main advantage (or disadvantage, depending on your perspective) or Thiopental (Pentothal)?**

It is very short acting, 5-10 minutes.

○ **Your patient has been placed on a mechanical ventilator in preparation for transport. How long after the initial ventilatory settings have been made should an arterial blood gas analysis be completed?**

After fifteen minutes.

○ **What is the purpose of administering Lidocaine in RSI?**

To reduce ICP.

○ **During mechanical ventilation the effectiveness of ventilation and oxygenation must be verified using what laboratory test?**

Arterial blood gas analysis.

○ **When using a volume-cycled ventilator, what is the recommended tidal volume that should be delivered to the patient?**

8 - 10 ml/kg.

○ **How often should the blood pressure of a hemodynamically unstable child be assessed?**

Blood pressure should be assessed every 5 minutes until stable and every 15 minutes thereafter. Attention to the patient's heart rate must also be closely monitored.

○ **List two primary advantages of using noninvasive monitoring devices such as pulse oximeters, transcutaneous oxygen and carbon dioxide monitors, and exhaled carbon dioxide monitors.**

These tools are very useful because they allow continuous assessment of oxygenation, ventilation, or both.

○ **Noninvasive monitoring devices such as those referenced in the above question may provide inaccurate data as a result of what types of medical conditions or equipment problems?**

Inaccurate results may occur as a result of hypothermia, poor peripheral perfusion, or endotracheal tube obstruction or displacement.

○ **Urine output often correlates with the effectiveness of renal and systemic perfusion. What is the preferred method of monitoring urine output?**

An indwelling catheter.

○ **As an ER resident working 16 hours on the late shift you are evaluating a child with some type of circulatory instability. What blood lab tests should be included in your assessment data?**

Laboratory evaluation of the circulatory state includes arterial blood gas and pH analysis and evaluation of serum electrolytes, lactic acid, calcium, glucose, urea nitrogen, and creatinine levels.

○ **Why is blind nasogastric tube placement contraindicated in the patient with serious facial trauma?**

Intracranial tube placement may result.

○ **What are two causes of acid-base imbalance?**

Respiratory failure and circulatory failure.

○ **What is the most common cause of shock in children?**

Hypovolemic shock.

○ **What are three causes of (volume loss) hypovolemic shock?**

1. GI losses through vomiting and diarrhea.
2. Diabetic ketoacidosis through increased urination (diuresis).
3. Trauma

○ **What kind of shock is caused by peripheral vasodilatation resulting in venous pooling of blood and a decrease of blood returning to the central circulation?**

Neurogenic shock.

○ **What types of shock result from both vasodilatation and increased capillary permeability causing plasma losses out of the vascular space and into the interstitium caused?**

Septic shock and anaphylactic shock.

○ **What is shock resulting from inadequate heart (pump) function called?**

Cardiogenic shock.

○ **What are the three types of fluids that may be used in volume resuscitation in children with hypovolemic shock?**

Isotonic crystalloid, colloid and blood products.

○ **Name three types of colloid solutions.**

Albumin 5%, fresh frozen plasma and synthetics.

○ **Name two examples of synthetic colloid preparations.**

Hetastarch and dextran.

○ **T/F: Blood products are considered the first choice treatment for the management of hypovolemia.**

False. Crystalloids should be tried first.

○ **When is blood considered the ideal fluid replacement in volume loss?**

When trauma victims in hypovolemic shock do not respond to crystalloid management or trauma patients present in decompensated shock.

○ **What is the blood type that may be administered without crossmatch?**

O-negative.

○ **Rapid infusion of cold blood or blood products containing citrate in large volumes may result in what two major complications?**

Hypothermia and hypocalcemia.

○ **When is volume therapy indicated?**

When the child demonstrates signs and symptoms of shock.

○ **What are five significant signs of hypovolemic shock in a child?**

Tachycardia, pale, mottled, cool skin, delayed capillary refill, diminished peripheral pulses and altered mental status.

○ **T/F: Optimum vascular access in a child requires only one large bore peripheral line.**

False. At least two are required.

○ **What is the fluid bolus dose of crystalloid for the management of the symptomatic hypovolemic child?**

20ml/kg IV in less than 20 minutes.

○ **How many times may fluid boluses of crystalloid be repeated during the first hour of trauma to manage volume losses in a hypovolemic child before giving blood?**

Twice.

○ **T/F: It is more efficient to administer bolus fluid infusions by IV push with a syringe than with an IV drip.**

True. In children the volumes are smaller than in adults, and the fluids can be pushed faster.

○ **T/F: A child in septic shock may require 60 to 80 ml/kg during the first hour of resuscitation.**

True.

○ **What should you do following each volume bolus?**

Reassess perfusion status of the child. Evaluate for effectiveness of therapy.

○ **T/F: Large volumes of dextrose containing solutions are particularly useful during volume resuscitation.**

False. They can be harmful because of their hypertonic effects.

○ **What would be the appropriate management of a patient with a respiratory acidosis?**

Adequate oxygenation and appropriate ventilation.

○ **What would be the appropriate management of a patient with a metabolic acidosis secondary to poor perfusion?**

Correct the perfusion problem.

○ **How do you determine a base deficit in the setting of a metabolic acidemia?**

Calculate the difference between the predicted pH (7.40) and the measured pH.
Multiply the difference by 67 (constant).
This will give you the patient's base deficit.

Example: Measured pH 7.18
Predicted pH 7.40
Difference: -0.22

-0.22 x 67 = -14.7 Base Deficit

○ **How do you calculate the appropriate $NaHCO_3$ to correct the base deficit for a 18kg baby in metabolic acidosis (pH 7.18)?**

Multiply the BASE DEFICIT x Pt. kg. wt. x 0.3 (constant) = $NaHCO_3$ dose (mEq)
Example: 14.7 Base Deficit x 18kg. x 0.3 = 79mEq $NaHCO_3$

○ **If a peripheral vein is utilized to administer a drug, it is recommended to flush the line with what volume of normal saline?**

5 ml of normal saline should be used to move the drug along.

○ **What are the indications for the administration of epinephrine?**

Cardiac arrest (Alpha), symptomatic bradycardia that will not respond to oxygenation and ventilation, and hypotension not responding to volume resuscitation.

○ **How often should epinephrine be administered in a cardiac arrest resuscitation?**

Every 3 - 5 minutes.

○ **What happens if epinephrine is added to or given through a line with bicarbonate?**

The epinephrine will become inactivated.

○ **What are two post epinephrine administration side effects?**

Hypertension and tachycardia.

○ **What narcotic agent is recommended in kids?**

Fentanyl citrate (Sublimaze) 2-4 mcg/kg IV or IM.

○ **What is the duration of action of Fentanyl?**

1-2 hours.

○ **What is the advantage of Fentanyl over other opioids?**

Less histamine release and associated hypotension.

○ **What is the dosing regimen for Midazolam?**

0.1-0.2mg/kg (maximum 4mg) IV or IM, 1-2 hours.

○ **What is the most significant side effect of Midazolam?**

Respiratory depression.

○ **T/F: Midazolam has analgesic as well as sedative properties.**

False. That is why it is important to always give an analgesic in addition when performing painful procedures.

○ **What is the therapeutic effect of sodium bicarbonate (NaHCO$_3$)?**

Sodium bicarbonate buffers the blood and reverses metabolic acidosis.

○ **Why is it important to be able to adequately ventilate a patient who has received sodium bicarbonate?**

NaHCO$_3$ (Sodium Bicarbonate) generates an increase in CO$_2$ production as the hydrogen ion is buffered – adequate ventilation is necessary to remove the additional load to CO$_2$.

○ **When should sodium bicarbonate be considered for administration?**

When severe acidosis is associated with prolonged cardiac arrest, shock, hyperkalemia or tricyclic antidepressant toxicity.

○ **What is the initial dose for sodium bicarbonate when a base deficit cannot be determined?**

1 mEq/kg IV or intraosseous.

○ **What is the subsequent dose of sodium bicarbonate when a base deficit cannot be determined?**

0.5mEq/kg IV.

○ **How fast should sodium bicarbonate be administered?**

Slowly over 1-2 minutes.

○ **T/F: Excessive administration of sodium bicarbonate may result in metabolic alkalosis.**

True.

○ **T/F: Administration of sodium bicarbonate can result in lowering serum potassium.**

True.

○ **What is the standard pediatric concentration of sodium bicarbonate?**

4.2%.

○ **What should be done with the IV tubing before and after sodium bicarbonate has been given?**

The IV tubing should be flushed with normal saline.

○ **What are two cardiovascular conditions for which atropine administration is indicated?**

Asystolic cardiac arrest and hemodynamically significant bradycardia.

○ **What is the benefit of atropine administration to a child during endotracheal intubation attempts?**

Atropine can prevent vagally mediated bradycardia.

○ **What is the recommended dose of atropine?**

0.02mg/kg IV or intraosseous (IO).

○ **What is the minimum IV/IO single dose of atropine for a child?**

0.1mg.

○ **What is the maximum IV/IO single dose of atropine for a child?**

0.5mg.

○ **What is the maximum total dose of atropine for a child?**

0.04 mg/kg.

○ **How often may atropine be repeated?**

3 - 5 minutes after initial administration if symptoms persist.

○ **What may atropine administrated at lower than recommended doses do to the heart rate?**

Cause a paradoxical slowing of the heart rate.

○ **What is the recommended dose of atropine to be administered endotracheally?**

Two to three times the IV/IO dose.

○ **T/F: The pupillary dilatation associated with atropine will not react (constrict) to light reflex.**

False. The pupils will still constrict.

○ **Naloxone (Narcan) is indicated for what condition?**

Narcotic (opiate) toxicity induced symptoms.

○ **What are three significant symptoms associated with narcotic (opiate) intoxication?**

Respiratory depression, CNS depression, and hypoperfusion.

○ **What is the onset of effect for naloxone (Narcan)?**

< 2 minutes.

○ **What is the duration of activity for naloxone (Narcan)?**

Around 45 – 120 minutes.

○ **By what routes may naloxone (Narcan) be administered?**

IV, IO and ETT.

○ **What is the recommended IV/IO dose of naloxone (Narcan) for infants and children up to 20kg?**

0.1mg/kg.

○ **What is the recommended infusion rate for Narcan?**

0.04 - 0.16 mg/kg/hour.

○ **What may occur after administration of naloxone (Narcan) if the narcotic effect is abruptly reversed?**

Acute narcotic withdrawal.

○ **What are the symptoms of acute narcotic withdrawal?**

Nausea and vomiting, tachycardia, hypertension, seizures and cardiac dysrhythmias.

○ **Why is hypoglycemia bad?**

Because it is important for cells to function normally especially in the brain. Hypoglycemia can precipitate seizure activity and depress myocardial function.

○ **When should glucose administration be considered?**

When hypoglycemia is present or the infant or child fails to respond to standard resuscitation measures.

○   **What is the dosage range of glucose?**

0.5 - 1.0 gm/kg IV or IO.

○   **What is the maximum recommended concentration of glucose for administration to children?**

25% (D25W) for children, D10W for neonates and infants, D50W for adolescents.

○   **What is the dilution to reduce the concentration to 10% (D10W)?**

1:4 with sterile water.

○   **What are four conditions that can lead to poor outcomes if high concentration glucose (D50/D25) is administered to children?**

Children with head injuries, near drowning (submersion), stroke, and shock.

○   **What are four indications for administration of calcium?**

Documented or suspected hypocalcemia, hyperkalemia, hypermagnesemia and calcium channel blocker overdose.

○   **Calcium chloride 10% is equal to how many milligrams per milliliter?**

100 mg/ml.

○   **What is the recommended dose of calcium chloride?**

20 mg/kg IV.

○   **How fast should calcium chloride be infused?**

Not to exceed 100 mg/min.

○   **Why should you avoid mixing calcium chloride with sodium bicarbonate?**

It forms a precipitate.

○   **What may happen if calcium is administered too fast?**

Bradycardia or asystole may occur.

○   **Why should calcium only be administered through a large, well-secured intravenous line?**

Calcium can cause significant chemical damage if it infiltrates into surrounding tissue.

○   **What does prostaglandin E1 do?**

Prevents closure of the ductus arteriosis in newborns.

○   **What are the indications for administration of prostaglandin E1?**

Infants with congenital cardiovascular disease with ductal dependent lesions.

○ **What are the signs and symptoms, in the newborn, associated with congenital cardiovascular abnormalities that could indicate the need for administration of prostaglandin E1?**

Cyanosis or shock.

○ **How should prostaglandin E1 be administered?**

Continuous intravenous infusion.

○ **Why should prostaglandin E1 be administered by continuous intravenous infusion?**

It has a very short half-life.

○ **What is the effective dose range of prostaglandin E1?**

0.05 - 0.10 mcg/kg/min.

○ **Because prostaglandin E1 may cause apnea, what should you be prepared to do during its administration?**

Secure the airway with an endotracheal tube and oxygenate/ventilate the infant.

○ **What is the infusion range for IV continuous infusion of epinephrine?**

0.01 mcg/kg/min. - 1.0 mcg/kg/min. titrated to desired response.

○ **What is the recommended preparation formula for IV continuous epinephrine infusion?**

0.6 x patient weight (kg) = amount of epinephrine (mg) added to 100 ml crystalloid.

○ **When mixed appropriately, how may the epinephrine infusion rate be calculated?**

By setting the infusion rate to 1ml/hour the delivery of epinephrine will equal 0.1 mcg/kg/min.

○ **What are five potential adverse reactions associated with epinephrine infusion?**

Tachycardia, ventricular dysrhythmias, profound peripheral vasoconstriction, compromised renal and hepatic blood flow, and local infiltration may cause ischemic tissue damage.

○ **What are three indications for the administration of lidocaine by IV bolus?**

Ventricular dysrhythmias, ventricular tachycardia, and ventricular fibrillation (after defibrillation).

○ **What is the recommended dose of lidocaine IV bolus?**

1mg/kg (not to exceed 3mg/kg).

○ **When should lidocaine infusion be started?**

Following effective lidocaine bolus administration.

○ **What are three potential adverse reactions associated with lidocaine administration?**

Myocardial depression, hypotension, and central nervous system manifestations, such as drowsiness, disorientation, muscle twitching and seizures.

○  **What are the indications for the administration of adenosine?**

Supraventricular tachycardia (heart rates >220 BPM) with or without evidence of poor perfusion.

○  **What is the recommended dose of adenosine?**

0.1 - 0.2mg/kg IV rapid bolus.

○  **What are the indications for the use of Amiodarone in children?**

Wide range of atrial and ventricular arrhythmias, particularly ectopic atrial tachycardia, junctional ectopic tachycardia, and ventricular tachycardia.

○  **What are the two main precautions when using Amiodarone?**

Hypotension and a prolonged QT interval.

○  **With what antiarrhythmic should you avoid using Amiodarone?**

Procainamide.

○  **What is the half-life of Amiodarone?**

Up to 40 days!

○  **What is the dosing of Amiodarone in refractory pulseless VT, VF?**

5mg/kg rapid IV/IO bolus.

○  **What is the dosing of Amiodarone for perfusing supraventricular and ventricular arrhythmias?**

Loading dose: 5mg/kg IV/IO over 20 to 60 minutes (repeat to a maximum of 15mg/kg per day IV).

○  **List the six ways the pediatric airway differs from the adult airway.**

1. The airway is smaller.
2. The tongue is relatively larger.
3. The larynx is more cephalad in position.
4. The epiglottis is short, narrow and angled away from the trachea.
5. The vocal cords attach lower anteriorly.
6. In children less than 10 the narrowest portion of the airway is subglottic.

○  **Why should a straight laryngoscope blade be used in children?**

The high position of the larynx makes the angle between the tongue and glottis more acute.

○  **Should endotracheal tube size be based on the size of the glottic opening or the size of the cricoid ring?**

The cricoid ring, as this is the narrowest part of the trachea in children.

○  **How is airflow resistance related to airway radius?**

Inversely proportional to the fourth power of the airway radius during laminar flow (quiet breathing), and inversely proportional to the fifth power of airway radius during turbulent airflow.

○ **Why should the child with airway obstruction be kept calm?**

To prevent the generation of turbulent airflow.

○ **What happens to functional residual capacity when respiratory effort is diminished?**

It is reduced.

○ **On what does tidal volume in infants and toddlers depend?**

Movement of the diaphragm.

○ **Why is the pediatric airway susceptible to dynamic collapse during airway obstruction?**

High compliance of the airway.

○ **Why do children have a high oxygen demand per kilogram?**

Their metabolic rate is high.

○ **Does hypoxemia occur more quickly in the child or adult in response to apnea?**

The child, secondary to high oxygen consumption.

○ **Why should children in respiratory distress be allowed to maintain a position of comfort?**

This position usually allows the maximal airway patency and minimizes respiratory effort.

○ **What does anxiety do to oxygen consumption?**

Increases it.

○ **What can occur if breaths with a bag-valve-mask are not coordinated with the child's breathing efforts?**

Coughing, vomiting, laryngospasm, and gastric distension.

○ **Why is pulse oximetry an important technique for monitoring respiratory insufficiency?**

It provides continuous evaluation of arterial oxygen saturation.

○ **T/F: Pulse oximeters reflect the effectiveness of ventilation.**

False, they only evaluate level of oxygenation.

○ **When is the pulse oximeter's accuracy limited?**

In the presence of methemoglobinemia, carbon monoxide poisoning or in shock states.

○ **Why is the pulse oximeter not useful during shock or poor perfusion?**

It requires pulsatile blood flow to determine oxygen saturation.

○ **Where may the oximeter probe be placed if a signal is not detected at the fingertip?**

Ear lobe, nares, cheek, tongue and foot.

○ **What is the most accurate method of determining arterial oxygen concentration?**

Arterial blood gas.

○ **Why is a low flow oxygen delivery system insufficient to meet all inspiratory flow requirements?**

Because with low flow systems room air is entrained and mixed with the oxygen decreasing the concentration of oxygen to be inhaled by the patient.

○ **What is the maximum inspired oxygen concentration achieved with a nonrebreather mask?**

95%.

○ **What inspired oxygen concentration can be achieved with an oxygen hood?**

80-95%.

○ **What is the indication for use of an oral airway?**

In an unconscious child with airway obstruction after usual airway maneuvers have failed.

○ **Why should an oral airway not be used in a conscious child?**

May stimulate gagging or vomiting.

○ **How is the appropriately sized oral airway chosen?**

Measure from the level of the central incisors, the bite block segment is parallel to the hard palate and the curved portion should reach the angle of the jaw.

○ **What is the appropriate length for a nasal airway?**

Distance from the tip of the nose to the tragus of the ear.

○ **Why should the space under the mask used for ventilation be small?**

To decrease dead space and minimize rebreathing of exhaled gases.

○ **From where to where should the appropriately sized ventilation mask extend?**

The bridge of the nose to the cleft of the chin.

○ **When performing bag-valve-mask ventilation, why should pressure on the submental area be avoided?**

Can cause the tongue to be pushed into the posterior pharynx leading to obstruction or airway compression can occur.

○ **Where should the fingers be placed during BVM ventilation?**

On the jaw.

○ **What patient position is appropriate during BVM of infants and toddlers?**

Supine and head and neck in the neutral sniffing position.

○ **What should be done if effective BVM ventilation cannot be achieved?**

Reposition head, make sure mask is snug, lift jaw, consider suctioning, ensure bag is functioning and connected to gas source.

○ **How can gastric inflation be minimized in the unconscious child?**

Use appropriate sized equipment, only inflate the lungs with a volume necessary to initiate chest rise. Ventilate at an age appropriate rate, apply cricoid pressure.

○ **How can the pop-off valve be occluded in a self-inflating bag?**

Either by depressing the valve or twisting the valve into a closed position.

○ **What can sudden decreases in lung compliance indicate?**

Right main bronchus intubation, obstructed endotracheal tube, and pneumothorax.

○ **What are some of the advantages of ventilation via an endotracheal tube?**

The airway is isolated, potential for aspiration is reduced, ventilations and chest compressions can be interposed efficiently, inspiratory time and peek pressures can be controlled and PEEP can be delivered.

○ **What are six indications for intubation?**

1. Inadequate CNS control of ventilation.
2. Loss of protective airway reflexes.
3. Respiratory failure.
4. Need for high ventilatory pressures or PEEP.
5. Need for mechanical ventilatory support.
6. Allows for stabilization of an airway that has the potential to deteriorate in transport or during special procedures at a hospital.

○ **When should a cuffed endotracheal tube be used?**

In children over 8 to 10 years old.

○ **At what pressure should an air leak occur in the intubated patient?**

20 to 30 cm $H_2O$.

○ **What does the absence of an air leak indicate?**

The cuff is inflated excessively, the ET tube is too large, or laryngospasm is occurring around the tube.

○ **If visual inspection is used for choosing the endotracheal tube size, what part of the child's anatomy should be chosen for approximating the appropriate diameter?**

The width of a child's little fingernail.

○ **What formula can be used to choose ET tube size in children over two?**

(Age [years]/4)+4.

○ **What is the most accurate way of determining ET tube size?**

Using a length–based tape for weight estimate and then reading the appropriate tube size for that weight.

○ **How can the ET tube size be used to estimate the depth of insertion of the tube?**

Internal diameter x 3 = depth of insertion (cm).

○ **How should a stylet be placed in an ET tube?**

Lightly lubricated with tip inside distal end of ET tube.

○ **What should be done if bradycardia occurs during an intubation attempt?**

The procedure should be interrupted and the patient should be ventilated with 100% oxygen via bag-valve-mask.

○ **Why and in whom should atropine be administered during intubation attempts?**

To prevent bradycardia in an infant or young child.

○ **When should an intubation attempt be interrupted?**

If the patient develops hypoxemia, cyanosis, pallor, or decreased heart rate.

○ **To directly visualize the glottis, what three structures must be aligned?**

The axes of the mouth, pharynx and trachea.

○ **How should children less than two years old without trauma be placed for intubation?**

On a flat surface with the chin in sniffing position.

○ **Why is orotracheal intubation preferred during resuscitation?**

It can be performed more rapidly than nasotracheal intubation and often with greater success.

○ **Why should the blade not be inserted into the esophagus and withdrawn to visualize the epiglottis?**

This practice increases the risk of laryngeal trauma.

○ **Where should the tip of the curved blade be placed?**

In the vallecula.

○ **What is done with the tip of the straight blade?**

Used to lift the epiglottis to visualize the glottic opening.

○ **From which direction should the endotracheal tube be inserted?**

From the right corner of the mouth.

○ **How can an assistant make intubation easier?**

By displacing the right corner of the mouth to visualize the passage of the endotracheal tube, and applying cricoid pressure to facilitate visualization of the glottis.

○ **Where is the black glottic marker on the endotracheal tube placed?**

At the level of or just below the vocal cords.

○ **How is the position of the endotracheal tube assessed after intubation?**

Observation of symmetrical chest movement, auscultation of equal breath sounds, documentation of absent gurgling sounds over the stomach, and rotation of end-tidal carbon dioxide level.

○ **When can endotracheal carbon dioxide levels be low?**

In low cardiac output states.

○ **What problems should be considered when intubation is confirmed but oxygenation or ventilation is inadequate?**

The endotracheal tube is too small, the pop off valve on the resuscitation bag is not depressed, A leak is present in the connections of the bag-valve device, inadequate tidal volume is provided by the operator, and lack of lung expansion or lung collapse is occurring for other reasons.

○ **How can displacement of the endotracheal tube be detected?**

By noting the distance marker number at the lips, by noting a deterioration in patient status, by use of end tidal CO2 device, by decreased oxygen saturation, by clinical assessment that the tube is in the right mainstem (decreased breath sounds on the right versus the left) or by noting gurgling sounds in the stomach indicating esophageal displacement of the tube.

○ **Should esophageal obturator airways be used in children?**

No. They are too long and do not come in pediatric sizes.

○ **Why shouldn't oxygen powered breathing devices be used in children?**

High airway pressures may produce gastric distension or tension pneumothorax.

○ **When should a tension pneumothorax be suspected?**

When any intubated patient deteriorates suddenly during positive pressure ventilation.

○ **What are the clinical signs of tension pneumothorax?**

Severe respiratory distress, hyperresonance to percussion, diminished breath sounds on the affected side, JVD and deviation of the trachea and mediastinum away from the affected side.

○ **What is the treatment for tension pneumothorax?**

Immediate needle decompression.

○ **For what clinical conditions might cricothyroidotomy be effective?**

Airway obstruction caused by foreign body, severe orofacial injuries, infection and laryngeal fracture.

○ **What age can you perform a cricothyroidotomy?**

Greater than 12 years of age.

○ **What size needle should initially be placed through the cricothyroid membrane?**

20 gauge.

○ **What signifies entry into the trachea?**

Aspiration of air.

○ **What size cannula should eventually be placed?**

At least a 14 gauge.

○ **How is the cannula connected to a bag valve device?**

Using a 3 mm endotracheal tube adapter.

○ **What gas flow rate should be used for oxygenation in needle cricothyroidotomy?**

1 to 5 l/min (100cc/kg).

○ **If a patient on a ventilator experiences a problem, what should be done?**

Patient should be manually ventilated with resuscitation bag using 100% oxygen.

○ **If the artificial airway is obstructed, what should be done first?**

Suction it with a large catheter.

○ **If the endotracheal tube is occluded and patency can't be restored, what should be done?**

Remove tube and ventilate with bag-valve-mask until reintubation.

○ **What equipment should be kept at the bedside of a patient with a tracheostomy?**

A pair of scissors and a new tracheostomy tube.

○ **If recannulation of a patient's tracheostomy stoma cannot be accomplished, what should be done?**

Try a smaller size stoma first: if this doesn't work orally intubate, or perform bag-valve-mask ventilation with gauze occluding the stoma. If there is no chest rise try placing a small mask over the stoma and performing mask to stoma ventilation using a bag-valve device.

○ **Why is a cricothryoidotomy contraindicated in a child < 12 years of age?**

High incidence of subglottic stenosis.

O   **Decompensated shock is characterized by what conditions?**

Hypotension and low cardiac output.

O   **In an unconscious, non-breathing patient with suspected cervical injury, which maneuver should be used to open the airway?**

Jaw thrust with cervical spine immobilization.

O   **Why shouldn't blind finger sweeps of the mouth be performed for manual removal of a foreign body?**

Because the foreign body may be pushed back into the airway, resulting in further obstruction.

O   **What do the indications for calcium therapy include?**

Documented or suspected hypocalcemia, hyperkalemia, hypermagnesemia, and calcium channel-blocker overdose.

O   **When should atropine be used to treat bradycardia?**

Only after adequate ventilation and oxygenation have been established, since hypoxemia is the most common cause of bradycardia in children.

O   **T/F: Defibrillation is indicated for the treatment of asystole.**

False.  Defibrillation is the definitive treatment for ventricular fibrillation or pulseless ventricular tachycardia.  The treatment for asystole is epinephrine.

O   **Name some complications associated with intraosseous cannulation and infusion.**

Tibia fracture, compartment syndrome, skin necrosis and osteomyelitis.  This has been reported in less than 1% of patients.

O   **What are the most common causes for deterioration of ventilatory status in a stable, intubated patient?**

Endotracheal tube dislodgment, occlusion, pneumothorax and equipment failure.

O   **Hypoxemia with a normal alveolar-arterial oxygen difference is the result of what?**

Hypoventilation.

O   **What is the narrowest part of the respiratory tract in children?**

The inferior ring portion of the cricoid cartilage.

O   **In what phase of respiration is stridor observed.**

Inspiration.

O   **What causes stridor?**

With extrathoracic airway obstruction, the pressure inside the extrathoracic part of the airway is negative relative to the level of atmospheric pressure. This results in further narrowing of the larynx during inspiration and therefore, stridor.

○ **A neonate has Apgar scores of 8 and 8. He is actively crying, but cyanosis and retractions appear when he is quiet. What is the most likely diagnosis?**

Choanal atresia.

○ **Which anomalies of the great vessels result in airway obstruction?**

1) Right aortic arch with or without a left ligamentum arteriosum.
2) Double aortic arch.
3) Anomalous innominate or left carotid artery.
4) Aberrant right subclavian.
5) Anomalous left pulmonary artery.

○ **What is the most common causes of pulseless electrical activity (PEA)?**

Pneumothorax, pericardial tamponade, hypoxemia, acidosis, hypovolemia.

○ **To achieve more than 90% $FIO_2$ in a non-intubated patient, which oxygen device should be used?**

Non-rebreather mask.

○ **Name some skin manifestations of shock/hypoxemia.**

Circumoral pallor/cyanosis, mottled skin, distal cyanosis, prolonged capillary refill, diminished distal pulses.

○ **A three-year-old presents with signs/symptoms of epiglottitis. Should intravenous access be a priority?**

No. Intravenous access is an absolute contraindication in suspected epiglottitis. The procedure is to put the patient in a comfortable position with supplemental oxygen and minimize the level of anxiety in the patient. All invasive procedures are to be done in the operating room.

○ **In a child who is hypoglycemic and hypotensive, is it appropriate to use a solution containing dextrose for fluid resuscitation?**

No. The use of a glucose containing solution for fluid resuscitation will result in an osmotic diuresis secondary to hyperglycemia.

○ **What is the appropriate treatment for a hypoglycemic child?**

D50W, 1.0 ml/kg through a central line, or D25W, 2.0 ml/kg through a central or peripheral line, use D10 in infants.

○ **What are the relative contraindications to the use of a nasopharyngeal airway?**

Suspected airway trauma, adenoidal hypertrophy, and bleeding diatheses.

O   **After intubating a 1 month old baby for respiratory failure, you confirm appropriate tube placement by auscultation. However, CXR reveals the tube is the right mainstem bronchus. Why were you able to hear breath sounds bilaterally?**

In small infants, it is not uncommon to hear transmitted breath sounds. In the patients, the physician is advised not only to auscultate, but also to visualize adequate chest rise bilaterally.

O   **What is the amount of $FiO_2$ each device can deliver?**

Nasal cannula: 30-40%.
Oxygen hoot/tent: up to 80-90%.
Simple mask: up to 40%.
Partial rebreathing mask: up to 60%.
Nonrebreathing mask: 100%.

O   **What comprises the assessment of the circulatory system in the pediatric patient?**

Blood pressure, heart rate, peripheral and central pulses, capillary refill, and skin color.

O   **What is the time-frame for a normal capillary refill?**

Two to three seconds.

O   **Renal output is a good indicator of adequate cardiac output. What can the physician do to assess recent urinary output in a patient?**

Assessment of simple things, like the color of the urine (dark color indicating concentrated urine) and the number of wet diapers can provide the physician with a general idea of recent urinary output.

O   **What are some major complications of endotracheal intubation?**

Esophageal intubation/perforation, trauma to the teeth, emesis and aspiration, and bradycardia.

O   **What are the major side effects of lidocaine?**

Dizziness, confusion, nausea, CNS depression, seizures, hypotension and heart blocks.

O   **What are the indications for calcium?**

Suspected hypocalcemia, hyperkalemia, hypermagnesemia, and calcium channel blocker overdose.

O   **Is there a difference between calcium chloride and calcium gluconate, in an emergency situation?**

Yes. The liver must first metabolize calcium gluconate before elemental calcium is available. Therefore, calcium chloride is the preferred drug during an emergency.

O   **What is the dose of calcium chloride?**

0.2 – 0.3ml/kg (5 - 10ml) of a 10% solution (100mg/ml). If a peripheral route is used, the drug should be given slowly. Extravasation of calcium can lead to tissue damage and necrosis.

O   **What is the catecholamine of choice when treating small infants with heart failure?**

Dopamine. In small infants, cardiac output is more dependent on heart rate than stroke volume. Dopamine is an excellent chromotrope, and will have a profound effect on blood pressure and cardiac output by increasing the heart rate. Unlike in adults, dopamine causes little renal vasoconstriction or vasodilatation.

○ **When inserting an intraosseous needle into the tibia, in which direction should the needle be placed?**

Caudal, away from the epiphysial plate. This will avoid damage to the growth plate of the tibia.

○ **When is isoproterenol indicated?**

Bradyarrhythmias and heart block. It can also be used in small infants with heart failure, because of its chronotropic properties.

○ **You are asked to assist in a precipitous delivery. The newborn is lethargic and unresponsive to tactile stimulation. The mother admits to recent heroin use. How should you proceed?**

The infant is most likely suffering from narcotic induced respiratory depression. Treatment is naloxone given either intravenously, intratracheally, intraosseously, subcutaneously, or intramuscularly, at a dose of 0.1 mg/kg.

○ **While hand-bagging a 14-year-old patient, you notice the stomach is getting distended. What steps should you take to remedy the situation?**

Apply gentle cricoid pressure to occlude the esophagus. Insertion of nasogastric or orogastric tube can also be used to decompress the stomach.

○ **In the previous patient, why not just push on the epigastric area to deflate the stomach?**

Pressure applied to the stomach for decompression can lead to emesis and aspiration.

○ **What is the normal systolic pressure in a neonate?**

Greater than 60 mm Hg.

○ **What are the signs of hypovolemia in a newborn?**

Poor response to resuscitation, persistent pallor after appropriate oxygenation, weak pulses, hypotension.

○ **Which actions are appropriate to provide tactile stimulation on a newborn in order to encourage the patient to cry?**

Flick or slap the sole of foot, or rub the back (preferably with a towel while drying the baby).

○ **What three signs suggest that a newborn is responding to resuscitation?**

Increasing heart rate, spontaneous respirations, improving color.

○ **Failure to respond to cardioversion is due to what?**

Hypothermia, hypoglycemia, acidosis, or hypoxia.

○ **How can it be determined that an endotracheal tube is in the right place?**

Symmetrical chest rise during inspiration; bilateral breath sounds on auscultation; presence of vapor in the tube; check for placement with a laryngoscope; improved oxygenation detection of $CO_2$ during expiration, with a $CO_2$ detector attached to the tube; CXR.

○ **If a newborn fails to respond to epinephrine, what should be the next step?**

Repeat epinephrine, volume expansion, and sodium bicarbonate. Unlike older pediatric patients where bicarbonate is indicated only in documented metabolic acidosis, the use of bicarbonate is indicated when the patient is not responding to epinephrine, even if there is no documented acidosis.

○ **Which sedatives are recommended for routine intubation?**

Valium 0.1 mg/kg, midazolam 0.1 mg/kg, lorazepam 0.1 mg/kg, morphine 0.1 mg/kg, fentanyl 1 mcg/kg.

○ **A 4-year-old is brought to the emergency room with suspected foreign body aspiration. The patient is alert, cyanotic, and gasping for air. What should be the immediate treatment?**

Provide oxygen. As long as the patient is awake medical personnel should not intervene. Patient should be encouraged to continue coughing and breathing.

○ **After a few minutes, the patient described in the previous question becomes unconscious. What should be the next step?**

Administer 5 back blows, followed by 5 abdominal thrusts until object is dislodged. When treating infants, administer 5 back blows, followed by 5 chest thrusts.

○ **Despite repeated efforts, the object has still not been dislodged. What should be the next procedure?**

An emergency needle cricothyrotomy or tracheostomy.

○ **Which medications cannot be given intraosseously?**

Phenytoin and chloramphenicol.

○ **Which site is used to evacuate a pneumothorax by using needle thoracentesis?**

The second intercostal space at the midclavicular line, or the fourth intercostal space at the anterior or midaxillary line.

○ **Which drug overdoses are associated with cardiac arrhythmias?**

Cocaine, heroin, tricyclic antidepressants, digitalis, calcium channel-blockers, and beta-blockers.

○ **Which laboratory studies can be obtained through an intraosseous needle?**

Electrolytes and blood cultures.

○ **Are there any differences in the "ABC" approach to cardiopulmonary arrest in children (as compared to adults)?**

Only one. The airway and breathing are relatively more stressed in children than is circulation. Except in the child with congenital cardiovascular anomalies, there are few purely cardiac causes of cardiopulmonary arrest.

## PEDIATRIC LIFE SUPPORT

○ **What is the normal IV maintenance amount for a 25 kg child?**

1600 cc/day or 65 cc/hr. The formula is: 4 ml/kg/hr or 100 ml/kg/day for the first 10 kg, 2ml/kg/hr or 50 ml/kg/day for the second 10 kg, and 1 ml/kg/hr or 20 ml/kg/day for all further kg.

○ **What is the fluid deficit in a child with mild (<5%), moderate (5-10%) and serve (>10%) dehydration?**

40-50 ml/kg, 60-90 ml/kg, and 100 ml/kg/respectively.

○ **What are high yield criteria for clinical determination of dehydration >5%?**

Capillary refill > 2 seconds, dry mucous membranes, absent tears, and general ill appearance.

○ **How does the urine specific gravity help you determine the level of dehydration in a child?**

<1.020 is found in mild dehydration, ~1.030 in moderate, and >1.035 in severe.

○ **What is cardiopulmonary arrest?**

Cardiopulmonary arrest refers to an apneic, pulseless state with cardiac standstill (asystole) or a dysrhythmia producing no cardiac output (ventricular fibrillation, ventricular tachycardia).

○ **Describe progression to non-traumatic cardiopulmonary arrest in children?**

Within the pediatric age group a cardiopulmonary arrest from a non-traumatic cause is rarely a sudden event. It occurs following an often-prolonged period of time during which a child's clinical condition deteriorates from a compensated state (respiratory distress or compensated circulatory failure) to a decompensated state (respiratory failure or decompensated shock) and finally to cardiopulmonary failure (global deficit in oxygenation, ventilation and perfusion). Once in cardiopulmonary failure, cardiopulmonary arrest is imminent.

○ **What is the outcome of cardiac arrest in infants and children?**

The outcome of cardiac arrest in children is dismal. Most (greater than 90%) of pediatric patients who present to an Emergency Department in asystole cannot be resuscitated. Only a very small percentage of those who survive are neurologically intact.

○ **What is shock?**

Shock is the clinical state of inadequate perfusion to meet the body's metabolic needs. Delivery of oxygen and important substrates (glucose) is impaired.

○ **Does shock occur exclusively in low cardiac output states?**

Shock can occur in the setting of low, normal or increased cardiac output.

○ **What is the difference between compensated and decompensated shock?**

In compensated shock, compensatory mechanisms (increased heart rate, increased peripheral vascular resistance) act to maintain adequate perfusion. Compensated shock is associated with an adequate blood pressure. Decompensated shock occurs when compensatory mechanisms have failed, perfusion is poor, and hypotension develops.

○ **What three factors determine oxygen delivery?**

Cardiac output, hemoglobin concentration and oxyhemoglobin saturation.

○ **What are clinical signs of cardiopulmonary failure?**

Respiratory failure (cyanosis, pallor), altered level of consciousness (irritability, lethargy), and hypoperfusion (tachycardia, hypotonia, weak pulses, and prolonged capillary refill). Bradycardia, hypotension and hypoventilation are seen late in cardiopulmonary failure and are signs of an imminent cardiopulmonary arrest.

○ **How does the normal respiratory rate vary in infants and children?**

A normal respiratory rate is inversely related to a child's age. It is normally fastest in the neonate and decreases throughout infancy and childhood.

○ **What is the respiratory rate of an infant?**

30-60 breaths per minute.

○ **What is the respiratory rate of a toddler?**

24-40 breaths per minute.

○ **What is the respiratory rate of a preschooler?**

22-34 breaths per minute.

○ **What is the respiratory rate for a school-age child?**

18-30 breaths per minute.

○ **What is the respiratory rate of an adolescent?**

12-16 breaths per minute (same as an adult).

○ **What is tidal volume?**

Tidal volume is the amount or volume of air that is moved with each breath. The total tidal volume increases with age (and size), but the tidal volume/kilogram remains constant throughout life.

○ **How is tidal volume assessed?**

Tidal volume is best assessed clinically by observation of chest wall movement (chest rise) with ventilation and by listening to air movement throughout the lungs.

○ **What is minute ventilation?**

Minute ventilation = tidal volume x respiratory rate.

○ **How is minute ventilation compromised with respiratory distress or failure?**

Abnormalities in the respiratory rate, tidal volume or both will compromise minute ventilation. For example, a very slow respiratory rate (bradypnea) with an adequate tidal volume or a rapid respiratory rate (tachypnea) with a very small tidal volume will both result in abnormally low minute ventilation.

MV=RR X TV
MV ↓ when RR↓ as TV↓
MV↓ when RR↓ as TV cannot ↑ to compensate

○ **What should the initial assessment of respiratory function include?**

Respiratory rate (tachypnea, bradypnea, apnea), respiratory mechanics (retractions, nasal flaring, grunting, head bobbing), color of the skin and mucous membranes (cyanosis, pallor). Patients who are developing respiratory failure present with symptoms of hypoxia or hypercarbia (decreased level of consciousness, poor muscle tone, and cyanosis).

○ **What is tachypnea?**

Tachypnea is an abnormally elevated respiratory rate. It is an early sign of respiratory distress in infants and children.

○ **Is tachypnea always caused by respiratory problems?**

Tachypnea is a compensatory mechanism seen with metabolic acidosis, abdominal disorders and some toxic ingestion as well.

○ **What is bradypnea?**

Bradypnea is an abnormally slow respiratory rate. An abnormally slow or decreasing respiratory rate is caused by fatigue and is an ominous sign of respiratory failure and decompensation.

○ **What are "seesaw or rocky" respirations?**

Seesaw respirations or abdominal breathing is characterized by chest retractions accompanied by abdominal distention. It is an ineffective form of ventilation seen with severe respiratory distress and impending respiratory failure.

○ **What is grunting?**

An ominous respiratory sound heard at the end of exhalation. It is an involuntary reflex in infants and is caused by exhalation against a prematurely closed glottis. Infants and children grunt in order to maintain or increase positive end expiratory pressure.

○ **With what conditions is grunting associated?**

Grunting is associated with conditions that result in hypoxia such as pulmonary edema and pneumonia.

○ **Grunting is observed during what phase of respiration?**

Expiratory-exhalation against a closed glottis.

○ **What is stridor?**

High-pitched inspiratory sound caused by extra-thoracic upper airway obstruction.

○ **What are common causes of upper airway obstructions in infants and young children that may present as stridor?**

Congenital anomalies (macroglossia, tracheomalacia, cysts, tumors or hemangiomas of the airway, vocal cord paralysis), infections (croup, epiglottitis, pharyngeal abscess, bacterial tracheitis), upper airway inflammation (allergy, post intubation), and esophageal or airway foreign body.

O **What is wheezing?**

A musical sound caused by pathology in the lower airway usually due to an obstruction from inflammation or swelling at the bronchial or bronchiolar level. This type of obstruction causes air trapping and in addition to wheezing, prolonged expiration can also be appreciated on physical examination.

O **What are common pediatric diagnoses that can cause prolonged expiration?**

Bronchiolitis, asthma, intrathoracic foreign body and rarely pulmonary edema.

O **During positive pressure ventilation how should the effectiveness of ventilation be assessed?**

Auscultation of breath sounds and observation of chest wall movement.

O **What should be observed regarding chest wall expansion?**

The chest wall should expand symmetrically with each breath.

O **Is central cyanosis an early indicator of hypoxemia?**

No. Central cyanosis is a late sign of hypoxemia. It is generally associated with marked respiratory distress and/or respiratory failure.

O **Is central cyanosis always seen with hypoxemia?**

No. For cyanosis to be clinically apparent, 5 grams desaturated hemoglobin per deciliter of blood must be present. Therefore, cyanosis may not be observed in an anemic child who is hypoxic.

O **What is the heart rate range of a newborn to 3 months?**

80 (with sleep)-160 beats per minute.

O **What is the heart rate range from 3 months to 2 years?**

75-190 beats per minute.

O **What is the heart rate range from 2 to 10 years?**

60-140 beats per minute.

O **What is the heart rate range >10 years?**

50-100 beats per minute.

O **What is the formula for estimating blood pressure in children 1-10 years of age (50$^{th}$ percentile)?**

80mm Hg + (child's age in years/2) mm Hg.

O **What is the difference between compensated and decompensated shock?**

Compensated and decompensated shocks occur in a continuum. In early or compensated shock, hypoperfusion of vital organs (decreased urine output, abnormal mental status) is present but compensatory mechanisms are sufficient to sustain adequate perfusion. Decompensated shock occurs when these compensatory mechanisms fail and organ perfusion worsens and hypotension develops.

○ **How is shock related to cardiac output?**

Shock is usually associated with a decreased cardiac output (hypovolemia), however the hypoperfusion seen with sepsis and anaphylaxis can occur with an increased cardiac output.

○ **What compensatory mechanisms occur when shock is associated with a low cardiac output state?**

Peripheral vascular resistance increases, the skin become cool and mottled and blood is diverted away from nonessential organs, such as the skin and mesentery. This redistribution of cardiac output and increased peripheral vascular resistance allows for an adequate blood pressure to be maintained.

○ **What occurs in shock with high cardiac output?**

In a high cardiac output state such as anaphylaxis, low peripheral vascular resistance results in increased blood flow to the skin and periphery. The skin may appear pink and well perfused and peripheral pulses may be full or bounding.

○ **Which compensatory mechanism maintains adequate cardiac output in the face of circulatory failure?**

Heart rate to a much greater extent than stroke volume influences cardiac output in infants and young children.

○ **What happens to the heart rate in older children in response to hypoxemia?**

The initial response to hypoxemia in older children is tachycardia. As hypoxemia persists, tachycardia is followed by bradycardia.

○ **What compensatory mechanisms come into play to maintain normal blood pressure despite falling cardiac output?**

Tachycardia, increased cardiac contractility (does not occur in young infants) and peripheral vasoconstriction.

○ **What is the significance of hypotension in a child with cardiopulmonary failure?**

Hypotension is a sign of endstage circulatory failure signaling depreciation of cardiovascular reserves and failure of compensatory mechanisms. It is rare but, when seen signifies an immanent cardiopulmonary arrest.

○ **T/F: Heart rate and blood pressure are of limited value in the recognition of circulatory failure in children.**

True. Heart rate and blood pressure are of limited value in determining the presence and degree of circulatory failure.

○ **What is the relationship between compensatory tachycardia and blood pressure?**

Because of compensatory tachycardia and peripheral vasoconstriction, the blood pressure is almost always found to be within the normal range in pediatric patients with progressing but still compensated circulatory failure.

O   **Is blood pressure reliable for the diagnosis or estimate of degree of shock?**

Blood pressure alone is unreliable for the diagnosis or estimate of degree of shock.

O   **How should the clinician evaluate circulatory failure in children?**

A carefully performed physical examination of end-organ perfusion as well as evaluation of vital signs will allow circulatory failure to be properly assessed.

O   **As the cardiac output drops in the setting of hypovolemia, how do the peripheral pulses feel?**

The volume of the pulse seems diminished or thready. As hypoperfusion progresses, peripheral pulses may become absent.

O   **What is the significance of the loss of central pulses in a child in cardiopulmonary failure?**

Loss of central pulses is a serious sign of an impending cardiopulmonary arrest.

O   **What is the importance of an examination of the skin of a child who is in circulatory failure?**

Because of the high surface area to volume ratio in young children and infants, the skin is a relatively large organ as compared to adults. Decreased skin perfusion is a common and early sign of circulatory failure.

O   **What are early signs of abnormal CNS perfusion?**

Signs of an abnormal mental status include confusion, irritability, lethargy, agitation and inappropriate behavior. An abnormal mental status in an infant or baby may be most easily assessed by observing the child's response to his parents, anxiety at parental separation and response to painful stimuli.

O   **What are clinical signs of severe and prolonged abnormal CNS perfusion?**

More profound change in mental status, loss of consciousness, abnormal muscle tones, seizures, and pupillary dilatation. A classification of a child's level of consciousness might include awake, responsive to voice, responsive to pain, and unresponsive.

O   **What are the causes of respiratory failure in a child who has suffered trauma?**

Respiratory failure may occur as a result of an injury to the brain, upper airway obstruction, injury to the lung or chest wall or even intra abdominal injury with restriction of movement of the diaphragm.

O   **What traumatic chest injuries may result in respiratory failure?**

Pneumothorax, hemothorax, pulmonary contusion, flail chest.

O   **What are the major causes of hemorrhagic shock?**

Trauma injuries to solid organs (liver or splenic laceration, hemothorax), fractures of large bones (femur fracture, pelvic fracture), and intracranial injury with hemorrhage or large soft tissue lacerations (scalp laceration) are all sources of significant blood loss.

O   **What are some of the complications associated with burns in young children?**

Significant fluid loss through the burn and extravascular tissue occurs in children with burns in excess of 10% of the total body surface area. Inhalation injury from toxins and thermal injury may cause upper airway obstruction or respiratory failure and carbon monoxide poisoning.

○ **What are causes of acute deterioration during positive pressure ventilation?**

Endotracheal tube obstruction (mucus, blood, secretions), displacement (into the esophagus, pharynx or right main stem bronchus) tension pneumothorax, and mechanical equipment failure.

○ **How does respiratory distress or failure develop during seizures?**

Poor chest wall movement occurs during generalized tonic seizures leading to hypoventilation. Upper airway obstruction may be caused by tongue displacement and secretions. The effect of the above factors can be compounded by medications that cause respiratory depression. It is important to continuously monitor a child (especially heart rate and oxygen saturation) during, and following seizures.

# INFECTIOUS DISEASES

○ **How quickly do patients infected with HIV become symptomatic?**

Five to ten percent develop symptoms within three years of seroconversion. Predictive characteristics include a low T4 count and a hematocrit less than 40. The mean incubation time is about 8.23 years for adults and 1.97 years for children less than 5 years old. When AIDS develops, the survival duration is about 9 months.

○ **An HIV+ patient presents with a history of weight loss, diarrhea, fever, anorexia, and malaise. She is also dyspneic. Lab studies reveal abnormal LFTs and anemia. What is the most likely diagnosis?**

*Mycobacterium avium-intracellulare.*

○ **Which drugs are used to treat CNS toxoplasmosis in AIDS patients?**

Pyrimethamine plus sulfadiazine.

○ **What is the most common cause of focal encephalitis in AIDS patients?**

Toxoplasmosis.

○ **The differential diagnosis of ring-enhancing lesions in AIDS patients is what?**

Lymphoma, cerebral tuberculosis, fungal infection, CMV, Kaposi's sarcoma, toxoplasmosis, and hemorrhage.

○ **What is the presentation of an AIDS patient with tuberculous meningitis?**

Fever, meningismus, headache, seizures, focal neurologic deficits, and altered mental status.

○ **On physical exam, what is the most common eye finding in AIDS patients?**

Cotton-wool spots. It has been proposed that the cotton-wool spots are associated with PCP.

○ **What is the most common opportunistic infection in AIDS patients?**

PCP.

○ **How is *Candida* of the esophagus diagnosed in the ED?**

An air-contrast barium swallow shows ulcerations with plaques. In contrast, herpes esophagitis produces punched-out ulcerations with no plaques.

○ **What is the risk of contracting HIV infection after an occupational exposure?**

0.32%. Eighty percent of the occupational exposure-related infections are from needle sticks.

○ **A patient is infected with *Treponema pallidum*; what is the treatment?**

The type of treatment depends upon the stage (1°, 2°, 3°) of the infection. Stages 1° and 2° syphilis are treated with benzathine penicillin G (2.4 million units IM X 1 dose) or doxycycline (100 mg bid po for 14 day). Stage 3° syphilis is treated with benzathine penicillin G, 2.4 million units IM X 3 doses 3 weeks apart.

○ **What is the cause of chancroid?**

*Hemophilus ducreyi*. Patients with this condition present with one or more painful necrotic lesions. Suppurating inguinal lymphadenopathy may also be present.

○ **What is the cause of granuloma inguinale?**

*Calymmatobacterium granulomatis*. Typically the onset occurs with small papular, nodular, or vesicular lesions that develop slowly into ulcerative or granulomatous lesions. Lesions are painless and are located on mucous membranes of the genital, inguinal, and anal areas.

○ **What is the causative agent in tetanus?**

*Clostridium tetani*. This organism is a Gram-positive rod, vegetative, and a spore former. *C. tetani* produces tetanospasmin, an endotoxin, which induces the disinhibition of the motor and autonomic nervous systems and thus the exhibition of tetanus clinical symptoms.

○ **What is the incubation period of tetanus?**

Hours to over 1 month. The shorter the incubation period, the more severe the disease.

○ **What is the <u>most</u> common presentation of tetanus?**

"Generalized tetanus" with pain and stiffness in the trunk and jaw muscles. Trismus develops and results in risus sardonicus (i.e., a sardonic smile).

○ **List 3 common protozoa that can cause diarrhea.**

1. *Entamoeba histolytica*. Occurs worldwide. Although half of the infected patients are asymptomatic, the usual symptoms consist of N/V/D/F, anorexia, abdominal pain, and leukocytosis. Determine the presence of this organism by ordering stool tests and performing an ELISA for extraintestinal infections. Treatment is with metronidazole or tinidazole followed by chloroquine phosphate.

2. *Giardia lamblia*. Occurs worldwide. This organism is one of the most common intestinal parasites in the U. S.. Symptoms include explosive watery diarrhea, flatus, abdominal distention, fatigue, and fever. The diagnosis is confirmed via a stool examination. Treatment is with metronidazole.

3. *Cryptosporidium parvum*. Occurs worldwide. Symptoms are profuse watery diarrhea, cramps, N/V/F, and weight loss. Treatment is supportive care. Medications may be needed for immunocompromised patients.

○ **Explain the pathophysiology of rabies.**

Infection occurs within the myocytes for the first 48 to 96 hours. It then spreads across the motor endplate and ascends and replicates along the peripheral nervous system, axoplasm, and into the dorsal root ganglia, spinal cord, and CNS. From the gray matter, the virus spreads by peripheral nerves back to tissues and organ systems.

O   **What is the characteristic histologic finding associated with rabies?**

Eosinophilic intracellular lesions found within the cerebral neurons called Negri bodies are the sites of CNS viral replication.

O   **What are the signs and symptoms of rabies?**

Incubation period of 12 to 700 days with an average of 20 to 90 days. The initial signs and systems begin with fevers, headache, malaise, anorexia, sore throat, nausea, cough, and pain or paresthesias at the bite site.

During the CNS stage, agitation, restlessness, altered mental status, painful bulbar and peripheral muscular spasms, bulbar or focal motor paresis, and opisthotonos are exhibited. 20% develop ascending, symmetric flaccid and areflexic paralysis. In addition, hypersensitivity to water and sensory stimuli to light, touch, and noise may occur.

The progressive stage includes lucid and confused intervals with hyperpyrexia, lacrimation, salivation, and mydriasis along with brainstem dysfunction, hyperreflexia, and extensor plantar response.

In the final stages, coma, convulsions, and apnea occur, followed by death between the fourth and seventh day for the untreated patient. The treated patient may survive for 14 days.

O   **How is rabies treated?**

Prevention is the most effective treatment. Wound care of a suspected rabies bite should include debridement and aggressive irrigation. The wound must not be sutured; it should remain open. This will decrease the rabies infection by 90%. RIG 20 IU/kg, as much as possible at wound site and the remainder in the deltoid muscle, should be administered along with HDCV, 1-mL doses IM on days 0, 3, 7, 14, and 28, also in the deltoid muscle.

O   **What is the second most common tick borne disease?**

Rocky Mountain spotted fever (RMSF). The causative agent is *Rickettsia rickettsii* and the vectors are the female Ixodi ticks, *Dermacentor andersoni* (wood tick) and *D. variabilis* (American dog tick). Lyme disease is the most common tick borne disease.

O   **Which test should be performed to confirm RMSF?**

Immunofluorescent antibody staining of a skin biopsy or a serologic fluorescent antibody titer. The Weil-Felix reaction and complement fixation tests are no longer recommended.

O   **Which antibiotics are prescribed for the treatment of RMSF?**

Tetracycline or chloramphenicol. Antibiotic therapy should not be withheld pending serologic confirmation.

O   **Which is the most deadly form of malaria?**

*Plasmodium falciparum.*

O   **What is the vector for malaria?**

The female Anopheline mosquito.

○ **What lab findings are expected for a patient with malaria?**

Normochromic normocytic anemia, a normal or depressed leukocyte count, thrombocytopenia, an elevated sed rate, abnormal kidney and LFTs, hyponatremia, hypoglycemia, and a false-positive VDRL.

○ **What is the drug of choice for treating *P. vivax*, *ovale*, and *malariae*?**

Chloroquine.

○ **Which type of parasite infections do not typically result in eosinophilia?**

Protozoa infections, such as *Amoeba*, *Giardia*, *Trypanosoma*, and *Babesia*.

○ **Which is the most common intestinal parasite in the US?**

*Giardia*. Cysts are obtained from contaminated water or passed by hand-to-mouth transmission. Symptoms include explosive foul-smelling diarrhea, abdominal distention, fever, fatigue, and weight loss. Cysts reside in the duodenum and upper jejunum.

○ **How is Chagas disease transmitted?**

The blood-sucking Reduviid "kissing" bug, blood transfusion, or breast feeding. A nodule or chagoma develops at the site of the bite. Symptoms include fever, headache, conjunctivitis, anorexia, and myocarditis. CHF and ventricular aneurysms can occur. The myenteric plexus is involved and may result in megacolon. Lab findings include anemia, leukocytosis, elevated sed rate, and ECG changes, such as PR interval, heart block, T-wave changes, and arrhythmias.

○ **What are two diseases that the deer tick, *Ixodes dammini*, transmits?**

Lyme disease and *Babesia*.

○ **How do patients present with *Babesia* infection?**

Intermittent fever, splenomegaly, jaundice, and hemolysis. The disease may be fatal in patients without spleens. Treatment is with clindamycin and quinine.

○ **When are patients most likely to acquire Lyme disease?**

Late spring to late summer with the highest incidence in July.

○ **How is Lyme disease diagnosed?**

Immunofluorescent and immunoabsorbent assays identify the antibodies to the spirochete. Treatment includes doxycycline or tetracycline, amoxicillin, IV penicillin (V in pregnant patients), or erythromycin.

○ **Which type of paralysis does tick paralysis cause?**

Ascending paralysis. The venom that causes the paralysis is probably a neurotoxin. A conduction block is induced at the peripheral motor nerve branches and thereby prevents the release of acetylcholine at the neuromuscular junction. Forty-three species of ticks have been implicated as causative agents.

○ **What is the most common sign of tularemia?**

Lymphadenopathy, usually cervical in children and inguinal in adults. It is caused by *Francisella tularensis* and is transmitted by the vectors *Dermacentor variabilis* and *Amblyomma americanum*.

○   **A patient presents with a sudden onset of fever, lethargy, headache, myalgias, anorexia, nausea, and vomiting. She describes the headache as retro-orbital and is extremely photophobic. The patient has been on a camping trip in Wyoming. What tick-borne disease might cause these symptoms?**

A virus of the genus *Orbivirus*, of the family, Reoviridae, causes Colorado tick fever. The vector is the tick *D. andersoni*. The disease is self-limited and treatment is supportive.

○   **What is the most common cause of cellulitis?**

*Streptococcus pyogenes*. *Staphylococcus aureus* can also cause cellulitis though it is generally less severe and more often associated with an open wound.

○   **What is the most common cause of cutaneous abscesses?**

*Staphylococcus aureus* is the most common aerobe in cutaneous abscesses; two-thirds are found in the upper torso, 97% are resistant to penicillin G.

○   **What is the probable cause of an infection arising from an animal bite that develops in less than 24 hours? More than 48 hours?**

Less than 24 hours is typically *P. multocida* or streptococci. More than 48 hours is usually *Staphylococcus aureus*.

○   **A patient who was involved in a work-related crush injury to his foot is brought to your office a day after the injury in shock. The patient has a fever, severe pain, and a horrible smell coming from his foot. On palpation you feel crepitus. Diagnosis?**

Gas gangrene. Gas from the infection quickly invades the fascial planes accounting for the crepitus. Treatment is with wound debridement and systemic antibiotics. The drug of choice is penicillin G; an alternative is chloramphenicol.

○   **What is the most common cause of gas gangrene?**

*Clostridium perfringens*.

○   **What is the most common site of herpes simplex I virus infection?**

The lower lip. First the lip itches and burns. Then the small vesicle with the red base appears. These lesions are painful and can frequently recur since the virus remains in the sensory ganglia. Recurrences are generally triggered by stress, sun, and illness.

○   **What are the most common causes of otitis media?**

*S. pneumoniae*, nontypeable *H. influenza*, and *M. catarrhalis*.

○   **An infant is brought to your office with fever and lethargy. On physical exam, you notice purulent rhinitis and an adherent membrane. The pt also has some shallow ulcers on the upper lip. What is your diagnosis?**

Diptheria in nares. This is more common in infants.

○   **What are the 3 stages of pertussis? How long does each last?**

Catarrhal, paroxysmal, and convalescent. Each stage lasts about 2 weeks.

○ **How do you calculate dosages for antibiotics in obese children?**

Calculate their ideal weight from height and use that.

○ **What are the most common viral causes of pneumonia in the otherwise healthy child?**

RSV, influenza, parainfluenza, and adenovirus.

○ **What viral cause of pneumonia can lead to acute fulminant pneumonia?**

Adenovirus.

○ **What is the treatment of choice for gastroenteritis caused by *Shigella* in an 8-year-old child?**

TMP/SMX or cefixime if resistant.

○ **The "red man syndrome" is classically associated with what antibiotic?**

Too rapid an infusion of vancomycin.

○ **What is the drug of choice in a child with the signs and symptoms of whooping cough?**

Erythromycin estolate (10 mg/kg QID PO for 14 days).

○ **In a child with the typical facial features of classic mumps, where else on the body should you look for suggestive signs?**

Look for sternal edema (classic) and examine the testicles.

○ **An 11-year-old child stepped on a nail on his way home from school. The nail pierced through his sneaker and into his foot. His tetanus status is up to date. What is your main concern?**

Infection with *Pseudomonas* that can lead to osteomyelitis. Pseudomonal infection is soon most commonly in association with hot, moist environments, such as sneakers.

○ **What would be your empiric antibiotic of choice for the boy in the preceding question?**

Ceftazidime (100mg/kg/day as TID) AND nafcillin (150mg/kg/day as QID). Debridement with culture is a cornerstone of therapy.

○ **What is the most common cause of infectious arthritis in patients with sickle cell disease? What joint is most commonly affected?**

*Staph. aureus* remains the most common cause, as in otherwise healthy children. However, *Salmonella* is more commonly seen in septic arthritis in children with hemoglobinopathies. The hip is most commonly affected.

○ **In a child with the clinical signs and symptoms of encephalitis, what non-invasive test can be used to determine whether herpes simplex is the causative agent?**

An EEG with patterns of periodic lateralized epileptiform discharges (PLEDs). An MRI of the brain is more sensitive.

○ **If the test above is positive, what test can be used to confirm your diagnosis of herpes simplex encephalitis?**

Polymerase chain reaction (PCR) analysis of CSF.

○ **Infection with what agent is commonly seen in children with liver transplants?**

CMV infection is seen in up to 60% of these patients.

○ **What is the antibiotic regimen of choice after an appendectomy?**

Cefoxitin or clindamycin and gentamicin.

○ **In the US what is the recommended time of isolation for a dog or cat to rule out rabies?**

10 days.

○ **A 15-year-old boy is brought to the ED with a complaint of joint pains and general weakness. On physical exam, he has a slight fever and hepatosplenomegaly. The father states that the boy has been really depressed lately for no known reason: "why look how happy he was just 2 weeks ago when he shot his first elk!" The father shows a picture of the son holding onto his kill. What possible diagnosis is the picture a clue to?**

It should make you consider brucellosis from handling the carcass or from ticks.

○ **What is the easiest way to distinguish residual formula in the mouth from thrush in an infant?**

Formula is easily scraped away with a tongue depressor, while the same maneuver in a child with thrush might lead to minute bleeding points.

○ **Cerebral calcifications are most commonly associated with what 3 congenital infections?**

Toxoplasmosis, herpes simplex and cytomegalovirus.

○ **Minimal to severe brain dysfunction can be a sequelae of what intrauterine infections?**

Toxoplasmosis, rubella, CMV, and herpes.

○ **Which is the most common congenital infection?**

CMV, though only about 5% will show any symptoms.

○ **How is neonatal herpes usually contracted?**

Contact with genital secretions at delivery.

○ **What is the treatment of choice for the neonate with an HSV infection?**

Acyclovir, but Vidarabine may be just as effective.

○ **What test should be ordered to insure that a pregnant woman does not have an active hepatitis B infection?**

HBsAg.

○ **What is the characteristic triad of manifestations for late congenital syphilis?**

Hutchinson's triad consists of Hutchinson's teeth, interstitial keratitis, and eighth nerve deafness.

○ **What is the most effective method of reducing fever in a child?**

Acetaminophen (and NSAIDs) can return the set-point to normal.

○ **What organism is responsible for most cases of occult bacteremia in infants and toddlers?**

*Streptococcus pneumoniae.*

○ **A child with a positive blood culture to what organism is most likely to develop meningitis?**

Meningococcus.

○ **How can the distribution of petechiae help one to evaluate the risk of a serious bacterial infection?**

Petechiae found only above the line of the nipples is rarely found in systemic disease.

○ **What is necessary for the diagnosis of fever of unknown origin?**

1) History of fever over 1 week,
2) Documentation of fever by health provider,
3) Lack of a diagnosis after one week of investigation.

○ **A pediatric AIDS patient with enlargement of salivary glands, digital clubbing, and generalized lymphadenopathy and an x-ray that reveals a nodular, reticular pattern most likely has what disease?**

Lymphoid interstitial pneumonitis (LIP).

○ **Which has a worse prognosis for the pediatric AIDS patient, PCP or LIP?**

PCP.

○ **What is the current treatment of choice for LIP therapy?**

Systemic steroid therapy.

○ **Why should a child with suspected idiopathic thrombocytopenic purpura (ITP) be tested for HIV?**

Thrombocytopenia may be the presenting sign for HIV infection.

○ **How do viral meningitis and bacterial meningitis differ with regards to CSF pressure? CSF leukocytes? CSF glucose?**

The pressure in bacterial infection is increased, whereas it is normal or slightly increased in viral. The leukocytosis is greater than 1000 (up to 60K) in bacterial, and rarely over 1000 in viral meningitis. The glucose concentration is decreased in bacterial meningitis and is generally normal in viral.

○ **What is the most common cause of bacterial meningitis in a child greater than 2 months old?**

*Strep. pneumoniae.*

○ **What antibiotic agent(s) should you start immediately in a toxic, febrile infant that is less than 3 months old?**

Ceftriaxone or cefotaxime and ampicillin.

○ **What is the most common cause of death in children with HbSS?**

Infection.

○ **A premature infant is delivered at 32 weeks of age. How long after delivery should the infant be given his first vaccine?**

Same schedule as a full-term baby.

○ **Why do so many patients with meningitis become hyponatremic?**

Because a majority of patients with this disease develop some degree of SIADH.

○ **What is the *sine quo non* of botulism poisoning presentation?**

Bulbar palsy.

○ **If the mother of a child with erythema infectiosum is infected, what would be her most likely presentation?**

Arthralgia and arthritis.

○ **Which cephalosporins cover *Listeria monocytogenes*?**

None. That is why ampicillin is usually added to the antibiotic regimen when infection with this organism is a possibility.

○ **Where does the rash of Rocky Mountain Spotted Fever usually start?**

On the wrists and ankles, spreading to the trunk and extremities within hours.

○ **A worried mother calls the ED concerned that her daughter was exposed to chickenpox at the day care center. If she were exposed, how long would it take for the symptoms to appear?**

Ten to twenty one days.

○ **What is the most common cause of nosocomial bacteremia?**

Coagulase negative *Staphylococcus*. This is usually successfully treated with methicillin.

○ **A child is diagnosed with impetigo from group A streptococcus. What sequelae do you have to keep an eye out for?**

Acute post-streptococcal glomerulonephritis. Impetigo does not lead to rheumatic fever.

○ **What is the usual etiologic agent of a hordeolum (stye)?**

*Staph. aureus.*

○ **For a hordeolum from a *Staph*. infection, what is the therapy of choice?**

Hot soaks, and I & D, if necessary. Routine antibiotic use is not recommended.

○ **What is considered to be the best therapy for patients with uncomplicated cat-scratch disease?**

Symptomatic relief. The use of antibiotic is controversial.

○ **A 10-year-old boy presents to your office with fever, tonsillopharyngitis, and lymphadenopathy. What laboratory tests will confirm your presumed diagnosis?**

CBC and Monospot should be all you need to confirm your suspicion of EBV (infectious mononucleosis).

○ **What would you expect to find on a peripheral blood smear of a patient with an acquired CMV infection?**

Absolute lymphocytosis and atypical lymphocytes.

○ **What is the drug of choice for meningococcal disease?**

Aqueous penicillin G is the ideal, though patients can be started effectively on empiric cefotaxime or ceftriaxone for suspected cases and in patients with penicillin allergy.

○ **How often are fever and a bulging fontanelle present in an infant less than 2 months old with meningitis?**

Only about half have a fever, and only a third will have a bulging fontanelle.

○ **How is CNS hemorrhage differentiated from a traumatic tap?**

A traumatic tap will have a decreasing RBC count in each successive tube and will not have crenated RBCs or xanthochromia of the supernatant.

○ **Of bacterial, viral, fungal and tubercular meningitis, which typically presents with the greatest concentration of WBCs?**

Bacterial meningitis.

○ **Meningitis due to what organism most commonly presents with a sub-dural effusion?**

*H. influenzae.*

○ **Should people who have had contact with patients with meningococcal meningitis be given prophylactic antibiotics?**

Yes. Rifampin is recommended.

○ **What is, overall, the most common cause of aseptic meningitis?**

Enteroviruses.

○ **Generally speaking, how do exudates of viral conjunctivitis differ from bacterial conjunctivitis?**

Viral is serous, and bacterial is mucopurulent or purulent.

○ **What is the cause of epidemic keratoconjunctivitis?**

Adenovirus.

○ **What is the initial therapy of gonococcal ophthalmia neonatorum?**

Ceftriaxone or cefotaxime and saline irrigation of the eye until resolution of the discharge.

○ **Clinically, how can you distinguish orbital cellulitis from periorbital cellulitis?**

Extra-ocular muscle dysfunction, decreased pupillary reflexes, decreased visual acuity and changes in globe position are seen only in orbital cellulitis.

○ **With a child you suspect has an otitis media from the history, but are unable to visualize the lumen secondary to cerumen obstruction, how should you proceed?**

Remove the cerumen and visualize the membrane.

○ **What is the most common cause of hearing deficits in children?**

Secretory otitis media.

○ **What is the drug of choice for streptococcal pharyngitis?**

Penicillin V.

○ **After initiation of therapy for streptococcal pharyngitis, when should children be allowed back into school?**

After 24 hours have elapse.

○ **What is the classic cause of herpangina?**

Coxsackievirus A16.

○ **Does trismus more commonly occur with a peritonsillar abscess or peritonsillar cellulitis?**

Peritonsillar abscess.

○ **Currently, what is the most common cause of epiglottitis?**

Group A strep. The widespread use of the HiB vaccine has brought the number of *Haemophilus* induced epiglottitis cases down dramatically.

○ **Are steroids effective in acute laryngotracheobronchitis?**

Yes. The use of dexamethasone (0.15-0.6 mg/kg, max 10 mg) can lead to decreased need for intubation and more rapid improvement.

○ **How often is sinus tenderness found in patients with sinusitis?**

Almost never.

○ **What sinuses are most commonly involved in sinusitis?**

Ethmoid and maxillary sinuses.

○ **What are the most common causes of acute sinusitis in children?**

*Pneumococcus*, *H. influenzae* nontypeable, and *Moraxella catarrhalis* (same as otitis media).

○ **Why does therapy for TB take several months, when other infections usually clear in a matter of days?**

Because the mycobacteria divide very slowly and have a long dormant phase, during which time they are not responsive to medications.

○ **What is the most common side effect of rifampin?**

Orange discoloration of urine and tears.

○ **What negative outcome can be avoided by supplementing pyridoxine in patients receiving isoniazid?**

Peripheral neuritis and convulsions.

○ **Name at least three infectious diseases that give false positive treponemal tests (FTA, MHA-TP, TPI) for syphilis.**

Yaws, pinta, leptospirosis, rat-bite fever (*Spirillum minus*) and Lyme disease.

○ **Name at least three diseases that give false positive non-treponema (VDRL, RPR) tests for syphilis.**

Infectious mononucleosis, connective tissue diseases, tuberculosis, endocarditis, and intravenous drug abuse.

○ **What are the organisms most commonly thought to be associated with Guillain-Barré Disease?**

CMV, EBV, Coxsackievirus, *Campylobacter jejuni*, and *Mycoplasma pneumoniae*.

○ **What is the appropriate diagnostic study to perform in order to distinguish lung sequestration from other changes on the pediatric chest x-ray?**

Angiography.

○ **Children who have cellular immunodeficiencies tend to get infections due to what organisms?**

Mycobacteria, *Nocardia*, cytomegalovirus, varicella zoster virus, *Cryptococcus*, *Candida*, and *Pneumocystis carinii*.

○ **Children with hypogammaglobulinemia tend to get infections with what organisms?**

The usual bacterial pathogens and *Pseudomonas*.

○ **Children with sickle cell disease most commonly are affected with what organisms?**

*Streptococcus pneumoniae*, *Haemophilus influenzae* B, and particularly severe *Mycoplasma pneumoniae* infections.

○ **What is the evaluation of foreign body in the lung?**

Chest x-ray and bronchoscopy.

○ **What is the evaluation for *Candida* of the lung?**

Fresh sputum or transtracheal aspirate should reveal yeast and pseudohyphae. Mycelia and blastospores will be seen in established colonization, so a tissue exam is needed for definitive proof.

○ **What are some of the most convenient ways to make the diagnosis of *Mycoplasma pneumoniae*?**

Cold agglutinin levels of >=1:32 with consistent clinical findings will make presumptive diagnosis. A complement fixation level to *Mycoplasma pneumoniae* may be seen of >= than 1:256, *or Mycoplasma pneumoniae* specific lgA or lgM will be elevated.

○ **What are the most common causes of non-infectious stomatitis?**

Behcet's syndrome, Stevens-Johnson syndrome, cancer chemotherapy, and Kawasaki syndrome.

○ **What culture media are used to grow *Neisseria gonorrhoeae*?**

Thayer-Martin or chocolate agar.

○ **What culture medium is used to isolate *Corynebacterium diphtheriae* and what antibiotic should be used for treatment?**

Loeffler's medium, tellurite agar, or silica gel pack. Patients should be treated with equine diphtheria antitoxin and either erythromycin or penicillin.

○ **What is the differential diagnosis for a patient who on first consideration appears to be suffering from tetanus?**

Dental abscess, rabies, hypocalcemic tetany, antipsychotic drugs, or the extrapyramidal effects of compazine.

○ **Name at least five causes of parotitis in pediatric patients.**

An incomplete list of causes of parotitis include bacteria in general, viruses, especially mumps, echovirus, coxsackie A, lymphocytic choriomeningitis virus, parainfluenza 1 and 3, cytomegalovirus, Epstein-Barr virus, and HIV. Other causes include mycobacteria, histoplasmosis, post-typhoid fever, cat scratch disease, dehydration, collagen-vascular disease, cystic fibrosis, ectodermal dysplasia, familial dysautonomia, sarcoidosis, drugs, poisoning (including lead, copper and mercury), sialolithiasis, and tumors.

○ **What organisms are known to cause renal and perinephric abscesses?**

The most common organisms are *Staphylococcus aureus*, *Escherichia coli*, *Proteus* spp., *Pseudomonas* spp., and *Enterococcus*.

○ **What are the common bacterial causes of parotitis in newborns?**

*Staphylococcus aureus*, *Escherichia coli*, and *Pseudomonas aeruginosa*.

○ **What are the most common etiologic agents of parotitis in older children?**

*Staphylococcus aureus* and streptococci.

○ **What is the differential diagnosis of a renal abscess in a neonate?**

Renal hamartoma or congenital cyst.

○ **What is the differential diagnosis of a renal abscess in an older infant or child?**

A Wilm's tumor, a lymphoma, an angiomyolipoma, hemorrhagic infarct, hematoma, and acute focal pyelonephritis (acute lobar nephronia).

○ **When a child presents with more than one infected joint simultaneously, what organisms should be considered as the likely culprits?**

*Staphylococcus aureus*, *Salmonella* or gonorrhea.

○ **When a child has an underlying cardiac condition which predisposes him/her to endocarditis, what events and procedures do not require endocarditis prophylaxis?**

Dental procedures without gingival bleeding; injection of local intraoral anesthetic (except intraligamentary injections); shedding primary teeth; tympanostomy tube insertion; endotracheal intubation; flexible bronchoscopy, with and without biopsy; cardiac catheterization; gastrointestinal endoscopy, with and without biopsy; cesarean section; and, if there is no infection present, urethral catheterization; dilation and curettage; uncomplicated vaginal delivery, therapeutic abortion; sterilization procedures and insertion or removal of an intrauterine device.

○ **Name at least five infectious agents associated with erythema nodosum.**

Erythema nodosum has been associated with many infectious and some non-infectious processes. Some of its better known associates are Group A streptococcus, meningococcus, syphilis, *Mycobacterium tuberculosis*, and *Mycobacterium leprae*, as well as histoplasmosis, coccidioidmycosis, blastomycosis and herpes simplex virus. Some of the less common associates of erythema nodosum include *Chlamydia trachomatis*, *Chlamydia psitacci*, *Corynebacterium diphtheriae*, *Campylobacter*, *Haemophilus ducreyi*, yersinia, *Bartonella henselae*, *Trichophyton*, filariasis, sarcoidosis, and various drugs.

○ **The inflammation associated with tuberculous meningitis classically affects what cranial nerves?**

Cranial nerves 3,6,7, and the optic chiasm.

○ **Pediatric patients that have received transplantations have an increase in what infections?**

*Staphylococcus, pseudomonas, Klebsiella, Candida, Aspergillus, Nocardia, Pneumocystis carinii,* cytomegalovirus, and varicella zoster virus.

○ **Children with malignancies are known to have an increase in infections due to what agents?**

*Pseudomonas, Klebsiella, Escherichia coli, Cryptococcus,* varicella zoster virus, *Pneumocystis carinii,* mycobacteria.

○ **A child has a pericardial tap and hemorrhagic fluid is withdrawn. What are the most likely possibilities?**

Trauma, tumor, tuberculosis, or histoplasmosis.

○ **What characteristics categorize a pleural fluid as empyema?**

Greater than 50,000 white cells, glucose <= than 30 mg.%, and a low pH.

○ **Name three common causes of pleural effusion without empyema in the pediatric age group.**

*Staphylococcus aureus, Streptococcus pneumoniae,* HiB, *Streptococcus pyogenes,* and *Mycoplasma pneumoniae.*

○ **Name two of the most common infectious causes of an empyema in the pediatric age group.**

*Staphylococcus aureus, Streptococcus pneumoniae,* anaerobes, and tuberculosis.

○ **What is the most common complication of otitis media?**

Effusion and hearing loss.

○ **What is the most common intracranial complication of otitis media?**

Meningitis. Other intracranial complications include epidural abscess, subdural abscess, brain abscess, encephalitis, lateral sinus thrombosis, communicating hydrocephalus, CSF otorrhea, and petrositis.

○ **What is the most common extracranial complication of otitis media?**

Labyrinthitis, mastoiditis, facial nerve paralysis, subperiosteal abscess, labyrinthine fistulas, perilabyrinthitis, ossicular destruction, cholesteatoma and temporal osteomyelitis.

○ **What are the indications for the prophylaxis of otitis media?**

Prophylaxis should be given after the third episode of otitis media under six months of age, or the fourth episode of otitis media before twelve months of age.

○ **How does the perforation of the tympanic membrane associated with chronic supporative otitis media differ from the perforation associated with acute otitis media?**

Tympanic membrane perforation in chronic suppurative otitis media can be permanent.

○   **What are the most common causes of acute mastoiditis?**

Group A streptococcus, *Streptococcus pneumoniae*, *Staphylococcus aureus*, and non-typeable *Haemophilus influenzae*.

○   **What are the most common intracranial complications of mastoiditis?**

Epidural empyema, brain abscess, meningitis, venous sinus thrombosis, and cerebellar abscess.

○   **What are the most common causes of chronic mastoiditis?**

The most common causes of chronic mastoiditis are *Staphylococcus aureus*, *Pseudomonas aeruginosa* and other gram negative rods, anaerobes and tuberculosis.

○   **What are the most common extracranial complications of mastoiditis?**

A subperiosteal abscess, a Bezold abscess (an abscess in the submastoid space), facial nerve paralysis, temporal bone osteomyelitis and hearing loss.

○   **What malignancies in children are most likely to present as a fever of unknown origin?**

Leukemia, lymphoma, neuroblastoma, hepatoma, sarcoma, and atrial myxoma.

○   **Name two immunizations that are associated with post-vaccine aseptic meningitis.**

Measles, polio, rabies, and vaccinia.

○   **If Creutzfeldt-Jakob disease (CJD) is a disease whose average age of presentation is 60 years, why has it suddenly become a concern in children?**

CJD was first described int he 1920's. It can be sporadic (no know cause), environmentally acquired (including pituitary hormones or dura mater grafts) or familial (due to mutations on chromosome 20). The recently diagnosed 21 patients in England were all under 50 years of age with and average age of 27 years. The "new variant" (nv) of CJD has in common with the classic CJD the features of progressive dementia, ataxia, and mild clonus. The unique characteristic of nvCJD are onset with psychiatric and/or sensory symptoms and an absence of characteristic electroencephalograph findings. The nvCJD seems to be associated with consumption of prion-contaminated beef.

○   **What four classes of contacts of a patient with meningococcal disease require prophylaxis?**

People who live in the same household, attendees of the same child care or nursery school in the previous seven days, those who have been directly exposed to the index case's secretions, such as by kissing or sharing of food, and health care providers whose mucous membranes were unprotected during resuscitation or intubation of the patient.

○   **Why isn't the meningococcal vaccine in routine use in the United States?**

Serogroups B and C meningococci each cause approximately 50% of the meningococcal disease in the United States. The highest risk age group for meningococcal disease is in children under two years of age. The reason meningococcal vaccine is not routinely used in this country is because serogroup B polysaccharide is not represented in the vaccine and the serogroup C that is present is very poorly immunogenic in children under two years of age.

○   **What is the most common infectious disease problem in patients with lupus who are not on steroid therapy?**

Urinary tract infections and urosepsis.

○ **How often is herpes simplex virus cultured from the cerebrospinal fluid of a pediatric patient or an adult with HSV encephalitis? How often is it cultured from the cerebrospinal fluid of a neonate with HSV encephalitis?**

Herpes simplex virus may be cultured from the cerebrospinal fluid of a child six months of age or older or an adult with herpes encephalitis only 5% of the time, whereas a neonate with HSV encephalitis will grow the virus from the CSF 50% of the time.

○ **What percent of school age children with classic symptoms (dysuria, frequency, urgency) actually have a urinary tract infection?**

10%. The remainder have urethral irritation from such things as pinworms, masturbation, bubble baths or poor hygiene.

○ **What is the only reliable result from a culture of urine collected by the bag method?**

No growth.

○ **Any organisms that grow in the culture of a urine specimen obtained by suprapubic aspiration can be considered to represent true infection. In symptomatic children, how many colonies in a urine culture are required to make the diagnosis when the urine specimen is obtained by catheterization?**

At least 10,000 colonies per ml of a single organism.

○ **What simple measures can be taken to prevent urinary tract infections in children?**

Taking showers instead of baths, avoiding bubble baths, treating pin worms, treating constipation and in sexually active females, post-coital voiding.

○ **What children are candidates for influenza vaccine?**

Any child six months of age or older who is a resident of a chronic care facility; who has a chronic cardiovascular condition; or who has pulmonary, metabolic, hematologic, or an immunologic disorder (including asthma, diabetes, renal failure, sickle cell disease, immunosuppression and HIV infection). Also, children who are receiving aspirin therapy, or are the siblings of children who are in any of these high risk group, should have the influenza immunization as well.

○ **Do bite wounds caused by humans usually become infected with one or with multiple organisms?**

The average human bite wound contains 5.4 organisms per wound.

○ **What are the most common organisms found in human bite wounds?**

*Staphylococcus aureus*, *Streptococcus* species, and *Eikenella corrodens*. Anaerobes are also commonly seen.

○ **Children with sickle cell disease are started on prophylactic penicillin by two to three months of age. This should be continued until what age?**

Routine prophylaxis with penicillin has been shown to have no effect on reduction of the risk of invasive pneumococcal infections for children older than five years of age.

○ **In a pediatric patient who is suspected of having meningitis, cranial computed tomography (CT) of the brain should be performed before lumbar puncture under what circumstances?**

When the patient is in a coma, has papilledema or focal neurologic findings. When head CT is performed, patients should have blood cultures taken and then appropriate empiric anibiotic therapy started prior to the CT.

○ **Is it necessary to treat the male sexual partner of women with bacterial vaginosis?**

No.

○ **If a pediatric patient with an acute illness who is receiving a third generation cephalosporin becomes secondarily infected and bacteremic, what organism would be the usual offender?**

Enterococcus.

○ **In the United States, which domestic animal is most commonly infected with rabies: the cat, or the dog?**

The cat. Among wild animals, rabies are most commonly found among raccoons, skunks, foxes, coyotes, and bats.

○ **Would a child be likely to receive a rabies vaccine following a wild rat bite?**

No. Bites from rodents rarely pose a risk of rabies.

○ **Since 1980, in the United States, what percentage of the 32 cases of human rabies has an associated history of animal bite?**

25%.

○ **There are twenty indigenously derived cases of rabies in the United States between 1980 and 1996. How many series of post exposure rabies prophylaxis were given in the United States during that same time period?**

40,000 people received post exposure prophylaxis during that time period. Post exposure prophylaxis for rabies consists of 20 international units per kilogram of Human Rabies Immune Globulin (HRIG) and five doses of vaccine.

○ **How many hours must *Ixodes scapularis*, the deer tick, feed on a human before being able to transmit Lyme disease?**

Transmission rarely occurs if the infected tick feeds for less than 48 hours.

○ **Neonates with HSV infection may present with a localized skin, eye and mouth (SEM) infection, a disseminated infection or an encephalitis. What is the mortality rate of infants with disseminated HIV infection who are treated with acyclovir?**

Fifty percent.

○ **What percentage of patients with localized skin, eye and mouth infection survive and what is the neurological outcome?**

All neonates with SEM treated with acyclovir survive and greater than 90% develop normally.

○ **What agent is the major cause of parenterally transmitted non-A, non-B hepatitis?**

Hepatitis C virus (HCV).

○ **What type of *Haemophilus influenzae* most commonly causes otitis media, conjunctivitis, and sinusitis?**

Nontypeable *Haemophilus*.

○ **Does nontypeable *Haemophilus influenzae* ever cause pneumonia, meningitis, septicemia, endocarditis, epiglottitis, septic arthritis, post-partum bacteremia, or neonatal sepsis?**

While *Haemophilus influenzae* B and other typeable *Haemophilus influenzae* infections are more likely causes of these invasive diseases, nontypeable *Haemophilus influenzae* may infrequently cause them as well.

○ **What impact does breast feeding by the mother have on immunizations of the baby?**

None. All vaccines may be given to a baby who is breast feeding and all vaccines may be given to a mom who is breast feeding a baby.

○ **T/F: A culture from a patient is reported as growing coagulase negative staphylococci. This should be interpreted to mean *Staphylococcus epidermidis*.**

False. There are 15 different coagulase negative staphylococci that have been reported to cause diseases in or to colonize humans.

○ **The laboratory report reads "*Streptococcus viridans*." What is wrong with that report?**

There is no such thing as *Streptococcus viridans*. The class of organisms being referred to is rightly called *Viridans* streptococci. *Viridans* streptococci are alpha hemolytic streptococci which are composed of at least eight separate species which cause diseases in man. Examples of *Viridans* streptococci include: *S. milleri*, *S. constellatus*, *S. anginosus* and *S. mutans*. While most laboratories will not normally speciate a Viridans streptococci for you because they may simply be contaminants, if they are seen in two or more blood cultures or grow in pure culture from a deep site, it is appropriate to ask for speciation. The species of the organism can point to the etiology of the disease. Certain *Viridans* streptococci are associated with endocarditis, while others are associated with such things as carcinoma and brain abscess.

○ **A six-year-old child presents with a history of having had a PPD placed three weeks ago which was 4 mm in induration, measured by a reliable colleague. A repeat PPD was placed one week ago and the child's forearm demonstrated 14 mm of induration. This PPD was measured by the same physician. Which PPD should be accepted as reflecting the correct amount of induration.**

The second, or "boosted" response, is accepted as the reliable response. It is routine for many institutions to test their employees with two PPD's, separated by two weeks, in order to take advantage of this phenomenon.

○ **An eighteen month old presents with an exudative pharyngitis, fever and mildly abnormal liver function tests. You suspect mononucleosis. What study would you send?**

An EBVlgG and IGM (lgG and lgM antibody to viral capsid antigen or VCA). The chances that a mono spot will be positive in the presence of mononucleosis between 0 and 2 years of age is practically zero. The chances that a mono spot is positive between the second birthday and the fourth birthday is approximately 30%. Specific Epstein-Barr virus antibodies are much more useful for making the diagnosis in the first four years of life.

○ **A ten month old presents with the signs and symptoms of pneumonia, which is confirmed by chest x-ray. What are the chances that this pneumonia is due to Mycoplasma pneumoniae?**

About 2%. *Mycoplasma pneumoniae* is hardly ever seen in the first year of life. It increases steadily as a cause of pneumonia in children into early adulthood. A convenient way to remember the chances of a child's pneumonia being due to mycoplasma is to assign a 2% chance per year of age into the twenties. By the mid-twenties, as many as 35-45% of all pneumonia is secondary to *Mycoplasma pneumoniae*.

○ **Pasteurella multocida infection from an animal bite is best treated with which antibiotic?**

Penicillin is the drug of choice.

○ **The intervention most likely to be successful in the treatment of onychomycosis of the toenail is: a) removal of the toenail or b) antifungal therapy for four to eighteen months.**

Drug therapy with itraconazole (Sporanox) is the easiest and shortest term of the various antifungal drug regimens. Treatment can be given for one week each month for three to four months. Other medications that are useful include terbinafine, ketoconazole, and griseofulvin. Therapy with griseofulvin can take as long as eighteen months.

○ **Name two common urinary pathogens that do not give a positive urine nitrate test.**

*Enterococcus* and *Staphylococcus saprophyticus*. *Acinetobacter* also fails to give a positive urine nitrate test.

○ **What unusual but important CNS side effect can be seen with ibuprofen usage?**

Aseptic meningitis.

○ **Group B streptococcus is known to have both an early and a late onset presentation in neonatal sepsis and meningitis. What other organism does the identical thing?**

*Listeria monocytogenes*.

○ **What common minor surgical procedure is associated with a decreased incidence of pyelonephritis in males?**

Circumcision.

○ **What percentage of the time do infants with documented pyelonephritis fail to demonstrate pyuria?**

Approximately 50% of the time.

○ **What is the incidence of occult bacteremia in infants between six and twenty-four months of age with temperature higher than 40 degrees centigrade and a white blood count >15,000/cu.mm?**

Approximately fifteen percent.

○ **How likely is it that a child with fever and petechiae has meningococcal sepsis or meningitis?**

Seven to ten percent.

○ **What could be concluded about the spinal fluid of a three day old infant with a CSF white count of 15 and a CSF protein of 90?**

That it is normal. At birth the CSF white count can be as high as 29. It may not fall to the expected "adult" normal of 6 or 7 until a month of age. The CSF protein can be up to 175 at birth and may take as long as three months to fall to the expected upper limit of normal of 45.

○ **What is the risk of *Salmonella* coming into a household in an ordinary package of a dozen eggs?**

In some studies, as many as 30% of commercial eggs are contaminated with *Salmonella*. The organism can be found on the surface of the shell, may penetrate the egg itself, or may contaminate the egg yolk, having been transmitted from an ovarian infection.

○ **What are the chances that *Salmonella* will be introduced into a household on contaminated meats?**

Up to 50% of poultry samples, 15% of pork and 5% of beef have been demonstrated to be contaminated with salmonella.

○ ***Bartonella henselae* is one of the causes of Parinaud's oculoglandular syndrome (a combination of conjunctivitis and ipsilateral preauricular adenitis) and is the most common cause of chronic lymphadenopathy in children. With what animal is this organism associated?**

The cat. It is the agent of cat scratch disease.

○ **While on the farm, *Coxiella burnetii* is most commonly associated with sheep. In the city a cat can aerosolize enough organisms in a closed space to be infective to people for days. What illness does *Coxiella burnetii* cause?**

Q Fever. This usually presents as an atypical pneumonia.

○ **One day after sitting in a hot tub, a three-year-old child and her mother develop papular and pustular skin lesions. What is the most likely explanation?**

*Pseudomonas aeruginosa* dermatitis has been reported to occur in healthy individuals following immersion in hot tubs. There may be a few scattered lesions or extensive involvement. Patients may also have malaise, fever, vomiting, sore throat, conjunctivitis, rhinitis, and swollen breasts.

○ **What are the two most common organisms known to be transmitted by unpasteurized Mexican cheese?**

*Brucella* and *Listeria*.

○ **What is the most productive source of positive cultures for patients with brucellosis?**

While blood, abscess and tissue cultures may be useful, bone marrow is the most productive source of positive cultures.

○ **Which hemoglobin provides the greatest innate resistance to falciparum malaria?**

Erythrocytes of patients that are heterozygous for sickle cell hemoglobin (sickle cell trait) are resistant to malaria.

○   **What is the most common infectious disease complication of both measles and influenza?**

Pneumococcal pneumonia.

○   **What rickettsial disease can be mistaken for chickenpox in inner city children?**

Rickettsialpox caused by *Rickettsia akari* is characterized by an initial skin lesion followed by headache, fever, chills and a vesicular rash. It is transmitted by the mouse mite.

○   **Which rickettsial infection is most common in the United States?**

Rocky Mountain Spotted Fever caused by *Rickettsia*.

○   **What is the most important therapeutic action to be taken in the teenager with infected abortion?**

Evacuation of the retained products of conception.

○   **In the treatment of a patient with cellulitis, what therapeutic maneuver is arguably as important as antibiotic therapy?**

Elevation of the affected part.

○   **What prophylactic antibiotic should be given systemically to burn victims?**

None. Prophylactic agents with antibacterial activity should be given topically. Chief among these is Silvadene.

○   **What is the most likely focus of infection in a patient who presents with gram negative enteric bacteremia?**

Urinary tract infection.

○   **What is the most likely focus of infection in a patient who presents with periorbital cellulitis unassociated with skin trauma?**

Sinusitis.

○   **A previously healthy child has had an accidental overdose of oral iron; she appears to be septic. What is the most likely organism to cause her sepsis?**

*Yersinia enterocolitica*. The growth of *Y. enterocolitica* appears to be enhanced after exposure to excess iron. This, combined with intestinal damage to the mucosa by the iron, may play a role in pathogenesis.

○   **A 3 month old infant presents with poor feeding, constipation, and hypotonia. There is a recent history of ingestion of honey. While you suspect infant botulism, you cannot rule out the possibility of sepsis. What class of antibiotics would you not give to this patient?**

Aminoglyosides. Gentamicin and related drugs can add to the blocked motor nerve terminals, and lead to respiratory failure in these patients with botulism.

○ **T/F: It is fairly common for children to become infected with tuberculosis following casual exposures.**

False. Primary infection in children usually occurs following a prolonged close contact with an untreated adult who has cavitary disease.

○ **A 7-year-old child is diagnosed with primary pulmonary tuberculosis and is treated appropriately with four drugs. An organism collected by gastric aspirate proves to be sensitive to three of the four drugs. Following six months of therapy, the chest x-ray appears unchanged from six months ago. What is wrong?**

Nothing. It can take many months for the chest x-ray abnormalities in pulmonary tuberculosis to show improvement. The child's symptoms, however, should have resolved and the sedimentation rate should be normal with effective therapy.

○ **In normal children, what is the most common clinical manifestation of disease due to non-tuberculous mycobacteria?**

The most common form of non-tuberculous mycobacteria is lymphadenitis of the submandibular or anterior cervical nodes. The usual agent is *M. avium intracellulare* complex and *M. scrofulaceum*.

○ **A teenager presents with an irritating cough which is becoming gradually worse. The boy's father had a similar problem, which was treated with erythromycin and resolved after seven days. PPD's on both the father and the son have been negative. What are the three most likely etiologic agents for this problem?**

*Mycoplasma pneumoniae*, *Chlamydia pneumoniae*, and *Bordetella pertussis*.

○ **What part of the body should you examine to confirm that a vesicular rash is related to chickenpox?**

The scalp. Vesicular and crusting lesions in the scalp are typical of chicken pox. It is extremely unlikely that other causes of vesicular lesions on the skin would be associated with scalp lesions.

○ **It is well known that children with chickenpox may eventually have an episode (or episodes) of herpes zoster. Will herpes zoster appear following an immunization with chickenpox vaccine?**

Yes. It occurs at approximately one-third to one-fifth the frequency that it does following the natural illness, but it is a distant complication of the vaccine as well.

○ **What is the earliest age at which a child may be immunized for influenza?**

At 6 months of age.

○ **While older infants and children with respiratory syncytial virus infection (RSV) usually present with cough and wheezing, some infants may present with what other symptom?**

Apnea.

○ **What is the name of the viral illness that presents predominantly with pharyngitis and conjunctivitis?**

Pharyngoconjunctival fever. It is caused by adenovirus.

○ **Since only a minority of children who present with fever and petechiae have meningococcemia, what etiologic agent accounts for the bulk of the remaining cases?**

The enteroviruses, including the Coxsackieviruses, and the ECHOviruses.

○ **A ten month old infant presents with fever, diarrhea, and mild irritability. A spinal tap shows 68 white cells, no red cells, normal protein, normal glucose, and a CSF latex agglutination that is negative for all bacterial pathogens tested. What is the most likely diagnosis?**

Rotavirus. A septic meningitis is not uncommon in children with rotavirus gastroenteritis.

○ **What parasitic agent should be included in the differential diagnosis when mononucleosis and CMV are considered?**

Toxoplasmosis. Everything EBV and CMV can do, toxoplasmosis can do.

○ **When itchy lesions are seen on the palms and/or soles, what blood sucking ecoparasite should be high in the differential diagnosis?**

Sarcoptes scabiei, the etiologic agent of scabies.

○ **Which strain of meningococcus is most commonly responsible for meningitis?**

Group B is the most common cause of non-epidemic meningococcal disease.

○ **Is there a vaccine available for group B meningococcus?**

No.

○ **What are the common pathogens for meningitis in the neonates?**

Streptococcus group B and *E. coli*.

○ **What is the most common neurologic sequel of pediatric bacterial meningitis?**

Hearing impairment.

○ **What other deficits may develop following bacterial meningitis?**

Mental retardation, seizure, and spastic weakness.

○ **What are the sequelae of viral meningitis?**

None, usually.

○ **What are the CSF characteristics of tuberculous meningitis?**

Lymphocytic pleocytosis, very high protein (several hundred to a thousand mg/dl), and very low glucose.

○ **What is the management of herpes simplex encephalitis?**

Early treatment with acyclovir, anticonvulsants for seizures and general supportive care.

○ **What is the most common cause of encephalitis in neonates?**

Enterovirus.

○ **What is the recommended treatment for neurosyphilis?**

Intravenous penicillin G. Follow up CSF examinations are mandatory.

○ **What complication may arise from aggressive penicillin treatment of neurosyphilis?**

Jarisch Herxheimer reaction.

○ **At which stage of Lyme disease does neurological involvement occur?**

The second and third stages.

○ **Which is the vector responsible for the transmission of Lyme disease?**

Deer tick (*Ixodes dammini*).

○ **What important feature in a patient's history should be sought when a diagnosis of Lyme disease is being considered?**

History of erythema chronicum migrans (ECM), which present in nearly 60-80% of patients early in this disease.

○ **What is the currently recommended treatment for Lyme disease?**

For early, localized disease in children over 7 years of age, doxycycline. Amoxicillin may be used for all ages. These same drugs are used for early-disseminated disease, facial palsy, and arthritis. Recurrent arthritis, carditis and CNS disease is treated with ceftriaxone or penicillin

○ **What is Weil's disease?**

A less common variety of leptospirosis. It presents with icterus, marked hepatic and renal involvement, along with a bleeding diathesis.

○ **How is brucellosis spread?**

Through the ingestion of contaminated milk and milk products. It may also be spread by contact with an infected animal (usually cattle), including respiratory.

○ **What are the typical features of zidovudine associated myopathy?**

AZT is known to cause myopathy when used in high doses over prolonged periods. There is typically severe myalgia, and striking atrophy of the gluteal muscles.

○ **Name some common causes of peripheral neuropathy in AIDS.**

Peripheral neuropathy has been postulated to be directly related to HIV, concomitant infections such as cytomegalovirus (CMV), side effects of drugs such as ddI, ddC, and 3TC, and nutritional deficiencies such as $B_{12}$ deficiency.

○   **What is the most common cause of intracranial mass lesions in HIV disease?**

Intracranial toxoplasmosis. About 20-30% of AIDS patients with positive serology for toxoplasmosis will develop toxoplasma encephalitis. The second most common intracranial mass lesion is lymphoma.

○   **What is the current recommended treatment for intracranial toxoplasmosis in HIV disease?**

This is usually a combination therapy with sulfadiazine, pyrimethamine, and folinic acid.

○   **What is the rationale for using folinic acid in the treatment of intracranial toxoplasmosis with pyrimethamine, and sulfadiazine combination?**

Folinic acid is thought to decrease the incidence of bone marrow suppression.

○   **What percentage of patients with HIV disease develop CNS lymphoma?**

Approximately 2% of AIDS patients will develop primary CNS lymphoma. Up to 0.6% will present with primary CNS lymphoma concurrent with a diagnosis of AIDS.

○   **What are the modes of transmission of HTLV-1?**

Vertical: Mother to child.

Horizontal: Through sexual contact, and blood transfusion.

○   **How is botulism contracted?**

Through the consumption of contaminated foods, by injury from non sterile objects (wound botulism), and (in infants) from intestinal colonization by *Clostridium botulinum*.

○   **What are botulism's principle clinical features?**

A descending paralysis with complete ophthalmoplegia, bulbar and somatic palsy.

○   **Which is the organism responsible for causing Bornholm's disease?**

Coxsackieviruses are a group of enteroviruses that are responsible for the epidemic myalgia (Bornholm's disease) where pleurodynia is also a common feature. Specifically the disease is thought to occur due to a Coxsackie group B virus.

○   **Name three paralytic diseases caused by an infectious agent other than polio?**

Paralytic rabies, botulism and tick paralysis.

○   **To which group of viruses does polio belong?**

The polio virus is an enterovirus like Echovirus and Coxsackievirus.

# CARDIOVASCULAR

○ **What are the most common causes of bradycardia in a newborn?**

Hypoxemia, hypoglycemia, hypothermia, exposure to narcotics, and sepsis.

○ **A seven day old baby is cyanotic. Physical exam reveals a holosystolic murmur. He remains cyanotic after treatment with 100% oxygen. What is the possible diagnosis and subsequent treatment of choice?**

The patient has a ductus dependent cyanotic congenital heart defect. The treatment of choice is prostaglandin E1.

○ **When is cardioversion indicated?**

During unstable SVT and ventricular Tachycardia (VT) and ventricular fibrillation. For SVT and VT, use synchronized cardioversion.

○ **A 5-year-old takes several KCL tablets. An EKG shows peaked T-waves, and the presence of U-waves. What is the indicated therapy?**

Calcium chloride, 10mg/kg IV; sodium bicarbonate, 0.5-1.0 mEq/kg IV; glucose and insulin intravenous drip; sodium polystyrene sulfonate (Kayexalate), 1 gm/kg/dose Q2-6 hours PR or PO.

○ **What is the most common cause of aortic regurgitation in children?**

Aortic valve prolapse associated with a congenital ventricular septal defect.

○ **What is the most common cause of atrial fibrillation in childhood?**

This is most often the result of a chronically stretched atrial myocardium. Atrial fibrillation occurs most commonly in older children with rheumatic mitral valve disease.

○ **What is the mechanism that most commonly produces SVTs?**

Re-entrant tachycardias using an accessory pathway in infants, though AV node re-entry becomes more common in childhood.

○ **What is the key feature of Mobitz I (Wenckebach) $2°$ AV block?**

A progressive prolongation of the PR interval until the atrial impulse is no longer conducted. If symptomatic, atropine and transcutaneous/transvenous pacing is required.

○ **Documentation of three BP results in a fully grown adolescent obtained at one week intervals must show an average greater than 140 mm Hg systolic or 90 mm Hg diastolic for the correct diagnosis of hypertension. What single reading can be considered sufficient for the diagnosis of hypertension without necessitating further investigations?**

When a patient's single reading is greater than 110 mm Hg diastolic, a diagnosis can be made. Another conclusive indicator of hypertension is when end organ damage occurs with a lower reading.

○ **What is Mobitz II 2° AV block, and how is it treated?**

A constant PR interval in which one or more beats fail to conduct. Treat with atropine and transcutaneous/transvenous pacing.

○ **Define a hypertensive emergency in a fully grown adolescent patient.**

An elevated diastolic blood pressure that is > 115 mm Hg with associated end organ dysfunction or damage.

○ **What are the signs and symptoms of hypertensive encephalopathy?**

Nausea, vomiting, headache, lethargy, coma, blindness, nerve palsies, hemiparesis, aphasia, retinal hemorrhage, cotton wool spots, exudates, sausage linking, and papilledema.

○ **What is the most common cause of myocarditis in US children?**

Viruses (especially adenovirus and Coxsackie virus group B). Other causes include bacteria (diphtheria, meningococcus and tuberculosis), fungi, protozoa (Chagas' disease), spirochetes (Lyme disease), and Kawasaki disease.

○ **What is the most common cause of mitral stenosis?**

Rheumatic heart disease.

○ **Is mitral valve prolapse (MVP) more common in males or in females?**

Females have a stronger genetic link to the disease. 2-5% of the population has MVP.

○ **What is the hallmark sign of mitral valve prolapse?**

A midsystolic click sometimes accompanied by a late systolic murmur. MVP is largely a clinical diagnosis. An ECG is performed to assess the degree of prolapse. Other clinical findings include a laterally displaced diffuse apical pulse, decreased S1, split S2, and a holosystolic murmur radiating to the axilla.

○ **What physical finding is usually indicative of acute pericarditis?**

Pericardial friction rub. The rub is best heard at the left sternal border or apex with the patient in a forward sitting position. Other findings include fever and tachycardia.

○ **Acute pyogenic pericarditis is most commonly caused by which organisms?**

*Staphylococcus aureus*, *Neisseria meningitidis* and *Haemophilus influenzae* type B.

○ **What does an x-ray of a pericardial effusion reveal?**

A water bottle silhouette.

○ **What are the most common signs and symptoms of a pulmonary emoblus?**

Tachypnea (92%), CP (88%), dyspnea (84%), anxiety (59%), tachycardia (44%), fever (43%), DVT (32%), hypotension (25%), and syncope (13%).

❍ **What is the most common CXR finding in PE?**

Elevated dome of one hemidiaphragm. This finding is caused by decreased lung volume, which occurs in 50% of patients with PEs. Other common findings include lack of lung markings in the area perfused by the occluded artery, pleural effusions, atelectasis, and pulmonary infiltrates.

❍ **Which test is considered the gold standard for a diagnosis of deep vein thrombosis (DVT)? Of pulmonary embolies (PE)?**

Venography. The gold standard for the diagnosis of PE is the pulmonary angiography.

❍ **Rheumatic heart disease is the most common cause of stenosis of what 3 heart valves?**

Mitral, aortic (along with congenital bicuspid valve), and tricuspid.

❍ **Which is most likely to be pathologic in children: an $S_3$ or an $S_4$?**

An $S_4$.

❍ **When measuring a pulsus paradoxus, what is considered a normal difference in systolic blood pressures (with inspiration versus expiration)?**

Up to 8-10 mmHg.

❍ **Which congenital heart lesions commonly present with cyanosis in an infant's first day of life?**

All the abnormalities that start with a T. Tetralogy of Fallot, Transposition of the great vessels, Total anomalous pulmonary circulation, Truncus arteriosus, and Tricuspid valve atresia (and Ebstein's malformation of the Tricuspid valve).

❍ **What is the usual presentation of children with a ventricular septal defect?**

A systolic murmur in the first days of life with no signs related to their condition. They usually resolve spontaneously.

❍ **How do infants with atrial septal defects usually present?**

The majority of these children are totally asymptomatic, and the defect usually is not diagnosed until they are school age.

❍ **A short PR interval and a delta wave are characteristic of what cardiac anomaly?**

Wolff-Parkinson-White (WPW) syndrome. This is due to a reentry phenomenon along the Bundle of Kent.

❍ **Which patients with mitral valve prolapse (MVP) should receive prophylactic antibiotics to protect against subacute bacterial endocarditis?**

Patients with MVP and a systolic murmur.

❍ **T/F: You can rule out subacute bacterial endocarditis (SBE) after you have obtained two negative blood cultures?**

False. False negatives occur 10-30% of the time in two cultures. For this reason, three blood cultures are recommended.

○ **How does the size of a VSD correlate with the risk of infective endocarditis?**

It doesn't. The risk is independent of size.

○ **How common do children with SBE present with cutaneous manifestations?**

Not very common. These manifestations are seen late in the disease, so they are not commonly seen in the appropriately treated patient.

○ **What test can be used to identify vasovagal neuroregulatory syncope as the cause of syncope in children with a history of "falling out"?**

The tilt-table test.

○ **What test can be used to differentiate congenital heart disease from primary pulmonary parenchymal disease in a newborn with cyanosis?**

The hyperoxia test. There is little to no difference in arterial oxygen content between breathing room air and 100% oxygen with cyanotic congenital heart disease

○ **On a chest x-ray of a child, what bony abnormality would lead you to suspect coarctation of the aorta?**

Bilateral rib notching.

○ **What bony abnormalities are seen in the chest x-rays of children with Down syndrome?**

You may see 11 ribs.

○ **What are the common cardiac complications of juvenile rheumatoid arthritis?**

Pericarditis and (rare) myocarditis.

○ **What are the common cardiac complications of Marfan syndrome?**

Aortic and mitral insufficiency, mitral valve prolapse (MVP), and dissecting aortic aneurysm.

○ **What are the common cardiac complications of sickle cell anemia?**

High output cardiac failure, cardiomyopathy and cor pulmonale.

○ **What congenital cardiac diseases will present with increased pulmonary markings on a chest x-ray?**

Transposition of the great vessels, total anomalous pulmonary venous return (and truncus arteriosus).

○ **An "egg shaped" heart is a characteristic x-ray finding for what congenital heart malformation?**

Transposition of the great arteries.

○ **What are the differential diagnoses for a widely split $S_2$?**

ASD, tetralogy of Fallot (TOF), pulmonary stenosis, right bundle branch block (RBBB), total anomalous pulmonary venous return.

❍ **In classifying a heart murmur's intensity, what differentiates a III from a IV?**

The absence (III) or presence (IV) of a thrill.

❍ **What are the auscultatory findings in an ASD?**

A loud first heart sound, sometimes a pulmonic ejection click, a second heart sound that is widely split and fixed in all phases of respiration, and a systolic ejection murmur (best heard at the left middle and upper sternal border). A short, rumbling mid-diastolic murmur may be heard at the left lower sternal border.

❍ **Describe the most common 'innocent' murmur?**

Medium-pitched, "musical" or vibratory systolic ejection murmur best heard at LLSB without radiation.

❍ **How common is an 'innocent' murmur?**

Very. Up to 30% of children have one, with peak incidence between 3-7 years of age.

❍ **What is the 13th lead in a 13 lead ECG?**

$V_3R$ or $V_4R$. These are right precordial leads which evaluate the extent of right ventricular hypertrophy.

❍ **What is the test of choice to examine for the presence of vegetations in a child with endocarditis?**

Transesophageal echocardiography.

❍ **An ECG shows the following findings: RSR' in $V_3R$ and $V_1$, prolonged P-R interval, tall P waves, a QRS axis of -60 degrees and signs of RVH. What is your diagnosis, doc?**

AV canal defect (a.k.a. AV septal defect, endocardial cushion defect).

❍ **What is the most common cardiac malformation?**

VSD. This accounts for about 25% of all heart diseases. Prognosis depends largely on size of the defect- if small it may close spontaneously (usually before 4 years of age).

❍ **A 10-year-old child with a history of VSD is about to have an impacted tooth removed. What antibiotic should he be given prophylactically to prevent endocarditis?**

Amoxicillin 50 mg/kg one hour before the procedure. If the patient has a penicillin allergy, use clindamycin 20 mg/kg one hour before the procedure.

❍ **What compound causes the ductus arteriosus to constrict right after birth?**

Oxygen, which is a vasoconstrictor.

❍ **When is it most effective to administer indomethacin to newborns with patent ductus arteriosus?**

During the first 24-48 hours of life, with a second and third dose at 12 and 36 hours, following the initial dose.

○ **What is the treatment of choice for a child with severe aortic stenosis?**

Balloon valvuloplasty if peak systolic gradient between the LV and aorta is > 60 mmHg.

○ **How does squatting help children with hypoxia secondary to their tetralogy of Fallot (TOF)?**

It increases their systemic vascular resistance.

○ **You are in the ED when a newborn with severe coarctation of the aorta suddenly starts deteriorating and is acidotic. What do you do initially?**

Infuse prostaglandin $E_1$ and administer oxygen.

○ **What test confirms the clinical suspicion of PDA?**

2-D echocardiogram detects up to 90%.

○ **What is the most reliable way to diagnose neonatal pulmonary hypertension?**

Right heart catheterization.

○ **What is the normal QRS axis in a newborn?**

+135 to +180 degrees. This reflects their right ventricular dominance.

○ **A 3-year-old child presents with premature atrial contractions (PAC's). Should this be a cause of concern?**

They are usually benign, except in children less than 1-year-old, or those on digitalis.

○ **Name the anomalies found in tetology of Fallot (TOF).**

Pulmonary stenosis, VSD, dextroposition of aorta with septal override and RVH.

○ **What are the most common complications of TOF prior to correction?**

Cerebral thromboses, brain abscess, bacterial endocarditis and CHF.

○ **What is the shunting procedure currently employed to correct the cyanosis in TOF?**

The modified Blalock-Taussig shunt. This aortopulmonary shunt is a Gore-Tex conduit which anastomoses the subclavian and pulmonary arteries (homolateral branch).

○ **What therapy can be instituted to decrease the incidence of coronary abnormalities in children with Kawasaki syndrome?**

IV immune globulin (2 g/kg given over 8 – 12 hours), and high dose aspirin.

○ **What medication has been shown to decrease the fever and discomfort associated with an acute attack of Kawasaki syndrome?**

High dose aspirin therapy (50 – 100 mg/kg/day).

○ **What laboratory findings differentiate Kawasaki disease from measles?**

Children with Kawasaki syndrome tend to have an increased WBC count, elevated ESR, elevated liver function and pyuria.

○ **What congenital cardiac defects are commonly seen in children with Down syndrome?**

Endocardial cushion defect, ASD, VSD.

○ **What congenital cardiac defects are commonly seen in infants with fetal alcohol syndrome?**

ASD, VSD.

○ **What congenital cardiac defects are commonly seen in patient with autosomal dominant polycystic kidney disease?**

Mitral valve prolapse (MVP).

○ **What is the 5 year survival rate of infants and children who undergo a complete heart transplantation?**

70-85% with immunosuppressive agents.

○ **What is the primary cause of congestive heart failure (CHF) in infancy and childhood?**

Congenital heart disease.

○ **A patient with congenital heart disease taking digoxin and Lasix, presents in CHF; what are the potential causes?**

1. Untreated or unrecognized infection
2. Anemia
3. Arrhythmias
4. Inadequate or excessive digitalis dose
5. Hypokalemia
6. Traumatic injury

○ **What diseases lead to a pulsus paradoxus greater than 20 mm Hg?**

Cardiac tamponade, asthma, CHF.

○ **What does a high pulsus paradoxus indicate?**

Circulatory compromise.

○ **What are the classic presenting features of pericarditis in children?**

Positional sharp substernal chest pain, abdominal pain, tachycardia, tachypnea, dyspnea, fever, friction rub.

○ **What are the potential complications of pericarditis?**

Myocarditis, pericardial effusion, pericardial tamponade.

○ **What is the mortality rate from myocarditis?**

35%.

○ **What are the ECG findings in myocarditis?**

1. Diffuse nonspecific ST-T wave changes.
2. AV blocks.
3. Ventricular ectopy.
4. Prolonged QT interval.

○ **What is the cause of sudden death in myocarditis?**

Dysrhythmias.

○ **How is acute myocarditis managed?**

Treat the CHF, restrict fluids, diuresis, oxygen, strict bed rest, and inotropic support if needed. Treat ventricular arrhythmias with lidocaine, supraventricular tachyarrhythmias with digoxin, and complete atrioventricular block with a temporary pacemaker.

○ **What are the ECG findings in a patient with a significant pericardial effusion?**

1. Low voltage.
2. Electrical alternans.

○ **What are the findings in an infant with acute CHF?**

1. Irritability
2. Poor feeding
3. Lethargy
4. Failure to thrive
5. Tachycardia
6. Tachypnea
7. Hyperactive precordium
8. Gallop rhythm
9. Rales
10. Hepatomegaly

Peripheral edema and neck vein distention are noted only in older children.

○ **What are the most common bacteria seen in a purulent pericardial effusion?**

1. *Staphylococcus aureus*.
2. *Streptococcus pneumoniae*.
3. *Haemophilus influenzae*.

○ **What condition in children is infective endocarditis most often associated with?**

Congenital heart disease (40% of cases).

○ **A patient is diagnosed with infective endocarditis. She has a history of recent dental surgery. What is the most likely organism?**

*Viridans* streptococcus. *Viridans* streptococcus is a family of organisms including such microbes of *Streptococcus mutans*, *Streptococcus salivarius*, etc.

○ **A child with congenital heart disease develops infective endocarditis postoperatively, what is the most likely organism?**

Staphylococcal species.

○ **In a previously healthy child without congenital heart disease, what is the most common cause of infective endocarditis.**

*Staphylococcus aureus.*

○ **In what percentage of cases of bacterial endocarditis will blood cultures be positive?**

90%.

○ **If antibiotics are required before the organism has been identified, which agents should be used?**

Aminoglycoside (gentamicin 5-7.5 mg/kg/day) + penicillinase-resistant penicillin oxacillin/ nafcillin.

○ **A child presents with chest pain and a new murmur. Which cardiac conditions should be suspected?**

Hypertrophic obstructive cardiomyopathy and aortic stenosis.

○ **What are the five major Jones criteria for diagnosing rheumatic fever?**

Carditis, migratory polyarthritis, chorea, erythema marginatum, and subcutaneous nodules.

○ **Which of the major criteria is the most commonly seen?**

Polyarthritis.

○ **Describe the rash present in rheumatic fever.**

Non-pruritic, fine, lacey in appearance with central blanching and a serpiginous pattern.

○ **What is the most common cardiac defect in children and adolescents with rheumatic heart disease?**

Mitral insufficiency.

○ **What are the cardiac complications of Kawasaki disease?**

Myocarditis and coronary artery aneurysms.

○ **What percent of untreated patients with Kawasaki's disease will develop coronary artery aneurysms?**

15% to 25%. The coronary artery damage can lead to thrombosis or sudden death after acute symptoms have resolved.

○ **What are the common causes of acquired third-degree AV block?**

Myocarditis, endocarditis, rheumatic fever, cardiac muscle disease, cardiac tumors, and postoperative cardiac surgery.

○ **What is the most common dysrhythmia seen in the pediatric age group?**

Supraventricular tachycardia (SVT).

○ **What is the dosage used in cardioverting a child?**

0.5 to 1 Joules/kg increasing up to 2 Joules/kg.

○ **What is the most common cause of SVT in infants?**

Congenital heart disease (30%). Other causes include fever, infection, or drug exposure (20%), and unknown etiology (50%).

○ **Twenty-five percent of SVT is associated with what syndrome?**

Wolf-Parkinson-White.

○ **What problem can occur by using digoxin to treat SVT in a patient with the WPW syndrome?**

Digoxin can shorten the refractory period in the bypass tract and enhance conduction in the accessory pathway, leading to a rapid ventricular response and ventricular fibrillation.

○ **What are the most common causes of atrial fibrillation and flutter?**

Congenital heart disease, rheumatic fever, dilated cardiomyopathy, hyperthyroidism.

○ **What is the treatment of choice in an unstable patient with atrial fibrillation and flutter?**

Immediate cardioversion with 0.5 J/kg.

○ **What is the treatment for stable atrial fibrillation?**

Digitalization.

○ **Why should atrial flutter be treated in a patient with congenital heart disease?**

Because this patient's risk of sudden death is four times higher than normal.

○ **What is the mortality in untreated congenital prolonged QT syndrome?**

80%.

○ **By what age should a child's ECG resemble an adults?**

> 3 years of age.

○ **What are the possible etiologies for ventricular tachycardia?**

Electrolyte imbalance, metabolic disturbances, cardiac tumors, drugs, cardiac catheterization or surgery, congenital heart disease, cardiomyopathies prolonged QT syndrome, and idiopathic.

○ **What is the normal QTc value?**

0.45 in infants, 0.44 in children, 0.43 in adolescents.

○ **What is the treatment for premature atrial contractions (PACs)?**

No treatment is required in an asymptomatic patient but frequent PACs should be evaluated to rule out myocarditis.

❍ **When should premature ventricular contractions (PVCs) be treated?**

Treat those that cause or are likely to cause hemodynamic compromise.

❍ **What is the initial treatment for symptomatic second and third degree heart block?**

Atropine 0.01 to 0.03 mg/kg. A minimum dose of 0.1 mg should be used in children to avoid atropine-induced paradoxical bradycardia.

❍ **What is the treatment for ventricular fibrillation (VF)?**

Defibrillation with 1 to 2 Joules/kg/dose.

❍ **What is the dose of epinephrine in ventricular fibrillation and asystole?**

0.1 mg/kg/dose q 3-5 minutes (1:10,000).

❍ **What is a "tet spell?"**

Episodes of paroxysmal hypoxemia which are usually self-limited and last less than 15 to 30 minutes, although they may last longer. The spells are seen more often in the morning but may occur during the day and may be precipitated by activity, a sudden fright, or injury or may occur spontaneously without apparent cause. The tachypnea and cyanosis are due to an increase in right-to-left shunting and concomitant decrease in pulmonary blood flow. The exact mechanism by which this occurs is unknown.

❍ **What is the treatment for a "tet spell?"**

Place in the knee-chest position which increases peripheral resistance in the lower extremities, which in turn, promotes increased pulmonary blood flow. Place the patient on oxygen and give morphine sulfate 0.1 mg/kg IV. If these measures fail, use propranolol to a maximum total dose of 0.1 mg/kg.

❍ **In the pre-term infant, what is the most common cause of congestive heart failure?**

Persistent patent ductus arteriosus.

❍ **What is the most common cause of cardiac chest pain in an infant or child?**

Anomalous pulmonary origin of a coronary artery.

❍ **What is the most common atrial septal defect seen and what does it involve anatomically?**

Most often involves the fossa ovalis, is midseptal, and is of the ostium secundum type.

❍ **What are the most notable cardiac auscultatory findings in children with atrial septal defects?**

Normal or split first heart sound, accentuation of the tricuspid valve closure sound, a midsystolic pulmonary ejection murmur and a wide, fixed split second heart sound.

❍ **What is the typical CXR findings of a patient with atrial septal defect?**

Enlargement of the right atrium and ventricle, dilated pulmonary artery and its branches, and increased pulmonary vascular markings.

○   **What is the confirmatory test of choice for atrial septal defect?**

Echocardiography with color Doppler flow and contrast echocardiography.

○   **T/F: In infants and children, life-threatening cardiac rhythm disturbances are more frequently the cause rather than the result of cardiovascular emergencies.**

False. In infants and children, life-threatening cardiac rhythm disturbances are more frequently the result rather than the cause of cardiovascular emergencies.

○   **Typically, what is cardiac arrest the result of in children?**

It is the end result of hypoxemia and acidosis resulting from respiratory insufficiency or shock.

○   **Toward what four things must attention first be directed when confronted with life-threatening cardiac arrhythmias in children?**

Toward establishment of a patent airway, effective ventilation, adequate oxygenation, and circulatory stabilization.

○   **Define the surface electrocardiogram.**

The surface electrocardiogram is a graphic representation of the electrical sequence of myocardial depolarization and repolarization.

○   **What are the two key factors in influencing differences in normal heart rate in children?**

Age and physical activity.

○   **What two primary pathological conditions may influence heart rate in children?**

Fever and volume loss (fluid loss, e.g. vomiting or diarrhea, and hemorrhage).

○   **T/F: A febrile infant with normal cardiovascular function can have a heart rate of 200 beats per minute or higher.**

True. These infants can have heart rates up to 200 + beats per minute, heart rates in infants and young children ≥ 220 often are caused a tachyarrhythmia (supraventricular tachycardia).

○   **When should you continuously monitor the ECG in children?**

When they have evidence of respiratory or cardiovascular instability, including children who have sustained a cardiopulmonary arrest.

○   **T/F: Never use adult ECG patches on children.**

False. Adult patches may be used by trimming excess tape from the electrodes to make them smaller.

○   **Why is it advantageous to avoid placing electrodes on the anterior chest?**

So they won't interfere with auscultation of the heart and lungs, and chest radiographs will be free of radiopaque artifact.

○ **What is the typical electrode placement on children?**

The shoulders or the lateral chest surfaces, and the ground electrode are usually placed on the abdomen or thigh.

○ **What is the most common cause of asystole on ECG?**

A loose electrode or wire.

○ **What are the four most common artifacts commonly observed on ECG?**

A straight line due to a loose lead.
A tall T wave counted as an R wave by the tachometer.
Absence of P waves due to lead placement.
60-cycle interference.

○ **When should a rhythm disturbance in a child be treated as an emergency?**

Only if it compromises cardiac output or has the potential to degenerate into a lethal (collapse) rhythm.

○ **What is the equation for determining cardiac output?**

Stroke volume times heart rate.

○ **Why can cardiac output diminish as a result of very rapid rates?**

Because they may compromise diastolic filling and therefore stroke volume.

○ **What are the two primary cardiac rhythms that result in excessively fast rates?**

Supraventricular and ventricular tachycardias.

○ **What is the most rapid and effective method of treating tachyarrhythmias that result in cardiovascular instability and signs of shock?**

Synchronized cardioversion.

○ **What is the cause of slow rhythms associated with cardiovascular instability in infants and children?**

AV block or suppression of normal sinus node impulse generation caused by hypoxemia or acidosis.

○ **What does the initial therapy for these slow rhythms consist of?**

Establishment of a patent airway, provision of adequate ventilation and oxygenation, and administration of medications to improve perfusion (i.e., sympathomimetics).

○ **With what dysrhythmias is the absence of palpable pulses associated?**

Asystole, ventricular fibrillation, pulseless ventricular tachycardia, or a pulseless electrical activity, such as electromechanical dissociation.

○ **Define sinus tachycardia in children.**

A rate of sinus node discharge higher than normal for age.

○ **What is the typical physiological cause of sinus tachycardia?**

The need for increased cardiac output or oxygen delivery.

○ **Is sinus tachycardia a true arrhythmia?**

No, it is often a nonspecific clinical sign rather than a true arrhythmia.

○ **Name six common causes of sinus tachycardia.**

Anxiety, fever, pain, blood loss, sepsis, shock.

○ **Is sinus tachycardia regular or irregular?**

Regular, but far less regular than SVT.

○ **Describe P wave morphology in sinus tachycardia.**

Normal, upright.

○ **What is the therapy for sinus tachycardia?**

Therapy is directed at treating the underlying cause.

○ **Why are attempts to decrease the heart rate by pharmacological means inappropriate in sinus tachycardia?**

Because it is a symptom, not a cause.

○ **What is the most common cause of SVT?**

A reentry mechanism that involves an accessory pathway and/or the AV conduction system.

○ **Which patient is least likely to tolerate SVT: small infants, infants, or older children?**

Although SVT is usually well tolerated in most infants and older children, it can lead to cardiovascular collapse and clinical evidence of shock in some small infants.

○ **What is the usual heart rate of infants in SVT?**

Greater than or equal to 220 bpm but often higher.

○ **What is the usual P wave morphology in SVT?**

P waves may not be visible, especially when the ventricular rate is high.

○ **What is the QRS duration in SVT?**

QRS duration is often normal (less than 0.08 seconds) in most (>90%) children.

○ **With what rhythm is SVT with aberrant conduction usually confused?**

Ventricular tachycardia, but this form of SVT is rare in infants and children.

## CARDIOVASCULAR

○ **What ST and T wave changes may be observed in SVT?**

ST and T wave changes consistent with myocardial ischemia may be observed if tachycardia persists.

○ **With what rhythm is narrow complex SVT in children easily confused?**

Extreme sinus tachycardia associated with sepsis or hypovolemia, particularly because either rhythm may be associated with poor systemic perfusion.

○ **What three things may help you distinguish SVT from sinus tachycardia?**

Heart rate, ECG, variability.

○ **How can heart rate help you distinguish SVT from sinus tachycardia?**

Sinus tachycardia is usually associated with a heart rate less than 200 bpm. In most (60%) infants with SVT, the heart rate is greater than 230 bpm.

○ **How can the ECG help you distinguish SVT from sinus tachycardia?**

P waves may be difficult to identify in both sinus tachycardia and SVT once the ventricular rate exceeds 200 bpm. If the P waves can be identified, the P wave axis is usually abnormal in SVT but normal in sinus tachycardia.

○ **How can variability help you distinguish SVT from sinus tachycardia?**

In sinus tachycardia, the rate may vary from beat to beat, but there is no beat-to-beat variation in SVT. Termination of SVT is abrupt, whereas the heat rate slows gradually in sinus tachycardia.

○ **In sum, what six indications would lead you to suspect sinus tachycardia?**

1. History compatible (fever, volume loss, hemorrhage or pain);
2. P waves present/normal;
3. HR often varies with activity;
4. Variable RR with constant PR;
5. Infants: rate usually <220 bpm;
6. Children: rate usually <180 bpm.

○ **In sum, what six factors would lead you to suspect this was supraventricular tachycardia?**

1. History incompatible (vague or nonspecific history or history of congenital heart disease);
2. P waves absent/abnormal;
3. HR not variable with activity;
4. Abrupt rate changes;
5. Infants: rate usually >220 bpm;
6. Children: rate usually >180 bpm.

○ **What are the first three things you should do when you encounter a child with a rapid heart rate with evidence of poor perfusion?**

1. Assess and maintain the airway;
2. Administer 100% oxygen;
3. Ensure effective ventilation.

○ **If the QRS duration is wide for the child's age, what dysrhythmia should you treat?**

Treat as presumptive ventricular tachycardia.

○ **Name two reversible causes of ventricular tachycardia in children.**

Electrolyte imbalance, drug toxicity.

○ **When should vagal maneuvers be attempted in children?**

In cases of stable SVT with a pulse. Do not delay adenosine therapy or cardioversion if poor perfusion is present.

○ **When should a 12-lead EKG be done?**

As soon as possible during treatment.

○ **What are the indications for amiodarone?**

Recurrent v-fib, recurrent hemodynamically unstable v-tach, sustained paroxysmal atrial fibrillation, paroxysmal SVT, and atrial flutter.

○ **If rapid vascular access is available, what is your first line of treatment in symptomatic wide complex tachycardia in children?**

Amiodarone 5mg/kg IV over 20-60 minutes, or Procainamide 15mg/kg IV over 30-60 minutes, or Lidocaine 1mg/kg IV bolus (no cardioversion delays).

○ **T/F: Amiodarone and procainamide should always be given together.**

False, do not routinely administer them together for they can lead to a prolonged QT interval.

○ **If the antiarrhythmic doesn't work, what do you do next?**

Synchronized cardioversion.

○ **Under what circumstance should you delay synchronized cardioversion in the symptomatic child with wide complex tachycardia?**

Never delay cardioversion.

○ **What is the dosage for synchronized cardioversion?**

0.5-1 Joules/kg. Repeat cardioversion as needed.

○ **If conversion with lidocaine was successful, at what rate should you start a lidocaine infusion?**

20-50 mcg/kg/minute.

○ **A two-month-old is brought into your ER by her mother, pale and with a capillary refill time of > 2 seconds. Mom says she hasn't been acting right all day. Her heart rate is too fast to count. Monitor shows a probable SVT at 260 bpm. No IV access is available. What do you do?**

Synchronized cardioversion 0.5-1 J/kg.

○    **You have the same patient, but with a patent IV. What do you do?**

Adenosine 0.1 mg/kg followed by rapid NS bolus 2-5ml (max dose of 0.25 mg/kg).

○    **What is unique about the way you administer adenosine?**

Proximal port.
Both medication and flush syringe in same port.
Very rapid sequential push.
Keep your thumb on both syringes while pushing.

○    **What do you do if the adenosine doesn't work?**

You may double the dose and repeat once.

○    **What is the maximum dose of adenosine?**

12 mg.

○    **A seven-year-old boy is brought by his father to your clinic. His father says that he complained of a fluttering in his chest, but otherwise feels fine. He is alert and oriented, skin is warm and dry, CRT is < 2 seconds. His pulse is strong but too rapid to count. What do you do?**

Obtain a 12-lead ECG and evaluate QRS duration, rate, and QTc interval.

○    **You obtain a 12-lead ECG and the rate is 240 bpm. What is the normal QRS duration?**

Approximately ≤ 0.08 seconds.

○    **The QRS is 0.05 seconds. What do you need to determine in order to treat this patient?**

Whether the rhythm is ST or SVT.

○    **In analyzing the ECG, you notice that P waves are absent, and the rate is sustained at 240 bpm. What rhythm is this?**

Probable SVT.

○    **The patient remains stable. What should you do?**

Establish vascular access and give adenosine.

○    **You administer 0.1 mg/kg adenosine rapid IV push. There is no change in rhythm. What now?**

Double the dose.

○    **You double the dose and still no change. The patient remains stable. What now?**

Call the cardiologist. Monitor the patient for deterioration or rhythm change and consider digoxin, beta blockers or amiodarone.

○  **Five minutes after you administer lidocaine, the rate suddenly drops to 88 and regular. The patient states the fluttering in his chest is gone. What now?**

Start a lidocaine infusion at 20-50 mcg/kg per minute. Keep waiting for the pediatric cardiologist.

○  **A 12 month-old male with history of congenital heart disease is brought to the ED by his mother for irritability. The boy is awake and you place the child on a monitor. A rate of 200 bpm is noted and the QRS complex is .15 seconds. How will the treatment for this patient be different than the previous patient?**

Do not administer adenosine. Because of the wide QRS complex treat as if it is ventricular in origin. First, identify and treat reversible causes, such as electrolyte imbalance and drug toxicity. Then, administer Amiodarone 5 mg/kg IV over 20 to 60 minutes or Procainamide 15 mg/kg IV over 30-60 minutes or Lidocaine 1mg/kg IV. May repeat Lidocaine twice as needed.

○  **What is the treatment of choice for patients with tachyarrhythmias (SVT, VT, atrial fibrillation, atrial flutter) who show evidence of cardiovascular compromise?**

Synchronized cardioversion.

○  **Why is synchronized cardioversion preferable to unsynchronized countershock?**

Synchronization of delivered energy with the ECG reduces the possibility of inducing VF, which can occur if an electrical impulse is delivered during the relative refractory period of the ventricle.

○  **What is the initial energy dose for synchronized cardioversion?**

0.5 J/kg.

○  **What is the second energy dose for synchronized cardioversion?**

1 J/kg.

○  **T/F: Ideally, infants and children should be ventilated with 100% oxygen before cardioversion.**

True.

○  **T/F: Secure vascular access should be achieved prior to cardioversion.**

True.

○  **What else should you consider before cardioversion?**

Vascular access and the administration of a sedative and analgesia. However, if shock is present, cardioversion should not be delayed while these therapies are instituted.

○  **What is adenosine?**

An endogenous purine nucleoside that slows conduction through the AV node and interrupts AV reentry pathways.

○  **What does adenosine cause?**

It causes transient sinus bradycardia, and usually terminates SVT rapidly, safely and effectively.

○ **What is the half-life of adenosine?**

Less than ten seconds.

○ **What is the duration of effect of adenosine?**

Less than two minutes.

○ **Why does adenosine have such a short half-life?**

It is rapidly sequestered by red blood cells.

○ **What are the primary indications for adenosine?**

It is the initial drug of choice for the diagnosis and treatment of SVT in infants and children.

○ **Why is adenosine so effective in terminating SVT in infants and children?**

Because SVT usually involves a reentrant pathway including the AV node in these patients.

○ **When may adenosine be ineffective in terminating SVT?**

If the arrhythmia is not due to a reentry rhythm involving the AV node or sinus node, e.g., atrial flutter, atrial fibrillation, or atrial or ventricular tachycardia.

○ **How may adenosine be of use in arrhythmias not involving reentry at the AV or sinus nodes?**

It will not terminate the arrhythmia but may produce a transient block at the AV node that may allow the health care provider to review the 12-lead ECG and determine the underlying rhythm.

○ **Why should you immediately push normal saline following adenosine?**

To push it quickly to the heart before the red blood cells have a chance to sequester it.

○ **Why is it important to use two hands to administer adenosine?**

One hand on the medication syringe, one on the flush. Maintain pressure on the plunger after pushing the drug to avoid having the flush pressure push the medication back into the medication syringe.

○ **T/F: Adenosine may not be administered intraosseously.**

False. It may be administered intraosseously if other IV access is not available.

○ **What are the common side effects of adenosine?**

Flushing, dyspnea, chest pain, bradycardia, and irritability.

○ **How quickly do these side effects usually resolve?**

Within 1 to 2 minutes.

❍   **With what group of patients should adenosine be used with caution?**

In children with denervated, transplanted hearts. Adenosine is contraindicated in patients taking dipyridamole (Persantine) or carbamazepine (Tegretol) because these medications can further prolong the AV block caused by the administration of adenosine.

❍   **What medications can block the receptor responsible for adenosine's electrophysiological effects?**

Therapeutic concentrations of theophylline or related methylxanthines (caffeine and theobromine).

❍   **Can you still use adenosine in a child on theophylline?**

Yes, but he or she may require a larger dose than usual.

❍   **What is verapamil?**

A calcium channel blocker.

❍   **How does verapamil exert its antiarrhythmic effect?**

By slowing conduction and prolonging the effective refractory period in the AV junctional tissue.

❍   **What effect of verapamil may cause myocardial depression?**

Its negative inotropic effect.

❍   **What negative consequences have been observed with verapamil?**

Profound bradycardia, hypotension, and asystole.

❍   **In what patients should verapamil not be used?**

It should not be used to treat SVT in an emergency setting in infants less than 1 year of age, in children with congestive heart failure or myocardial depression, in children receiving beta-adrenergic-blocking drugs, or in those who may have a bypass tract.

❍   **T/F: Ventricular tachycardia (VT) is common in the pediatric age group.**

False. It is uncommon.

❍   **What is the ventricular rate range of VT?**

The ventricular rate may vary from 120 to 400 beats per minute.

❍   **T/F: VT with a slow ventricular rate can be well tolerated.**

True.

❍   **Why is rapid VT not well tolerated?**

It compromises stroke volume and cardiac output and may degenerate into ventricular fibrillation.

○   **Which children are most likely to develop VT?**

Those with underlying structural heart disease or prolonged QT syndrome.

○   **What are some of the non-congenital causes of VT?**

Acute hypoxemia, hypothermia, acidosis, electrolyte imbalance, drug toxicity (e.g., tricyclic antidepressants, digoxin toxicity), and poisons.

○   **Describe the ventricular rate for VT.**

At least 120 beats per minute and regular.

○   **Describe the QRS in VT.**

The QRS is wide (greater than 0.08 seconds).

○   **Describe the P waves in VT.**

P waves are not identifiable. When present, they will not be related to the QRS (AV dissociation). At slower rates the atria may be depolarized in a retrograde manner, and therefore there will be a 1:1 VA association.

○   **Describe the T waves in VT.**

T waves are usually opposite in polarity to the QRS.

○   **What other dysrhythmia can look like VT?**

SVT with aberrant conduction. Fortunately, aberrant conduction is present in less than 10% of children with SVT.

○   **T/F: Previously undiagnosed wide QRS tachycardia in an infant or child should be treated as VT until proven otherwise.**

True.

○   **How should you treat VT without palpable pulses?**

Like ventricular fibrillation (VF).

○   **If VT is associated with signs of shock (low cardiac output, poor perfusion), but pulses are palpable, what is the indicated treatment?**

Synchronized cardioversion.

○   **What should be done if possible prior to cardioversion?**

Intubate and ventilate with 100% oxygen, secure vascular access, provide adequate sedation and analgesia.

○   **Why is lidocaine useful in defibrillation?**

It raises the threshold for VF.

❍ **Why should lidocaine be given prior to cardioversion?**

It suppresses postcardioversion ventricular ectopy.

❍ **What is the dose of lidocaine given prior to cardioversion?**

A loading dose of 1 mg/kg followed by an infusion at 20-50 mcg/kg/minute.

❍ **When is it inappropriate to give lidocaine prior to cardioversion?**

In an unstable child if the drug is not readily available or if vascular access has not been achieved.

❍ **When should a lidocaine drip be considered following the return of spontaneous circulation after VT or VF?**

If the ventricular arrhythmias are thought to be associated with myocarditis or structural heart disease.

❍ **To ensure adequate plasma concentration, what should you do prior to starting the infusion?**

Administer a bolus of 1mg/kg.

❍ **What effects can excessive plasma concentrations of lidocaine have?**

Myocardial and circulatory depression and possible central nervous system symptoms, including drowsiness, disorientation, muscle twitching, or seizures.

❍ **When should you consider a reduced lidocaine infusion?**

If reduced lidocaine clearance is suspected, such as might occur in patients with shock or chronic congestive heart failure.

❍ **In patients where reduced lidocaine clearance is suspected, what should be the infusion dose?**

A maximum of 20 mcg/kg/minute.

❍ **What are the most common terminal rhythms in children?**

Sinus bradycardia, sinus node arrest with a slow junctional or ventricular escape rhythm, and various degrees of AV block.

❍ **What is QRS duration in bradycardia?**

QRS duration may be normal or prolonged depending on the pacemaker focus.

❍ **If blood pressure is normal, should you treat bradycardia?**

If there is poor systemic perfusion, it should be treated regardless of blood pressure.

❍ **What is the treatment for bradycardia?**

Adequate ventilation with 100% oxygen must be ensured, chest compressions performed, and epinephrine and atropine are administered as necessary.

○   **What are the six possible causes of pediatric bradycardia identified by PALS?**

1. Hypoxemia;
2. Hypothermia;
3. Head injury;
4. Heart block;
5. Heart transplant;
5. Toxins/poisons/drugs.

○   **What are some of the other causes you can think of?**

Spinal shock.
Sepsis.
Toxicity/overdose.
Electrolyte imbalance.
Myocarditis.
Congenital cardiac anomaly.

○   **Is VF a common terminal event in the pediatric age group?**

No, it is documented in only about 10% of children in whom a terminal rhythm is recorded.

○   **What is defibrillation?**

The untimed (asynchronous) depolarization of a critical mass of myocardial cells to allow spontaneous organized myocardial depolarization to resume.

○   **What will happen if organized depolarization does not resume after defibrillation?**

VF will continue or will progress to electrical silence, at which point restoration of spontaneous cardiac activity may be impossible.

○   **How does synchronized cardioversion differ from defibrillation?**

Synchronized cardioversion also results in depolarization of the myocardium, but cardioversion provides depolarization that is timed (synchronous) with the patient's intrinsic electrical activity.

○   **Why is synchronized cardioversion inappropriate in the patient with VF?**

VF has no organized cardiac electrical activity with which to synchronize.

○   **Successful defibrillation requires the passage of sufficient electric current (amperes) through the heart. On what two factors does this current flow depend?**

The energy (joules) provided and the transthoracic impedance (ohms), which is the resistance to current flow.

○   **If transthoracic impedance is high, what must be done to achieve sufficient current for successful defibrillation or cardioversion?**

Increase the electrical current.

○ **What eight factors determine transthoracic impedance?**

1. Energy selected;
2. Electrode size;
3. Paddle-skin coupling material;
4. Number of shocks;
5. Time intervals between shocks;
6. Phase of ventilation;
7. Size of chest;
8. Paddle electrode pressure.

○ **What is the optimal energy dose for defibrillation in infants and children?**

Trick question: the optimal energy dose has not been established.

○ **Although available information does not demonstrate a relation between energy dose and weight, pediatricians are committed to that relationship, with or without evidence! So what starting dose has been arbitrarily recommended for defibrillation?**

2 joules/kg, until further notice (or data is available).

○ **What can the operator do to minimize transthoracic impedance?**

Apply firm pressure to the paddles. Use an appropriate conduction medium.

○ **What should you do if the initial dose doesn't work?**

Double it.

○ **Why should you deliver the second dose as soon as possible after the first?**

Because the first dose reduces transthoracic impedance. And VF isn't too good for the kid.

○ **If the second shock doesn't work, what should you do?**

Give a third at the same energy level as the second.

○ **How long should you delay between the first three shocks?**

Just long enough to charge the paddles and check the rhythm with the paddles in place.

○ **Should you pause for CPR between shocks?**

No, unless there will be a delay due to equipment malfunction or other calamity.

○ **If VF continues after three shocks, what should you do?**

Administer epinephrine.

○ **After administration of epinephrine, how many times should you shock?**

The AHA 2000 guidelines give you a choice. Either once or three times.

○ **T/F: If VF continues despite the three defibrillation attempts, energy levels may need to be increased further.**

True, but ventilation with 100% oxygen, chest compressions and epinephrine should precede further defibrillation attempts.

○ **After CPR, defibrillation, and epinephrine, what medications should you consider?**

Amiodarone, Lidocaine, or Magnesium.

○ **What is important to remember to do after administering each drug?**

Circulate with good CPR for 30-60 seconds before shocking.

○ **How soon after the administration of a medication should you shock?**

Between 30-60 seconds. Elevate the limb (if used) in which you injected the medication and perform CPR to distribute the drug prior to shocking.

○ **What is the relationship between paddle size and impedance?**

The larger the size, the lower the impedance.

○ **What is the optimal paddle size?**

The largest size that allows good chest contact over the entire paddle surface area and good separation between the two paddles.

○ **Up to what age should infant paddles (4.5cm) be used?**

Up to approximately one year of age or 10kg. Above this age and weight, adult paddles should be used.

○ **Why should bare paddles not be used?**

They result in very high impedance and can burn the skin.

○ **What should be used to help reduce impedance?**

Electrode cream or paste, saline-soaked gauze pads or self-adhesive defibrillation pads.

○ **Why should alcohol pads be avoided?**

They are a fire hazard and can produce serious chest burns.

○ **T/F: Sonographic gel is an acceptable alternative to defibrillation pads.**

False, it is not acceptable.

○ **Why must the interface medium under one electrode paddle not come into contact with the interface medium under the other electrode paddle?**

Bridging will occur, creating a short circuit and an inadequate amount of current will traverse the heart.

○ **How must electrode paddles be positioned?**

So that the heart is between them.

○ **What is theoretically the ideal paddle position?**

Anterior-posterior.

○ **Why is the anterior-posterior position impractical?**

It would interfere with CPR.

○ **What is the standard paddle position?**

One paddle is placed on the upper right chest below the clavicle and the other to the left of the left nipple in the anterior axillary line.

○ **What position should be used if dextrocardia is present?**

The mirror position of the standard.

○ **When might the anterior-posterior position be necessary?**

In an infant when only adult paddles are available.

○ **May the airway person continue to hold the BVM during defibrillation?**

No, all hands must be removed from all equipment in contact with the patient, including the endotracheal tube, ventilation bag and intravenous solutions.

○ **T/F: At the very low defibrillation dose settings required for infants, stored and delivered energies are usually identical.**

False. At these settings they may vary significantly.

○ **What special measures should be taken to ensure accurate defibrillation dosing in infants and children?**

Defibrillators should be checked at very low energy doses so that any variations between set and delivered energies could be prominently posted on the machine.

○ **A code is called in the trauma room of your ED. A ten-year-old child has become unresponsive and VF is observed on the ECG monitor. The patient is being effectively ventilated with 100% oxygen and chest compressions are being performed. You are in charge of defibrillating. What do you do first?**

Turn on the defibrillator. The synchronous mode should not be activated.

○ **What should be done next?**

Apply conductive medium to the paddles.

○ **Then what?**

Select the proper energy and charge the capacitor.

○ **What next?**

Have compressions stopped, place paddles, and recheck rhythm and patient.

○ **And now?**

Clear the area properly, apply firm pressure and defibrillate.

○ **What now?**

Reevaluate ECG and patient.

○ **What is an Automated External Defibrillator (AED)?**

Automated external defibrillators are external defibrillators that incorporate a rhythm analysis system and are commonly used in adults.

○ **Do AEDs have paddles like manual defibrillators?**

No, they use two adhesive pads that are placed on the patient's chest wall and attached to the AED unit by a cable.

○ **What two functions are served by the adhesive pads?**

They capture the surface electrocardiogram, transmitting it through the cables to the AED unit, where it is analyzed. If a defibrillation shock is indicated, the pads provide the contact to deliver the shock to the patient.

○ **What is a fully automated AED?**

A fully automated unit requires only that the operator apply the electrodes and turn the unit on. If the victim's rhythm is determined to be either ventricular tachycardia above a present rate or ventricular fibrillation, the unit will charge its capacitors and deliver a shock.

○ **How does a semi-automated unit differ from one fully automated?**

It requires additional operator steps, including pressing an "analyze" button to initiate rhythm analysis and pressing a "shock" button to deliver the shock. Semi automated devices use voice prompts to assist the operator.

○ **What shock level is delivered by most AEDs?**

200 J, although some devices have a switch to enable delivery of an alternative smaller shock (e.g. 50 J).

○ **Can AEDs be used in pediatric arrest?**

Because current units have been developed for adults, they may be considered when the child is 8 years old or older. At this age the child weights approximately 25-30kg, so that a shock of 200 J would likely deliver a defibrillating dose of approximately 8 J/kg.

○ **In a child 8 years old or older in cardiac arrest, what do you do until the AED arrives?**

CPR.

○ **T/F: Always attach the patches to the patient before turning on the power to an AED.**

False, always turn on the power first.

○ **After 3 shocks or after any "no shock indicated," what should you do?**

Check for signs of circulation.

○ **If, after checking for signs of circulation, there is no pulse, what do you do?**

Resume CPR for one minute.

○ **After one minute of CPR, what do you do?**

Check for signs of circulation.

○ **If there are no signs of circulation, what do you do?**

Press analyze and attempt defibrillation up to three times.

○ **If there are signs of circulation, but absent or inadequate ventilation, what should you do?**

Ventilate at a rate of one breath every 5 seconds.

○ **When is noninvasive (transcutaneous) pacing indicated in children?**

In cases of profound symptomatic bradycardia refractory to BLS and ALS.

○ **T/F: Transcutaneous pacing has been shown to be effective in improving the survival rate of children with out-of-hospital unwitnessed cardiac arrest.**

False. It has not been shown to be effective.

○ **Under what weight should pediatric pacing electrodes be used?**

Under 15 kg.

○ **Where should pacing electrodes be placed on the patient prior to initiating external pacing?**

The negative electrode is placed over the heart on the anterior chest and the positive electrode behind the heart on the back. If the back cannot be used, the positive electrode is placed on the right side of the anterior chest beneath the clavicle and the negative electrode on the left side of the chest over the fourth intercostal space, in the midaxillary area.

○ **Is precise placement of electrodes necessary to effective pacing?**

No, provided that the negative electrode is placed near the apex of the heart.

○ **What types of pacing may be provided noninvasively?**

Either ventricular fixed-rate or ventricular-inhibited pacing.

○   **T/F: If smaller electrodes are used the pacemaker output required to produce capture generally will be lower than if larger electrodes are used.**

True.

○   **How must pacemaker sensitivity be adjusted if ventricular-inhibited pacing is performed?**

It must be adjusted so that intrinsic ventricular electrical activity is appropriately sensed by the pacemaker.

○   **Why is it difficult to determine if ventricular capture and depolarization are taking place?**

Because of the large pacing artifact that often occurs with transcutaneous pacing.

○   **In this circumstance, how can you determine ventricular capture and depolarization?**

By palpating a pulse or from the pressure wave of an indwelling arterial cannula.

○   **You are at the triage desk when mom brings in her three-month old. She states her daughter has had a fever for two days and is not feeding well. Patient is conscious and alert, skin is warm and dry. P 180, R 34, T 38, BP 88/62, SAT 98%. You place the child on a cardiac monitor and this is what you see. What is this rhythm?**

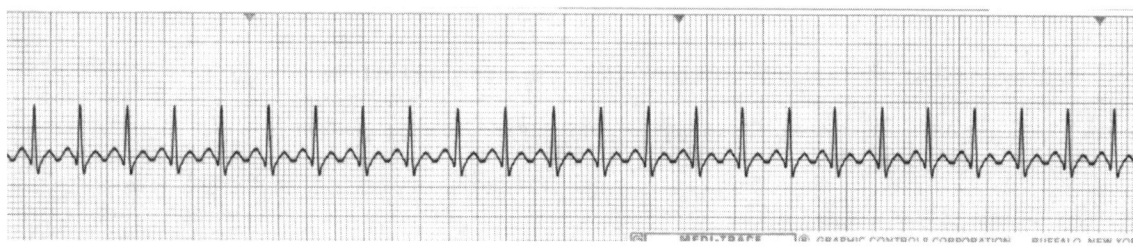

Sinus tachycardia at a rate of 180.

○   **What are the most likely causes of this rhythm?**

Fever, anxiety, dehydration.

○   **You are called to Room Eight to evaluate a three-week old infant. The child is conscious and alert, skin is cool, mottled and dry, capillary refill is delayed, R 64 and gasping, P 80, BP 60/40, SaO$_2$ 84%. The monitor shows the following rhythm. What is it?**

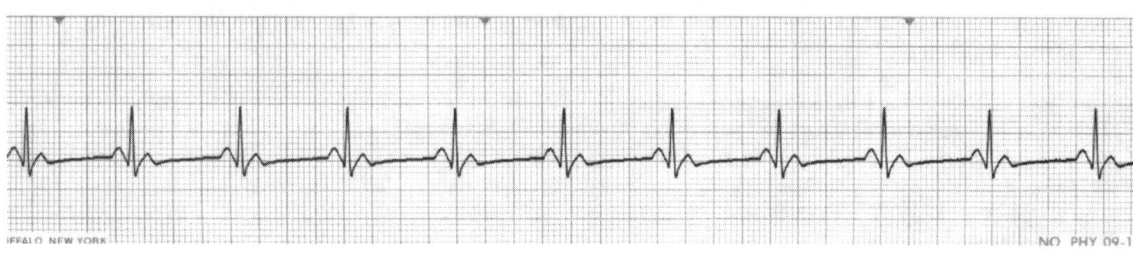

Sinus bradycardia.

○   **What is the probable etiology of this rhythm?**

Hypoxia.

○ **What is the immediate treatment priority?**

Administer 100% oxygen by non-rebreather mask. Assist ventilations with BVM as necessary.

○ **You are dispatched to the scene of a high school basketball game for a player down. When you arrive, you find a fifteen-year-old player on the court. CPR is being performed by bystanders. You place your paddles in "quick look" mode and this is what you see. What is this rhythm?**

Coarse ventricular fibrillation.

○ **What immediate action must you take?**

Three rapid, stacked shocks.

○ **After the third shock, the patient converts to the following rhythm. What is it?**

Ventricular tachycardia.

○ **What do you do now?**

Check for a pulse. If no pulse, defibrillate. If pulse, cardiovert.

○ **There is no pulse and you defibrillate at 360 joules. The patient converts to the following rhythm. What is it?**

Fine ventricular fibrillation.

○ **What now?**

Defibrillate and 360 joules.

○ **You defibrillate at 360 joules and the patient converts to the following rhythm. What is it?**

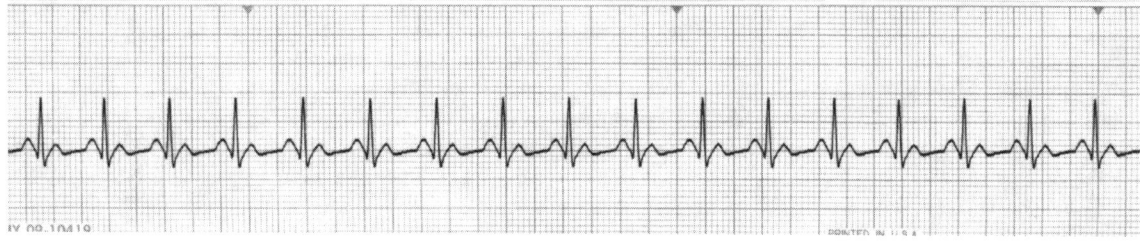

For a fifteen year-old, this would be a sinus tachycardia if accompanied by a pulse. If no pulse, pulseless electrical activity (PEA).

○ **Dad brings in his eight year-old son, who is conscious, alert and oriented. Dad states he was playing baseball with his son in the yard, who suddenly felt weak and dizzy. He had him rest and drink some water, but the symptoms persisted, so he brought him to the emergency department. Skin is warm and dry, PERRL, P 280, R 22, BP 110/72, $SaO_2$ 99%. The monitor shows the following rhythm. What is it?**

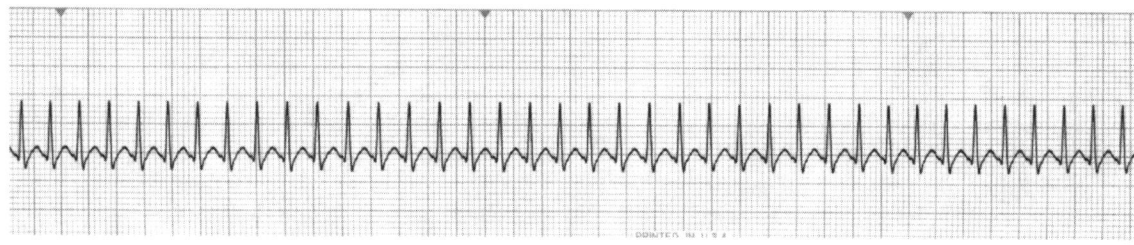

Supraventricular tachycardia.

○ **What do you do?**

As the patient is currently stable, obtain detailed history and physical, monitor closely, establish IV access, and administer adenosine 0.1 mg/kg rapid IVP followed by a 5 ml saline flush. Call for a cardiology consult.

○ **While waiting for the cardiologist, the patient lapses into unconsciousness. What should you do?**

Immediate cardioversion.

○ **If you saw this rhythm on the monitor but there was no pulse, what algorithm would you follow?**

The pulseless arrest algorithm.

# SEDATION AND ANALGESIA

○ **Explain the differences between the terms Opium, Opiate, and Opioid.**

Opium: From the Greek word for juice, applies to the juice extracted from the seeds of the poppy plant, the source for over 20 alkaloids.

Opiate: Any substance that is derived from the opium plant and can induce sleep, the naturally occurring medications from the opium plant are morphine and codeine.

Opioid: Any synthetic substance not derived from opium but that can induce narcosis. Synthetic opioids are meperidine (Demerol), and fentanyl (Sublimaze).

○ **What is the most common adverse reaction caused by local anesthetics?**

Contact dermatitis is the most common local adverse reaction and is characterized by erythema and pruritus that could progress to vesiculation and oozing.

○ **What is the half-life of acetaminophen (Tylenol)?**

Its half-life is 2-3 hours and is unaffected by renal disease as acetaminophen is metabolized in the liver.

○ **What is the indication for naloxone (Narcan) use?**

Naloxone (Narcan) is a narcotic antagonist used to treat or prevent respiratory depression or hypotension known or suspected to be caused by opioids/opiates.

○ **How may naloxone be administered?**

Although the intravenous route is preferred, the same dosage is effective almost as rapidly following endotracheal, intramuscular or subcutaneous administration at a dose of 0.1 mg/kg or 2.0 mg/dose if > 20 kg or 5 years, and can be repeated once in 2-3 minutes if there is no response.

○ **In what specific clinical situations should naloxone be used?**

Reverse CNS depression in suspected narcotic overdose, neonatal opiate depression and coma of unknown origin.

○ **What are the contraindications to using succinylcholine (Anectine)?**

History or a family history of malignant hyperthermia, skeletal muscle myopathies, or known hypersensitivity to the drug. It should not be used in patients with a history of pseudocholinesterase deficiency. It should be avoided in infants and children with ventricular arrhythmias in which you suspect hyperkalemia.

○ **On what specific sites in the CNS do the benzodiazepines act and where are they located?**

Thalamus, limbic structures and the cerebral cortex. They form part of a GABA receptor-chloride ion channel complex, and binding of benzodiazepines to this receptor facilitates the inhibitory actions of GABA, which are exerted through increased chloride ion conductance.

○ **Compare the three benzodiazepines commonly used.**

The clinical effects of diazepam are shorter than lorazepam because it dissociates more rapidly from receptor sites than diazepam, however the elimination half-times are longest for diazepam.

| Medication | Elimination half time in minutes |
|---|---|
| diazepam | 20-35 |
| lorazepam | 10-20 |
| midazolam | 1-4 |

○ **Describe the state induced with the use of ketamine (Ketalar)?**

Ketamine produces a state of dissociative anesthesia in which the patient remains conscious but has marked catatonia, analgesia and amnesia.

○ **What is the most commonly sited contraindication for ketamine use?**

Ketamine should not be used in patients with blunt head injury as causes an increase in intra-cranial pressure.

○ **How is intravenous ketamine administered in the pediatric patient?**

At a dose of 1-2 mg/kg per initial dose IV, given over 60 seconds, producing 5-10 minutes of anesthesia and used in increments of 1/2 of an initial dose if needed to maintain anesthesia.

○ **What are the common symptoms during recovery from intravenous ketamine?**

It causes disorientation and hallucinations during recovery. These symptoms are seen less in younger patients.

○ **How can the side effects of ketamine be lessened during recovery?**

The concomitant use of a benzodiazepine can lessen the side effects commonly seen during emergence.

○ **What is the dose and route of administration of fentanyl (Sublimaze) when used in the neonate?**

In the neonate, fentanyl can be given IV or IM at a dose of 1-2 micrograms/kg infused slowly over 1 minute.

○ **What is the fentanyl lollipop and what is its main side effect?**

The lollipop is a pediatric pre-anesthetic medication to be used by children as a self-administered drug. Some series report up to 50% incidence of vomiting making it impractical in children with "full stomachs" such as in an emergency department.

○ **When using midazolam (Versed) in patients with renal or hepatic dysfunction how should dosing be adjusted?**

If a patient has renal or hepatic dysfunction or is receiving concomitant narcotics, the dose should be decreased by 25-30%.

○ **What is the half-life of morphine?**

In neonates: 4.5-13.3 hours (mean of 7.6 hours). In children: 2-4 hours.

○   **Describe the pharmacokinetics of codeine.**

Codeine has adequate oral absorption and is metabolized in the liver to morphine. It has a half-life of 2.5-3.5 hours and is excreted in the urine.

○   **Why should IV fentanyl be infused slowly?**

Rapid IV infusion of fentanyl can result in skeletal muscle and chest wall rigidity, leading to impaired ventilation, respiratory distress and eventual apnea.

○   **How potent is fentanyl, when compared to morphine?**

Fentanyl is 100 times more potent.

○   **What are the contraindications to using eutectic mixture of local anesthetics (EMLA) cream?**

Contraindications include known hypersensitivity to lidocaine (Xylocaine), prilocaine or local anesthetics of the amide type. Also, patients with idiopathic or congenital methemoglobinemia should not be given these topical agents.

○   **What is the mechanism of action of acetaminophen?**

Acetaminophen inhibits the synthesis of prostaglandins in the central nervous system and peripherally blocks pain impulse generation. It also produces antipyresis by inhibiting the hypothalamic heat regulating center.

○   **Why should codeine not be given intravenously?**

When given intravenously, codeine causes a large histamine release which leads to palpitations, hypotension, bradycardia, and peripheral vasodilatation.

○   **Compare the cardiovascular adverse effects of fentanyl when compared to morphine.**

Fentanyl has less hypotensive effects than morphine due to minimal or no histamine release.

○   **Is it appropriate to use eutectic mixture of local anesthetics on mucous membranes?**

No, because it has increased absorption across mucous membranes which can lead to toxic levels.

○   **What is the maximum daily dose of ibuprofen (Motrin, Advil)?**

40 mg/kg, up to a 3 grams maximum.

○   **How much sugar, and what kind, is found in each 5 ml suspension of ibuprofen?**

2.5 gm of sucrose. This is important if you plan to use this suspension in a diabetic patient.

○   **What are some of the misconceptions about pain in children?**

One of the misconceptions about pain in children is that pain perception in children is decreased because of biologic immaturity and that children have a higher tolerance to pain. Other misconceptions are that children have little or no memory of pain and that not only are they more sensitive to the side effects of analgesics, but that they are at special risk for addiction to narcotics. These beliefs are false.

○ **Discuss pain conduction in the neonate.**

In the neonate, as in the adult, unmyelinated C fibers transmit nociceptive information peripherally. Nerve pulse transmission in incompletely myelinated A-d fibers is delayed, not blocked, until myelination has been completed postnatally. The shorter distances necessary for impulse travel offset any delay in conduction velocity.

○ **Which two common paralytic agents are non-depolarizing?**

Pancuronium (Pavulon) and vecuronium (Norcuron).

○ **How do non-depolarizing blocking paralytics exert their effects?**

The non-depolarizing blocking drugs compete with acetylcholine for cholinergic receptor sites on the postjunctional membrane, but lack the transmitter action of acetylcholine. They do not relieve pain and do not effect consciousness.

○ **In many prepubertal children, what appears in the urine after the patient receives succinylcholine?**

Myoglobinuria. About 40% of prepubertal children exhibit this effect; however, it is not related to the apparent severity of the fasciculations.

○ **How long does anesthesia last from a perineural injection of lidocaine?**

When used alone it lasts 60-75 minutes and when used in combination with epinephrine, anesthesia lasts up to two hours.

○ **How long does it take for a local injection of lidocaine to exert its effect?**

Its effect is immediate.

○ **What are endorphins?**

Endogenous morphine.

○ **What are the routes of administration of chloral hydrate?**

Never intravenous. Chloral hydrate may only be given PO or PR.

○ **What are the contraindications to using chloral hydrate?**

Chloral hydrate is contraindicated in patients with hepatic or renal impairment.

○ **What is the maximum dose of locally injected lidocaine?**

7.0 mg/kg/dose with epinephrine every 2 hours or 4.0-5.0 mg/kg/dose without epinephrine every 2 hours.

○ **Describe the anesthetic agent propofol (Diprivan).**

Propofol is chemically unrelated to any other anesthetic drugs, it most closely resembles the alcohol family and has sedative properties which are similar to the alcohols. It is anecdotally called *milk of amnesia*. It may cause apnea.

○ **Compare and contrast pancuronium (Pavulon) and vecuronium (Norcuron).**

Vecuronium (Norcuron) has a shorter duration of action that pancuronium (Pavulon). The vagolytic property of vecuronium is 20 times less than pancuronium.

|  | Duration of Maximum Effect | Half-life | Elimination | Dose |
|---|---|---|---|---|
| Pancuronium (Pavulon) | 60 minutes | 90-150 minutes | Renal | 0.1 mg/kg |
| Vecuronium (Norcuron) | 30 minutes | 70 minutes | Hepatic | 0.1 mg/kg |

# PULMONARY

○ **What should you suspect if a patient has symptoms similar to those associated with emphysema but he/she is very young and is not a smoker?**

α-1-antitrypsin deficiency. Without α-1-antitrypsin, excess elastase accumulates resulting in lung damage.

○ **A 14-year-old high school freshman attended three days of classes at his new high school last week before it was shut down because of the potential of asbestos exposure. The boy currently exhibits a non-productive cough and says his chest hurts. Does this boy have asbestosis?**

Although a non-productive cough and pleurisy are symptoms of asbestosis, other signs, such as exertional dyspnea, malaise, clubbed fingers, crackles, cyanosis, pleural effusion and pulmonary hypertension, should be displayed before making a diagnosis of asbestosis. In addition, asbestosis does not develop until 10-15 years after regular exposure to asbestos.

○ **What procedures should be performed to confine aspiration in a patient who is continuously vomiting and at risk for aspiration pneumonia?**

Lie the patient on his right side in Trendelenburg. This will help confine the aspirate to the right upper lobe.

○ **How can aspiration be prevented when intubating?**

By appropriate use of rapid sequence induction, including minimizing unnecessary ventilation and applying cricoid pressure during intubation.

○ **Where does aspiration generally occur as revealed by chest x-ray?**

The lower lobe of the right lung. This is the most direct path for foreign bodies in the lung.

○ **What pH of aspirated fluid suggests a poor prognosis?**

pH < 2.5.

○ **A 16-year-old triathlete develops wheezing when exercising. Describe a relevant treatment program for this individual.**

Beta agonist prior to exercise is the initial management therapy.

○ **What x-ray markings usually result in a patient with a long history of bronchial asthma?**

Increased bronchial wall markings and flattening of the diaphragm. The bronchial wall markings are caused by epithelial inflammation and thickening of the bronchial walls.

○ **What pulmonary function test is the most diagnostic for asthma?**

FEV1/FVC. The amount of air exhaled in 1 second, in comparison to the total amount of air in the lung that can be expressed, is determined by performing this test. A ratio of under 80% is diagnostic of asthma. Peak flow monitors are helpful in monitoring asthma at home.

○ **Is wheezing an integral part of asthma?**

No. Thirty-three percent of children with asthma will have only cough variant asthma with no wheezing.

○ **Which is more effective for relieving an acute exacerbation of bronchial asthma in a conscious patient, nebulized albuterol or albuterol MDI administered via an aerosol chamber?**

They are equally efficacious.

○ **A child is born to two parents who are both asthmatic. What is the risk factor of the child having asthma as well?**

Up to 50%.

○ **What are the <u>most</u> <u>common</u> extrinsic allergens that affect asthmatic children?**

Dust and dust mites.

○ **What treatment should be initiated for a patient with acute asthma who does not improve with humidified $O_2$, albuterol nebulizers, steroids, or anticholinergics?**

Subcutaneous epinephrine, 0.3 cc of 1:1,000. (0.01 cc/kg to a max of 0.3 cc)

○ **What kind of medical family history are asthmatic patients most likely to have?**

Asthma, seasonal allergies, and/or atopic dermatitis.

○ **Which type of exercise usually triggers an asthmatic episode in patients with exercise-induced asthma?**

High intensity exercise for more than 5-6 minutes.

○ **What is the role of salmeterol in the asthmatic patient?**

It is used for the long term management of these patients and not in the acute setting. Because of its long half-life, it may be ideal for chronic use in nocturnal break-through exacerbations.

○ **What effects do increased levels of cAMP have on bronchial smooth muscle and on the release of chemical mediators, such as histamine, proteases, platelet activation factor and chemotactic factors, from airway mast cells?**

Relaxes smooth muscle and decreases the release of mediators. Recall that the effects of cAMP are opposed by cGMP. Thus, another treatment approach can be provided by *decreasing* the levels of cyclic GMP via the use of anticholinergic (antimuscarinic) agents, such as ipratropium bromide.

○ **As discussed above, stimulation of ß-adrenergic receptors increases cAMP availability and results in smooth muscle relaxation. Which flavor of ß-adrenergic receptors primarily control bronchiolar and arterial smooth muscle tone?**

ß2-adrenergic receptors.

○ **Terbutaline is administered SQ for asthma in what dose?**

0.01 mL/kg of 1 mg/mL terbutaline up to 0.25 mL, (i.e., 0.25 mg), which may be repeated once in 20-30 minutes.

○ **Is theophylline useful in the emergency management of a severely asthmatic pediatric patient?**

No. It has not been shown to affect further bronchodilatation in patients fully treated with β-adrenergic agents. However, theophylline can be used successfully for inpatient management of asthma and may be started in the hospital.

○ **If corticosteroids are prescribed, how should prednisone be dosed?**

1-2 mg/kg/day in two divided doses; no tapering is necessary if duration of therapy is 5 day or less.

○ **What effect does acidosis have on treatments with β-adrenergic agonists?**

Decreased efficacy.

○ **If one prefers the most simplified algorithm for determining loading dose of theophylline, what are the appropriate doses for a patient who has not been given any theophylline recently? A patient who has recently been given a dose of theophylline?**

1) No recent dose: Load with 7 mg/kg theophylline.
2) Recent dose: Load with 5 mg/kg theophylline.

○ **What is the appropriate parenteral dose of methylprednisolone (Solu-Medrol) to administer to a pediatric patient with status asthmaticus?**

1-2 mg/kg every 6 hours.

○ **If mechanical ventilation is required for such a patient, what is an appropriate setting for the initial tidal volume?**

7 - 10 mL/kg.

○ **What is the most common postoperative respiratory complication?**

Atelectasis. Respiratory failure and aspiration pneumonia are other postoperative complications.

○ **What percentage of patients who have had abdominal surgery also develop atelectasis?**

> 25%.

○ **Atelectasis accounts for what percentage of postoperative fevers?**

90%.

○ **Why do we care about postoperative atelectasis?**

If it persists for more than 72 hours, pneumonia may develop. Perioperative mortality rates are then 20%. Incentive spirometry is an important therapy for the prevention of atelectasis.

○ **A chest x-ray shows "honeycombing," atelectasis, and increased bronchial markings. What is the diagnosis?**

Bronchiectasis. Bronchography will show dilations of the bronchial tree, but this method of diagnosis is not recommended for routine use.

O **Bronchiectasis occurs most frequently in patients with what conditions?**

Patients with cystic fibrosis, immunodeficiencies, lung infections, or foreign body aspirations.

O **Which is the most common type of pathogen in bronchiolitis?**

RSV. It generally affects infants younger than 2 years old.

O **A 2-year-old patient presents with a sudden harsh cough that is worse at night, wheezing, and rhonchi/inspiratory stridor. What is the diagnosis?**

Croup (also known as laryngotracheitis). This condition is usually preceded by an URI and most frequently caused by the parainfluenza virus. A barking seal cough is a characteristic of croup.

O **In treating a patient with a common cold, you prescribe an oral decongestant. Is it necessary to also suggest an antitussive?**

Most coughs arising from a common cold are caused by the irritation of the tracheobronchial receptors in the posterior pharynx by postnasal drip. Postnasal drip can be cleared up with decongestant therapy, thereby eliminating the need for cough suppressant therapy.

O **What are the most common etiologies of a chronic cough?**

Postnasal drip (40%), asthma (25%), and gastroesophageal reflux (20%). Other etiologies include bronchitis, bronchiectasis, bronchogenic carcinoma, esophageal diverticula, sarcoidosis, viruses, and drugs.

O **Which condition must be ruled out when childhood nasal polyps are found?**

Cystic fibrosis.

O **What age group is afflicted with the most colds per year?**

Kindergartners win the top billing with an average of 12 colds per year. Second place goes to preschoolers with 6-10 per year. School children get an average of 7 per year, and adolescents and adults average only 2-4 per year.

O **What is the duration of a common cold?**

3-10 day self-limited course.

O **Which age group usually contracts croup?**

6 months to 3 years. Croup is characterized by cold symptoms, a sudden barking cough, inspiratory and expiratory stridor, and a slight fever.

O **A newborn presents with poor weight gain, steatorrhea, and a GI obstruction arising from thick meconium ileus. What test should be performed?**

The "sweat test," which detects electrolyte concentrations in the sweat. The infant may have cystic fibrosis. Cystic fibrosis is an autosomal recessive defect affecting the exocrine glands. As a result, electrolyte concentrations increase in the sweat glands.

○   **What is the classic triad of cystic fibrosis?**

1) COPD.
2) Pancreatic enzyme deficiency.
3) Abnormally high concentration of sweat electrolytes.

○   **What is the most common presentation of newborns with cystic fibrosis?**

GI obstruction due to meconium ileus.

○   **Which age group typically gets epiglottitis?**

The 3-7 year age group, although any group can get epiglottitis.

○   **What is the difference between the "cough of croup" and the "cough of epiglottitis"?**

Croup has a seal like "barking" cough, while epiglottitis is accompanied by a minimal cough. Children with croup have a hoarse voice while those with epiglottitis have a muffled voice.

○   **What is the "thumb print sign"?**

A soft tissue inflammation of the epiglottis on a lateral x-ray of the neck.

○   **Should a 7-year-old who has never received her Hib vaccine be vaccinated now?**

No, most children are immune by the age of 5.

○   **Are aspirated foreign bodies more likely to be found in the right or left bronchus?**

Right.

○   **What is the definition for massive hemoptysis?**

Coughing, not vomiting, of more than 300 mL of blood in 24 hours.

○   **Life threatening hemoptysis should be suspected when there is:**

1) A large volume of blood.
2) The appearance of a fungus ball in a pulmonary cavity via chest x-ray.
3) Hypoxemia.

○   **What are Kerley B lines?**

X-ray findings found in pulmonary edema. Fluid in the lung causes waterlogged interlobular septa that become fibrotic with time. These show up as lines and shadows on an x-ray.

○   **Which type of bacteria is most commonly found in lung abscesses?**

Anaerobic bacteria.

○   **Which single antibiotic is the most effective for treating uncomplicated lung abscess?**

Clindamycin.

O   **T/F: Flora of lung abscesses are usually polymicrobial.**

True.

O   **Which age group is usually afflicted by pertussis?**

Infants younger than 2.

O   **Where does pain from pleurisy radiate?**

The shoulder, as a result of diaphragmatic irritation.

O   **Which is the most common community-acquired pneumonia?**

*Pneumococcal pneumonia.*

O   **Pneumatoceles, thin-walled air-filled cysts, on an infant's x-ray are a sign of which type of pneumonia?**

Staphylococcal pneumonia.

O   **What are the most common causes of Staphylococcal pneumonias?**

Drug use and endocarditis. This pneumonia produces high fever, chills, and a purulent productive cough.

O   **What are the extrapulmonary manifestations of mycoplasma?**

Erythema multiforme, pericarditis, and CNS disease.

O   **What is the most frequent etiology of nosocomial pneumonia?**

*Pseudomonas aeruginosa.* It most frequently occurs in immunocompromised patients or patients on mechanical ventilation.

O   **A 14-year-old comes to your office bragging, between coughs, about a 3 day Young Republicans convention she attended last week in Las Vegas. She is nauseous and coughing; she has chills and a fever of 103.5°F. She also has a minor gait problem and splints her chest when she breaths. Should you be concerned about your own health as she has just given a mighty cough in your direction?**

This patient most likely has Legionnaires' disease. Unless you attended the same convention in Las Vegas, you are unlikely to catch this pneumonia from her. *Legionella pneumophila* contaminates the water in air conditioning towers and moist soil. It is not spread from person to person.

O   **Describe the classic chest x-ray findings in a patient with mycoplasma pneumonia.**

Patchy diffuse densities involving the entire lung are most common. Pneumatoceles, cavities, abscesses, and pleural effusions can occur, but are uncommon.

O   **Describe the classic chest x-ray findings in *Legionella* pneumonia.**

Dense consolidation and bulging fissures. Expect elevated liver enzymes and hypophosphatemia.

○ **Describe the different presentations of bacterial and viral pneumonia.**

Bacterial pneumonia is typified by a sudden onset of symptoms, including pleurisy, fever, chills, productive cough, tachypnea, and tachycardia. The most common bacterial pneumonia is pneumococcal pneumonia. Viral pneumonia is characterized by gradual onset of symptoms, no pleurisy, chills or high fever, general malaise, and a non-productive cough.

○ **A 17-year-old college student is home for winter break and comes to your office complaining of a 1 1/2 week history of a non-productive dry hacking cough, malaise, a mild fever, and no chills. What is the diagnosis?**

*Mycoplasma pneumoniae*, also known as walking pneumonia. Although this is the most common pneumonia that develops in teenagers and young adults, it is an atypical pneumonia and is most frequently found in close contact populations (e.g., schools and military barracks).

○ **Match the pneumonia with the treatment.**

1) *Klebsiella pneumoniae*
2) *Streptococcal pneumoniae*.
3) *Legionella pneumophila*.
4) *Haemophilus influenza* pneumonia.
5) *Mycoplasma pneumoniae*.

a) Erythromycin, tetracycline, or doxycycline.
b) Penicillin G.
c) Cefuroxime and clarithromycin.
d) Erythromycin and rifampin.

Answers: (1) c, (2) b, (3) d, (4) c, and (5) a.

○ **What is the most common cause of pneumonia in children?**

Viral pneumonia. Infecting viruses include influenza, parainfluenza, RSV, and adenoviruses.

○ **What is the most common lethal, inheritable disease in the white population?**

Cystic fibrosis, an autosomal recessive disease occurring in 1/2,000 births.

○ **Which clase of antimicrobial agents are broadly effective against organisms that cause both typical and atypical pneumonias?**

Macrolides.

○ **What percentage of upper-respiratory infectious agents are non-bacterial?**

Non-bacterial agents account for over 90% of pharyngitis, laryngitis, tracheal bronchitis, and bronchitis.

○ **If a patient has a patchy infiltrate on a chest x-ray and bullous myringitis, what antibiotic should be prescribed?**

Erythromycin for mycoplasma.

○ **What secondary bacterial pneumonia often occurs following a viral pneumonia?**

*Staphylococcus aureus* pneumonia.

❍ **What 3 findings should be present to consider a sputum sample adequate?**

1. > 25 PMNs;
2. < 10 squamous epithelial cells per low powered field;
3. a predominant bacterial organism.

❍ **Should steroids be used in aspiration pneumonia?**

No.

❍ **What is the indication for a chest tube in pneumothorax?**

Over 15% pneumothorax or a clinical indication, such as respiratory embarrassment.

❍ **What therapy may increase the body's absorption of a pneumothorax or pneumomediastinum?**

A high inspired $FiO_2$.

❍ **What is the profile of a classic patient with a spontaneous pneumothorax?**

Male, athletic, tall, slim, 15-35 years of age. Pneumothorax does not occur most frequently during exercise.

❍ **What accessory x-rays may be obtained for the diagnosis of pneumothorax?**

Expiratory film and lateral decubitus film on the affected side.

❍ **Which types of pneumonia are commonly associated with pneumothorax?**

*Staphylococcus*, TB, *Klebsiella*, and PCP.

❍ **Primary pulmonary hypertension is most common in what population?**

Young females. It is rapidly fatal within a few years.

❍ **What heart sounds are heard with pulmonary hypertension?**

A shortened second heart sound split and a louder P2.

❍ **What is the major etiology of pulmonary hypertension?**

Chronic hypoxia.

❍ **T/F: Pulse oximetry is a reliable method for estimating oxyhemoglobin saturation in a patient suffering from CO poisoning.**

False. COHb has light absorbance that can lead to a falsely elevated pulse oximeter transduced saturation level. The calculated value from a standard ABG may also be falsely elevated. The oxygen saturation should be determined by using a co-oximeter that measures the amounts of unsaturated $O_2Hb$, COHb, and metHb.

○  **What is the half-life of COHb for a patient breathing room air? Breathing 100% oxygen? Breathing 100% oxygen at 3 atm of pressure?**

| $FIO_2 = 0.21$ | $FIO_2 = 1.0$ | $FIO_2 = 1.0$ @ 3 atm |
|---|---|---|
| 4–6 hours | 40–90 minutes | 20-30 minutes |

○  **A newborn is breathing rapidly and grunting. Intercostal retractions, nasal flaring, and cyanosis are noted. Auscultation shows decreased breath sounds and crackles. What is the diagnosis?**

Newborn respiratory distress syndrome, also known as hyaline membrane disease. X-rays show diffuse atelectasis. Treatment involves artificial surfactant and $O_2$ administration through CPAP.

○  **Which type of rhinitis is associated with anxious patients?**

Vasomotor rhinitis. This is a non-allergic rhinitis of unknown etiology that involves nasal vascular congestion.

○  **Which sinuses are fully formed in children?**

Only the ethmoid and the maxillary. Frontal sinuses form by age 10.

○  **Differentiate between transudate and exudate.**

1. Transudate: Serum protein is < 0.5 and LDH is < 0.6. Most common with CHF, renal disease, and liver disease.
2. Exudate: Serum protein > 0.5, LDH > 0.6. Most common with infections, malignancy, and trauma.

○  **Where do primary TB lesions most often occur in the lung?**

Primary lesions most often occur in the lower lobes of the lung. Reactivation occurs in the apices.

○  **What are the side-effects of INH?**

Neuropathy, pyridoxine loss, lupus-like syndrome, and hepatitis.

○  **What percentage of tuberculosis is drug-resistant?**

About 15%, but this mainly depends on the geographic location.

○  **What are the classic signs and symptoms of TB?**

Night sweats, fever, weight loss, malaise, cough, and a greenish-yellow sputum most commonly seen in the mornings.

○  **Where are some common extrapulmonary TB sites?**

The lymph node, bone, GI tract, GU tract, meninges, liver, and the pericardium.

○  **A patient presents with cough, lethargy, dyspnea, conjunctivitis, glomerulonephritis, fever, and purulent sinusitis. What is the diagnosis?**

Wegener's granulomatosis. This is a necrotizing vasculitis and pulmonary granulomatosis that attacks the small arteries and veins. Treatment is with corticosteroids and cyclophosphamide.

○ **Are sedatives beneficial for anxious asthmatic patients?**

Only if you are trying to kill them. However, sedatives are appropriate for use during Rapid Sequence Intubation (RSI).

○ **What is the prognosis of childhood asthma?**

50% of all asthmatic children are symptom free within 10-20 years. In mild asthma, the remission rate is 50%, with only 5% experiencing severe disease. 95% of children with severe childhood asthma, however, become asthmatic adults.

○ **Define extrinsic asthma.**

Asthmatic exacerbation following environmental exposure to allergens such as dust, pollens, and dander.

○ **Define intrinsic asthma.**

Asthmatic exacerbation not associated with an increase in IgE or a positive skin.

○ **When administering epinephrine in the treatment of asthma, how might the side effects of epinephrine be minimized?**

Side effects such as pallor, tremor, anxiety, palpitations, and headache can be minimized if doses of no more than 0.3 ml are given.

○ **What are the historical risk factors for status asthmaticus?**

Chronic steroid-dependent asthma, prior ICU admission, prior intubation, recurrent ER visits in past 48 hours, sudden onset of severe respiratory compromise, poor therapy compliance, poor clinical recognition of attack severity, and hypoxic seizures.

○ **What is the major side effect associated with the inhalation of N-acetylcysteine?**

Cough and bronchospasm, most likely due to irritation from the low pH (2.2) of the aerosol solution.

○ **What is the effect of macrolide antibiotics (erythromycin, clarithromycin) on mucus hypersecretion?**

Some macrolide antibiotics have the ability to down regulate mucus secretion by an unknown mechanism. This is thought to be due to an anti-inflammatory activity.

○ **What are the signs of a large obstructing foreign body in the larynx or trachea?**

Respiratory distress, stridor, inability to speak, cyanosis, loss of consciousness, death.

○ **What are the symptoms of a smaller (distally lodged) foreign body?**

Cough, dyspnea, wheezing, chest pain, fever.

○ **What is the procedure of choice for foreign body removal?**

Rigid bronchoscopy. Fiberoptic bronchoscopy is an alternate procedure in adults, not in children. If bronchoscopy fails, thoracotomy may be required.

○ **What are the common radiographic findings in foreign body aspiration?**

Normal film, atelectasis, pneumonia, contralateral mediastinal shift (more marked during expiration), and visualization of the foreign body

○ **T/F: Aspiration of fluids with pH less than 5 produces chemical pneumonitis.**

False. Aspirate pH less than 2.5 produces chemical injury.

○ **What is the antibiotic choice for gastric acid aspiration?**

None.

○ **What is the role of corticosteroids in gastric acid aspiration?**

None.

○ **What is the main priority in treating gastric acid aspiration?**

Maintenance of oxygenation. Intubation, ventilation, and PEEP (positive end expiratory pressure) may be required.

○ **What are the radiographic manifestations of acid aspiration?**

Varied, may be bilateral diffuse infiltrates, irregular "patchy" infiltrates, or lobar infiltrates.

○ **What is the usual source of infected aspirated material?**

The oropharynx.

○ **What pleuropulmonary infections may occur after aspirating infected oropharyngeal material?**

Necrotizing pneumonia, lung abscess, "typical" pneumonia, empyema.

○ **What is the predominant oropharyngeal flora in outpatients?**

Anaerobes. Community acquired aspiration is usually anaerobic. The most common aerobes involved are *Streptococcus* species.

○ **What is the antibiotic of choice for outpatient acquired infectious aspiration pneumonia?**

Clindamycin, high dose penicillin or unasyn.

○ **What is the bacteriology of patients with inpatient acquired infectious aspiration pneumonia?**

Mixed aerobic and anaerobic organisms. Unlike outpatients, *Staphylococcus aureus*, *E. coli*, *Pseudomonas aeruginosa*, and *Proteus* species are common.

○ **What are the consequences of aspirating small (non-obstructing) food particles?**

Inflammation and hypoxemia, may result in chronic bronchiolitis or granulomatosis.

○ **Name the commonly aspirated hydrocarbons.**

Gasoline, kerosene, furniture polish, lighter fluid.

O   **What are the effects of hydrocarbon aspiration?**

Hypoxemia, intrapulmonary shunting, pulmonary edema, hemoptysis, respiratory failure.

O   **What is the role of emesis induction or gastric lavage in hydrocarbon ingestion?**

These maneuvers are not recommended as the patient may aspirate during regurgitation.

O   **Lipoid pneumonia is associated with chronic aspiration of what?**

Mineral oil, animal or vegetable oils, oil-based nose drops.

O   **What is the annual U.S. mortality from drowning?**

9000. There are 500 near drowning for each drowning.

O   **What is the definition of drowning?**

Death due to suffocation by submersion in water.

O   **Can drowning occur without aspiration of water?**

Yes. 10% of victims die from intense laryngospasm.

O   **How much fluid can be drained from the lungs after drowning in fresh water?**

Little, as hypotonic fresh water is rapidly absorbed from the lung, unlike salt water which is hypertonic and is retained. There is no difference in outcome.

O   **What is the priority in treatment of near drowning?**

Maintenance of oxygenation.

O   **When is the Heimlich maneuver applied directly after a near drowning?**

When foreign body aspiration is suspected.

O   **What are the indications for intubation and ventilation after near drowning?**

Apnea, pulselessness, altered mental status, severe hypoxemia, respiratory acidosis.

O   **Resistance to airflow in the airway is inversely proportional to what?**

The fourth power of the airway radius.

O   **What is the most common etiology of croup or laryngotracheobronchitis?**

Parainfluenza virus.

O   **What is the most common organism isolated from patients with bacterial tracheitis?**

*Staphylococcus aureus.*

○ **How do retropharyngeal abscesses arise?**

Lymphatic spread of infections in the nasopharynx, oropharynx, or external auditory canal.

○ **What is the most common type of tracheo-esophageal fistula?**

Blind esophageal pouch with a fistulous connection of the trachea to the distal esophagus.

○ **The croup score is used to assess the degree of respiratory distress accompanying an illness. Which symptoms are evaluated in the score?**

Stridor, cough, air entry, flaring/retractions, and color.

○ **Why does a newborn with bilateral choanal astresia present with severe respiratory distress that is relieved by the insertion of an oral airway?**

Because the newborn is an obligatory nose breather.

○ **According to Poiseuille's law, if the radius of the conducting airway is reduced from 4 mm to 2 mm, by how much will the airflow resistance increase?**

Sixteen-fold.

○ **The funnel-shaped narrowing of the glottis and subglottic airway, commonly known as steeple sign, is observed in what type of extrathoracic airway obstruction?**

Croup or laryngotracheobronchitis.

○ **Name one of the conditions which makes a child a likely candidate for tonsillectomy.**

Recurrent tonsillar abscesses.

○ **A six-year-old male complains of dysphagia and fever. Tonsillar exudates and anterior cervical adenitis are noted. What sign differentiates Group A strep from other causes of pharyngitis?**

A sandpaper-like rash.

○ **A 4-year-old child has high fever, hoarseness, and increased stridor of 3 hours duration. He has a low fever and sore throat earlier in the day. He is ill appearing, with a temperature of 40 degrees C, inspiratory stridor, drooling and intercostals retractions. He prefers to sit up. What is the most likely diagnosis?**

Epiglottitis.

○ **Foreign body aspiration occurs most commonly in which age group?**

1-3 years of age, with slight male predominance.

○ **Name the most common offender in foreign body aspiration.**

Organic substances such as nuts and corn.

○ **What are the McConnochie criteria for the diagnosis of bronchiolitis?**

1) Acute expiratory wheezing.
2) Age 6 months or less,
3) Signs of viral illness, such as fever or coryza,
4) Without pneumonia or atopy,
5) The first such episode,

○   **What will be the predominant symptom of a child who has aspirated a foreign body which is lodged in his/her trachea?**

Stridor.

○   **The predominant auscultatory finding in a child with a foreign body lodged in the right mainstem bronchus:**

Expiratory wheezing.

○   **An 11-month old male presents with rhinorrhea, cough and increasing respiratory distress. Treatment with bronchodilators have produced equivocal results. He is now in obvious distress with retractions, grunting, prolonged expiratory time, inspiratory and expiratory wheezes. Chest x-rays shows a tracheal shift to the left and hyperexpansion of the right chest. What is the most likely diagnosis?**

Foreign body aspiration.

○   **The total work of breathing is divided into two parts. Name them.**

1) To overcome lung and chest wall compliance.
2) To overcome airway and tissue resistance.

○   **Total work of breathing in neonates and infants is lowest at what respiratory rate?**

35-40/minute.

○   **Why are infants more susceptible to inflammatory changes in the airway?**

Because the airway in infants is smaller, and is also much more compliant.

○   **Grunting is usually more prominent in what type of respiratory pathology?**

Typically in smaller airway disease such as bronchiolitis, or in diseases with loss of functional residual capacity such as pneumonia or pulmonary edema because grunting is an effort to maintain positive airway pressure during expiration.

○   **What is Sampter's Triad?**

Asthma, nasal polyps, and aspirin allergy.

○   **What are the criteria associated with severe asthma and likelihood of hospital admission?**

A pretreatment PEFR <25% predicted, pulsus paradoxus > 10 mm Hg on presentation, failure of PEFR to rise > 15% after treatment, or posttreatment PEFR <60% predicted or SaO2 <93%.

○   **What is the dose of epinephrine in acute asthma?**

0.01 mg/kg SC or epinephrine 1:1000, repeated q 20 minutes as needed; max 0.3 cc

○ **What is the dose of nebulized albuterol?**

0.1-0.15 mg/kg of a 2 mg/5 ml solution.

○ **What is the dose of Prelone (prednisolone) in acute asthma?**

1-2 mg/kg/day of a 15 mg/5 ml solution.

○ **What are the high yield indications for chest radiography in suspected pneumonia?**

Tachypnea, rales, decreased breath sounds, stridor, retractions, or cyanosis.

○ **What is the best single predictor of pneumonia in children?**

Tachypnea.

# GASTROINTESTINAL

O **Distinguish, by location, between anal cryptitis, anal fissure, anorectal abscess, and fistula in ano.**

Cryptitis, fissures, and perianal abscess typically occur in the posterior midline. Deep abscesses can point to areas far from the anus. Goodsall's rule declares that fistulas opening anteriorly go straight to the anal canal, while fistulas opening posteriorly may follow a circuitous route.

O **What are some common conditions that mimic acute appendicitis?**

Mesenteric lymphadenitis, PID, Mittlesmertz, gastroenteritis, and Crohn's disease.

O **What conditions are associated with an atypical presentation of acute appendicitis?**

Situs inversus viscerum, malrotation, hypermobile cecum, long pelvic appendix, and pregnancy (1/2200).

O **What are the most frequent symptoms of acute appendicitis?**

Anorexia and pain. The classical presentations of anorexia and periumbilical pain with progression to constant RLQ pain are present in only 60% of the cases.

O **What percentage of acute appendicitis cases have an elevated WBC count?**

An elevated leukocyte count and an elevated absolute neutrophil count are present in 86% and 89% of the cases, respectively.

O **What intraabdominal pathology should be assumed in a pregnant female with right upper quadrant pain until proven otherwise?**

Acute appendicitis.

O **What does an ultrasound show in acute appendicitis?**

A fixed, tender, non-compressible mass, but only in 75-90% of these cases.

O **Which method is more sensitive for locating the source of GI bleeding, a radioactive Tc-labeled red cell scan or an angiography?**

A bleeding scan can detect a site bleeding at a rate as low as 0.12 mL/minute, while angiography requires rapid bleeding (i.e., greater than 0.5 mL/min).

O **A patient with an "acid stomach" develops melena and vomits bright red blood. Is esophagitis a feasible cause?**

No. Capillary bleeding rarely causes impressive acute blood loss. Arterial bleeding—from a complicated ulcer, foreign body, or Mallory-Weiss tear—or variceal bleeding are much more probable.

O **Recurrent pneumonias, especially in the right middle lobe or the superior segments of the bilateral upper lobes, are indicative of what syndrome?**

Aspiration associated with motor diseases and gastroesophageal reflux.

○   **Repeated violent bouts of vomiting can result in both Mallory-Weiss tears and Boerhaave's syndrome. Differentiate between the two.**

1. Mallory-Weiss tears involve the submucosa and mucosa, typically in the right posterolateral wall of the GE junction.

2. Boerhaave syndrome is a full-thickness tear, usually in the unsupported left posterolateral wall of the abdominal esophagus.

○   **A 6 month old infant is constipated, flaccid, and only stares straight ahead. He is not running a fever. However, his mother is especially worried because he won't take his bottle—not even for her "honey on the tip of the bottle" trick. Diagnosis?**

Infantile botulism. Infants ingest spores that are in the environment, most commonly in honey. The spores then grow and produce toxins within the host.

○   **How does infantile botulism differ from food-borne botulism?**

Infantile botulism is caused by the spores of *C. botulinum* while adult food-borne botulism arises from the ingestion of *C. botulinum* neurotoxins.

○   **What is the antidote for botulism poisoning?**

Trivalent A-B-E antitoxin. This antidote is not required for infantile botulism.

○   **Gallbladder stones are generally formed of:**

Cholesterol. The diagnostic test of choice is ultrasound. This technique may show stones, sludge bile plugging, or dilated bile ducts.

○   **A patient with a history of gallstones presents with an acute, postprandial right upper quadrant pain. What's the KUB likely to show?**

Nothing specific. Only around 10% of gallstones are radiopaque. Complications of cholelithiasis, such as emphysematous cholecystitis, perforation, and pneumobilia are uncommon but useful findings.

○   **A child with sickle-cell disease presents with fever, shaking chills, and jaundice. What is the diagnosis?**

Charcot's triad suggests ascending cholangitis. The precipitating cause is probably pigment stones resulting from chronic hemolysis.

○   **A 12-year-old male complains of 2 days of rice water stools, muscle cramps and extreme fatigue. He looks pale, dehydrated, and very ill. The patient states that he has just returned from India. What is the diagnosis?**

Cholera. The incidence of cholera in the US is 1/10,000,000. Cholera usually develops in travelers returning from endemic areas, such as India, Africa, southeast Asia, southern Europe, Central and South America, and the Middle East. This disease can be prevented if the water ingested during the trip is purified and raw, and unpeeled fruits/vegetables and seafood are avoided altogether.

○   **How does the pathology of Crohn's disease differ from that of ulcerative colitis?**

Crohn's is a trans-mucosal, segmental, granulomatous process, while ulcerative colitis is a mucosal, juxtapositioned, ulcerative process.

○   **A young man with atraumatic chronic back pain, eye trouble, and painful red lumps on his shins develops <u>bloody diarrhea</u>. What is the point of this question?**

To remind you of the extraintestinal manifestations of inflammatory bowel disease, such as ankylosing spondylitis, uveitis, and erythema nodosum, not to mention kidney stones.

○   **At least one-third of the patients with Crohn's disease develop kidney stones. Why?**

Dietary oxalate is usually bound to calcium and excreted. When terminal ileal disease leads to decreased bile salt absorption, the resulting fattier intestinal contents bind calcium by saponification. Free oxalate is "hyper-absorbed" in the colon, resulting in hyperoxaluria and calcium oxalate nephrolithiasis.

○   **Complications of Crohn's include perirectal abscesses, anal fissures, rectovaginal fistulas, and rectal prolapse. What percentage of patients with Crohn's disease have perirectal involvement?**

Approximately 90%.

○   **What are the odds that a patient with severe ileal disease will be cured by surgery?**

Virtually zero. Crohn's invariably recurs in the remaining GI tract. In contrast, total proctocolectomy with ileostomy is curative procedure for ulcerative colitis.

○   **What hereditary diseases evident in infancy may cause cirrhosis?**

Glycogen storage disease, cystic fibrosis, galactosemia, fructose intolerance, tyrosinemia, and acid cholesterol esterhydrolase deficiency.

○   **What stool studies are crucial for evaluating acute diarrhea?**

Statistically speaking, acute diarrhea is so common and typically self-limited that most cases require no testing, just oral rehydration. In sick patients or those at risk for complications, (i.e., at the extremes of age, recently hospitalized, or the immunocompromised), enteroinvasive infection should be ruled out with a stool guaiac and test for fecal leukocytes. Gram's or methylene blue stains are comparable. Also consider checking for ova and parasites.

○   **Which diarrheal illnesses cause fecal leukocytes?**

The usual culprits are *Shigella*, *Campylobacter*, and enteroinvasive *E. coli*. Others include *Salmonella*, *Yersinia*, *Vibrio parahaemolyticus*, and *C. difficile*. Fecal WBCs are absent in toxigenic and enteropathogenic infection, even with such a virulent organism as *Vibrio cholera*. Viral and parasitic infections rarely produce fecal WBCs.

○   **Name the most probable cause of diarrhea in a 6-month old in day-care.**

Viral diarrhea caused by *Rotavirus* is the most common. Also test for *Giardia* and *Cryptosporidia* because these agents have recently been added to the list of day-care-associated diarrheal illnesses.

○   **What is the most common cause of bacterial diarrhea?**

*E. coli* (enteroinvasive, enteropathogenic, enterotoxigenic).

○   **Which is the most common form of acute diarrhea?**

Viral diarrhea. It is generally self limited, lasting only 1-3 days.

○ **Diarrhea that develops within 12 hours of a meal is most probably caused by what?**

An ingested pre-formed toxin.

○ **When does traveler's diarrhea typically occur?**

3-7 days after arrival in a foreign land.

○ **What is the treatment for traveler's diarrhea?**

Traveler's diarrhea is caused by *E. Coli*; the preferable treatment is with Bactrim.

○ **What is the definition of chronic diarrhea?**

Passage of greater than 200 g of loose stool per day for over 3 weeks.

○ **The most common symptom of esophageal disease is:**

Pyrosis (heartburn).

○ **What are the indications for the surgical removal of a GI foreign body?**

GI obstruction, GI perforation, the toxic properties of the material, and whether its length, size, and shape will prevent the object from passing safely.

○ **What size objects rarely pass through the stomach and require endoscopic retrieval?**

Objects longer than 5 cm and wider than 2 cm.

○ **Radiographs should be performed on all patients suspected of swallowing coins to determine the presence and location of the foreign body. How will the coin appear on a x-ray in the AP view?**

Coins in the esophagus lie in the frontal plane. Coins in the trachea lie in the sagittal plane.

○ **What is the management of button batteries that have passed the esophagus?**

In the asymptomatic patient, repeat radiographs. The symptomatic patient and patients in whom the battery has not passed the pylorus after 48 hours require an endoscopic retrieval.

○ **Foreign bodies lodge at what esophageal levels in the pediatric patient?**

Typically at levels of the cricopharyngeus muscles. The thoracic inlet, aortic arch, tracheal bifurcation, and lower esophageal sphincter are also possible lodging sites.

○ **X-rays are crucial for finding suspected swallowed foreign bodies. In kids, what physical findings can tip you off?**

Besides the child's distress, a red or scratched oropharynx, dysphagia, a high fever, or peritoneal signs may be evident. In addition, subcutaneous air suggests perforation.

○ **Which type of hepatitis is usually contracted through blood transfusion?**

Hepatitis C. Eighty five percent of post transfusion hepatitis is caused by hepatitis C.

○ **A poor prognosis is associated with which two LFTs in acute viral hepatitis?**

A total bilirubin > 20 mg/dL and a prolongation of the prothrombin time > 3 seconds. The extent of transaminase elevation is not a useful marker.

○ **Match the following hepatitis serologies with the correct clinical description.**

1. HBsAg (-), and antiHBs (+)
2. IgM HBcAg (+), antiHBs (-)
3. IgG HBcAg (+), antiHBs (-)
4. HBeAg (+)

a. Ongoing viral replication, highly infectious.
b. Remote infection, not infectious.
c. Recent or ongoing infection; a high titer means high infectivity, while a low titer suggests chronic, active infection.
d. Prior infection or vaccination, not infectious.

Answers: (1) d, (2) c, (3) b, and (4) a.

HBeAg (+): "e" = "Eeek! I'm infectious!" for e ANTIGEN, anti-HBe implies decreased infectivity.
IgG HBcAg (+): "G" = Gone.
IgM HBcAg (+): "M" = Might be contagious still.
ANTIHBs (+): "s" = Stopped. Patient has antibodies to surface antigen.

Warning! You must specify whether the antigen or the antibody is present when learning these letter codes; otherwise you will learn these the wrong way around! Go over it ten times in your text of choice so it will make sense. Then, remembering the letters won't be necessary.

○ **T/F: The "omega-agent" can cause hepatitis D in a patient without active hepatitis B.**

False. The omega-agent is an incomplete, "defective" RNA virus that is responsible for hepatitis D. It is an obligate covirus and requires hepatitis B for replication.

○ **You stick yourself with a needle from a chronic hepatitis B carrier. You've been vaccinated, but have never had your antibody status checked. What is the appropriate post exposure prophylaxis?**

Measure your anti-HBs titer. If it's adequate (> 10 mIU), treatment is not required. If it is inadequate, you need a single dose of HBIG as soon as possible and a vaccine booster.

○ **Which is more dangerous, a small hernia or a large one?**

Incarceration is more likely with small hernias.

○ **List three types of internal hernias.**

1. Diaphragmatic hernia.
2. Lesser sac hernia (i.e., through the foramen of Winslow).
3. Omental or mesenteric hernia.

○ **Distinguish between a groin hernia, a hydrocele, and a lymph node.**

Hydroceles transilluminate and are non-tender. Lymph nodes are freely moving and firm. Hernias don't transilluminate and may produce bowel sounds.

○ **A patient tells you that 2 days ago his groin bulged. He then developed severe pain with progressive nausea and vomiting. He also has a tender mass in his groin. What shouldn't you do?**

Don't try to reduce a long-standing, tender, incarcerated hernia! The abdomen is no place for dead bowel.

○ **What simple test can distinguish between conjugated and unconjugated hyperbilirubinemia?**

A dipstick test for urobilinogen, which reflects conjugated (water soluble) hyperbilirubinemia.

○ **In addition to conjugated hyperbilirubinemia, what liver function abnormalities suggest biliary tract disease?**

Elevated alkaline phosphatase out of proportion to transaminases.

○ **Currant jelly stool in a child is indicative of what?**

Intussusception.

○ **When does physiologic jaundice of infancy peak?**

$3^{rd}$ to the $5^{th}$ day of life.

○ **Why is it normal for neonates to have an elevated unconjugated bilirubin?**

Neonates have a higher hematocrit, shorter red cell half-life, lower levels of circulating albumin and reduced albumen binding reslting in less bilirubin being transported to the liver.

○ **What is the most common cause of bowel obstruction in children under 2?**

Intussusception. Usually the terminal ileum will slide into the right colon. The cause is unknown but suspected to be due to hypertrophied lymph nodes at the junction of the ileum and colon.

○ **What is the treatment for intussusception?**

An air, or barium, enema is both a diagnostic tool and curative (i.e. by reducing the intussusception). If the air enema is unsuccessful, surgical reduction may be required.

○ **Crampy abdominal pain with mucus in the stool is indicative of what syndrome?**

The irritable bowel syndrome. Patients are afebrile and often improve after passing flatus.

○ **What is the most common cause of small bowel obstruction?**

Adhesions are the most common cause of extraluminal obstruction, followed by incarcerated hernia. Conversely, gallstones and bezoars are the most common causes of intraluminal obstruction.

○ **What is the hallmark sign of a perforated viscus?**

Abdominal pain.

○ **What percentage of patients with a perforated viscus also have radiographic evidence of a pneumoperitoneum?**

60-70%. Therefore, one-third of patients will not have this sign. Keep the patient in either the upright or left lateral decubitus position for at least 10 minutes prior to performing x-rays.

○ **Name two endocrine problems that cause peptic ulcer.**

Zollinger-Ellison syndrome and hyperparathyroidism (hypercalcemia).

○ **A postprandial midabdominal pain is indicative of what ectopic syndrome?**

Peptic ulcer in a Meckel's diverticulum.

○ **T/F: Antibiotics are unnecessary after an uncomplicated perirectal abscess is incised and drained.**

True, assuming the patient has no underlying immunoincompetence, such as HIV, diabetes, or malignancy. The primary aftercare includes sitz baths beginning the next day.

○ **Do pilonidal abscesses communicate with the anal canal?**

No. They are virtually always midline and overlie the lower sacrum. Posterior-opening, horseshoe-type anorectal fistulas can find their way to the lower sacrum, but are rarely in the midline. Remember Goodsall's rule.

○ **Should pilonidal cysts be excised in the office?**

Probably not. Incision and drainage are okay, followed by a bulky dressing, analgesics, and hot sitz baths, which should be initiated the next day. Antibiotics are not typically necessary. Excision should be completed in the OR once the acute infection clears up.

○ **A patient with chronic and occasionally bloody diarrhea develops severe diarrhea and abdominal pain with marked distention. What "can't-miss" diagnosis is confirmed by these signs?**

Toxic megacolon. This condition is a life-threatening complication of ulcerative colitis.

○ **What are the peak ages for the onset of ulcerative colitis?**

15-35 years with a smaller incident rate in the seventh decade.

○ **What are potential gastro-intestinal causes of apnea and bradycardia in neonates?**

Oral feeding, bowel movement, G.E. Reflux, esophagitis and intestinal perforation.

○ **What substances can mimic upper GI bleeding?**

Red food coloring in cereals, Jell-O, drinks such as Kool-Aid and fruit juices and natural coloring in beets.

○ **What substance can mimic melena?**

Iron supplements, dark chocolate, spinach, cranberries, grape juice, bismuth, and blueberries.

○ **Name the infectious causes of hematochezia?**

*Salmonella, Shigella, Yersinia enterocolitica, Campylobacter jejuni, Escherichia coli, Clostridium difficile, Aeromonas hydrophila* and *Entamoeba histolytica*.

○ **A 10-year-old child presents with a three day history of episodic abdominal pain and hematochezia. Examination reveals a palpable purpuric rash mostly on the lower limbs. Platelet count is normal. What is the most likely cause?**

Henoch-Schonlein purpura (anaphylactoid purpura).

○   **What are the three most common causes of upper gastrointestinal bleeding in neonates?**

Swallowed maternal blood, gastritis (Sepsis/Hypoxia), duodenitis.

○   **What test can differentiate neonatal from swallowed maternal blood?**

Apt test (also known as Kleihauer-Betke Test) - which is based on the conversion of oxhemoglobin to hematin when mixed with alkali. Fetal hemoglobin is resistant to alkali (pink reaction) while maternal hemoglobin is denatured (dirty brown).

○   **Name the more common prescription drugs associated with gastric ulcers in children.**

Salicylates, nonsteroidal anti-inflammatory agents, digitalis, reserpine, aminophylline, anticoagulants, and antimetabolites.

○   **Is there an increased risk for GI bleeding in patients with Turner Syndrome?**

Yes. Turner syndrome is associate with GI vascular malformations and Inflammatory bowel disease.

○   **What is the recommended volume of normal saline for gastric lavage in pediatric patients with GI bleeding?**

3-5 cc/Kg.

○   **Vasopressin intravenously may be useful in the control of variceal bleeding in children. What are the side effects of this drug?**

Bradycardia, vasoconstriction, myocardial ischemia, elevation of systemic blood pressure, oliguria, tissue necrosis, hyponatremia and water intoxication.

○   **At what age does intussusception most commonly occur?**

60% of all cases occur by 12 months of age, and 80% by 24 months.

○   **Which test is best to diagnose a bleeding Meckel's diverticulum?**

Technetium pertechnetate scan, preferably with Pentagastrin or H2 antagonist stimulation.

○   **How common is infantile hypertrophic pyloric stenosis?**

Affects approximately 1:150 males and 1:750 females, and is more common in first born males.

○   **Name the three areas of physiologic narrowing in the esophagus, where an ingested coin is likely to lodge.**

Below the cricopharyngeal muscle, at the level of the aortic arch, and just below the diaphragm.

○   **What is the classical metabolic picture in infants with pyloric stenosis?**

Hypochloremic alkalosis.

○   **What is the incidence of intestinal obstruction in newborn infants?**

Approximately 1:1500.

○ **What is the most common mechanical reason for malrotation?**

Failure of the cecum to move into the right lower quadrant, so that the bands fixing it to the posterior abdominal wall cross over and may obstruct the duodenum.

○ **When does midgut volvulus usually present?**

50% of cases in 1st week of life and 80% within the first month.

○ **Do infants with malrotation, always present with bilious vomiting?**

No. About 25% of infants under 2 months, present with nonbilious emesis.

○ **What is the incidence of meconium ileus in newborn infants with cystic fibrosis?**

Meconium ileus is most commonly seen in infants with cystic fibrosis, but less than 10% of infants with cystic fibrosis have meconium ileus.

○ **What are the typical radiographic findings in meconium ileus?**

Lack of air in the distal colon; distended loops of small bowel associated with bubbles of stool and air-described as a ground-glass appearance or Neuhauser's sign.

○ **How common is diabetes mellitus in patients with cystic fibrosis?**

It is 40 to 200 times higher than in the general pediatric population. This may be very difficult to control, especially in DKA.

○ **How common is rectal prolapse in children with cystic fibrosis?**

It occurs in almost 20% of patients and is the presenting sign of CF in half of these.

○ **What could happen to patients with cystic fibrosis during periods of increased physical activity and heat stress?**

Hyponatremia dehydration due to the high losses of sodium in sweat.

○ **Name the 3 leading causes of acute pancreatitis in children.**

Viral infections, drugs and trauma.

○ **What is the most common clinical finding in children with acute pancreatitis?**

Epigastric tenderness with decreased bowel sounds.

○ **What is the age of patients when ulcerative colitis in childhood is usually diagnosed?**

Between 5 and 16 years of age.

○ **What are the most common presenting signs and symptoms of ulcerative colitis?**

Stool mixed with mucus and blood; lower abdominal cramping which is most intense during defecation.

○ **What is the most common organic causes of chronic/recurrent abdominal pain in children?**

Genitourinary-Approximately 10% of children age 5-10 years have chronic/recurrent pain. Of these less than 10% have an organic cause.

○ **How common is retrocecal appendix?**

19-20% - according to most recent reviews.

○ **Name the most common non-infectious causes of chronic diarrhea in children.**

Food allergy, food intolerance, chronic nonspecific diarrhea (CNSD), lactase deficiency, irritable colon, encopresis, metabolic/malabsorption disease, ulcerative colitis, regional enteritis, and Hirschsprung's disease.

○ **When you suspect that a child has CNSD, what are the "four Fs" to which you should pay special attention?**

Fiber, Fluid, Fat and Fruit juices.

○ **Pedialyte is frequently used for oral hydration in infants. What is the composition of this solution?**

| | | |
|---|---|---|
| Na | - | 45 meq/L |
| K | - | 20 meq/L |
| Cl | - | 35 meq/L |
| HCO3 | - | 30 meq/L |
| Glucose | - | 25 g/L |

○ **Is this oral solution appropriate for rehydration?**

Pedialyte is appropriate and may lead to less osmotic diarrhea. However, the American Academy of Pediatrics recommends a solution containing at least 75 to 90m Eq Na per liter for rehydration. REHYDRALITE and the WHO solution are two such solutions.

○ **What is the most common reason for "spitting up" in young infant?**

Overfeeding! Parents frequently report that the child is vomiting.

○ **A two week old male infant presents with persistent emesis and dehydration. Blood electrolytes reveal significant hyperkalemia. What potentially lesion must be ruled out?**

Congenital adrenal hyperplasia (CAH).

○ **What anti-emetic is recommended in the infant who presents with emesis?**

Trick question! Antiemetics are strongly discouraged because of the incidence of side effects.

○ **Two children from the same family present with severe nausea and vomiting about 4-6 hours after eating. What are the most likely causes?**

*S. aureus* toxins, *Bacillus cereus*, heavy metals.

○ **Two children from another family develop paraesthesias a few hours after eating. What causes should you consider?**

Fish (scombroid and ciguatera poisoning); Shellfish (neurotoxic & domoic acid poisoning); Monosodium glutamate. (Chinese Restaurant Syndrome).

○ **What is a common G.I. complication of nephrotic syndrome?**

Spontaneous bacterial peritonitis.

○ **Is perforation following appendicitis more common in children than in adults?**

Yes, because localization of abdominal pain is more difficult. Also, the omentum is not as well developed and cannot wall off the inflamed appendix.

○ **What are some lesions that can present as a mass protruding the rectum?**

Rectal polyp, rectal prolapse, and procidentia.

○ **Give the DDX of an inguino-scrotal mass.**

Inguinal hernia, hydrocele, hydrocele of a cord, and retractile testes.

○ **What are the common causes of unconjugated hyperbilirubinemia in the neonatal age group?**

Physiological jaundice, blood group incompatibility, and breast-milk jaundice.

○ **At what level of serum bilirubin will a newborn appear icteric?**

5-7 mg/dl.

○ **In older children?**

2-3 mg/dl.

○ **What are the most common causes of unconjugated hyperbilirubinemia in childhood?**

Sickle cell anemia and other hemolytic disorders, ie, hereditary spherocytosis, hereditary elliptocytosis.

○ **What clinical investigations would you consider for the initial work-up of a case of unconjugated hyperbilirubinemia?**

Serum bilirubin and direct fraction, Coombs' test, Hematocrit, and RBC morphology/Retic count.

○ **What is the span of the liver at birth?**

4.5 - 5 cm.

○ **What pathognomonic eye-sign is noted in almost all patients of Wilson's disease with neurological symptoms?**

Kayser-Fleischer rings.

○ **What is the best screening test for Wilson's disease?**

Serum Ceruloplasmin level (decreased).

○ **What agent is commonly used in the treatment of Wilson's disease?**

D-Penicillamine (chelates copper).

○ **Beyond what duration is the use of Total Parenteral Nutrition (TPN) in newborns, especially prematures, associated with cholestasis?**

Two weeks.

○ **The consumption of what agent has been implicated in the incidence of Reye's syndrome in children with an influenza-like illness?**

Aspirin.

○ **What age group is Reye's syndrome seen most commonly?**

4 - 12 years.

○ **What is the major lethal factor in children with Reye's syndrome?**

Increased intracranial pressure, secondary to cerebral edema.

○ **Name some drugs associated with hepatic injury in children?**

Acetaminophen, Sulfonamide, Erythromycin, Ceftriaxone, INH, Valproic acid, Phenytoin.

○ **What are some causes of fulminant hepatic failure?**

Viral hepatitis
Hepatotoxic drugs and chemicals
Circulatory shock
Metabolic liver diseases like Wilson's or galactosemia

○ **What are the common causes of biliary colic?**

Gall stones caused by hemolytic diseases like spherocytosis, infections like Salmonellosis, and parasitic infestations like ascariasis.

○ **What common NICU procedure might result in portal hypertension?**

Umbilical catheterization.

○ **What is the most common presentation of childhood portal hypertension?**

Bleeding from esophageal varices.

○ **What is the major risk associated with portocaval shunts, which divert blood flow away from esophageal varices?**

Hepatic encephalopathy.

○   **What is the major indication for liver transplantation in the pediatric age group?**

Biliary atresia.

○   **What metabolic condition manifests with jaundice, hypoglycemia, convulsions, cataracts, and mental retardation?**

Galactosemia.

○   **Do the levels of liver-dependent coagulation factors decrease after birth?**

Yes, they fall 48 - 72 hours after birth, and return to birth levels only by 7 to 10 days of life.

○   **A healthy three-week old female child is brought to the emergency room with complaints of spitting up blood. She was a full-term birth, who has been thriving well on breast milk, and has gained 15oz since birth. CBC and liver enzymes are normal, but the prothrombin time, and partial thromboplastin time are prolonged. What would you do next?**

Administer 1 to 5 mg of Vit K1 intravenously.

○   **Can a newborn manifest Vitamin K deficiency induced bleeding within the first 24 hours of life?**

Yes, if the mother has been on Phenobarbital or Phenytoin. Classic Hemorrhagic Disease of the Newborn is seen between 2 and 7 days of life.

○   **What is the most commonly occurring malignant liver neoplasm in the pediatric age group?**

Hepatoblastoma.

○   **What hepatic condition could manifest with hepatomegaly, failure to thrive, congestive cardiac failure, thrombocytopenia, and a bruit over the right upper abdominal quadrant?**

An angiomatous malformation like hemangioma-endothelioma.

○   **Of the hepatitis viruses A through E, which are transmitted by the feco-oral route?**

Hepatitis A and E.

○   **How would you distinguish a person who is immune to hepatitis B as a result of a past infection from one who is immune following a vaccination?**

Both anti-HBs and anti-HBc are seen in serum following an infection, while only anti-HBs is seen following immunization.

○   **Has the American Academy of Pediatrics recommended universal administration of Hepatitis A vaccine?**

No, it is used only in high-risk children, and in those considering travel to Hepatitis A-endemic areas.

○   **What is the chief sequel of untreated perinatal acquired Hepatitis B?**

Chronic infection, which might occur in close to 70- 90 % of the cases.

○ **What is the best indicator of the severity of liver damage, in a case of acetaminophen overdosage?**

Prothrombin time, done at 12-hourly intervals.

○ **What is breast-feeding jaundice?**

Elevated levels of serum bilirubin, approaching 15-20 mg/dl, seen in the second or third week of life in breast-fed infants who are otherwise healthy.

○ **What effect is encountered in an infant with conjugated hyperbilirubinemia who is subjected to phototherapy?**

"Bronze baby syndrome" caused by an unusual bronzing of the skin by bilirubin breakdown pigments. This is reversible.

○ **An infant with biliary atresia is noted on follow-up to be short-stature, and has round, bony prominence at the costochondral junctions. What is the pathology you suspect?**

Vitamin D deficiency, leading to rickets.

○ **6-12 hours after ingesting a wild mushroom, a child developed vomiting, diarrhea, and abdominal pain which has lasted for the past 3 days. Now the child is noted to be jaundiced. What do you suspect?**

Acute liver toxicity from *Amanita* mushroom poisoning.

○ **You see a 10-year-old boy in the ER, with ear ache, and diagnose him as having otitis media. The boy is clearly jaundiced, and his mother informs you that he has the Dubin-Johnson syndrome. What management would you like to offer for his jaundice?**

Nothing, the condition is benign. However, drugs capable of aggravating jaundice should be avoided.

○ **An 11-year-old girl with cystic fibrosis presents with a one-day history of fever. On examination she is noted to have equal breath sounds on both sides. She has right upper abdominal quadrant pain. Labs reveal leukocytosis, with an increase in serum bilirubin. What do you suspect?**

Acute calculous cholecystitis, seen in up to 4% of patients with cystic fibrosis.

○ **A patient with portal hypertension presents to the your office with a nose bleed. The patient insists that he lost only about 5cc of blood, yet looks quite pale. CBC reveals a Hb of 8.5 gm/dl with a platelet count of 25, 000cu.mm. How would you explain these hematological findings in this patient?**

Hypersplenism, in which one or more blood cell lines are decreased on blood counts.

○ **What are xanthomata?**

Depositions of lipid in the dermis and subcutaneous tissue, seen often in chronic cholestasis, when the serum cholesterol levels exceed 500 mg/dl.

○ **A neonate with neonatal hemochromatosis is awaiting liver transplantation. He is presently being managed with deferoxamine. His anxious mother calls you up, and informs you that her son's diapers are stained brown. What is your diagnosis?**

Deferoxamine chelates iron, which is then excreted in the urine. When such urine stands for some time, it turns brown in color.

○ **What are some poor prognostic factors for survival in a patient with hepatic encephalopathy?**

Jaundice for more than 7 days before the onset of encephalopathy; a prothrombin time more than 50 sec; a serum bilirubin level more than 17.5 mg/dl.

○ **Esophageal varices are a form of portal-systemic blood shunting. Name some other sites at which such shunts might develop.**

Around the umbilicus (caput medusae), between the middle and inferior hemorrhoidal veins.

○ **What is Charcot's triad?**

The triad of right upper quadrant abdominal pain, fever, and jaundice. This should lead you lead to the suspicion of cholangitis.

○ **Which infectious agents are commonly associated with necrotizing enterocolitis?**

Gram negative enteric bacilli, *E. coli*, *Klebsiella pneumonia*, and *Enterococcus*.

○ **What is the most common time of the day for colic to occur?**

Late afternoon and evening.

○ **What helps colic?**

Holding, correct positioning, gentle rocking.

○ **What is the normal range of infant crying in the first 3 months of life?**

<u>2 weeks</u>:   2 hours per day
<u>1 month</u>:   3 hours per day
<u>3 months</u>:  1 hour per day

○ **How many stools per day do breast fed infants have from 1 week to 2 months of life?**

4-10.

○ **What are the Wessel criteria for the diagnosis of infantile colic?**

33333! Crying or irritability lasting longer than 3 hours a day, 3 days a week, or 3 weeks total, all in an infant under 3 months old. Colic usually subsides after the age of 3 months.

○ **What percentage of infants have colic?**

25%. The etiology is unknown.

○ **When does physiological jaundice of the newborn occur?**

2–4 days after birth. Bilirubin levels may rise up to 6-9 mg/dl.

○ **A neonate presents with a history of poor feeding, vomiting, respiratory distress, has abdominal distention, and is found to have hyperbilirubinemia. What is the likely cause of this complex?**

This neonate is septic.

○ **Name some causes of jaundice occurring in the first day of life.**

Sepsis, congenital infections, ABO/Rh incompatibility.

○ **What is the most common cause of fulminant hepatic failure in the U.S.?**

Acute viral hepatitis.

○ **The liver dysfunction in fulminant hepatic failure is evidenced by what condition?**

Uncorrectable coagulopathy, jaundice and encephalopathy.

# TOXICOLOGY AND ENVIRONMENTAL

O   **Which metabolic pathway for acetaminophen predominates in childhood?**

Sulfonation.

O   **At what age does the predominant metabolism of APAP switch from sulfonation to glucuronidation?**

14-year-old.

O   **What is the volume of distribution for acetaminophen?**

1L/kg.

O   **What is the toxic dose of acetaminophen in acute ingestion?**

140 mg/kg.

O   **What percentage of a therapeutic dose of acetaminophen is normally metabolized by the cytochrome P450 system?**

3 to 15%.

O   **What are the symptoms in the first few hours after an acetaminophen overdose?**

None or mild gastrointestinal symptoms.

O   **T/F: Acetaminophen overdose may cause a depressed mental status in the first few hours after overdose.**

True. This only occurs in large overdoses.

O   **What is the oral dose of N-acetylcysteine in acetaminophen overdose?**

140 mg/kg po followed by 70 mg/kg po every four hours for 17 doses.

O   **T/F: The dose of N-acetylcysteine should be adjusted if it is given with activated charcoal.**

False.

O   **T/F: Charcoal hemoperfusion should be used in severe acetaminophen toxicity.**

False. N-acetylcysteine should be utilized since it is an effective antidote.

O   **For what toxic ingestions is N-acetylcysteine indicated?**

Acetaminophen, pennyroyal, carbon tetrachloride and chloroform.

○ **What complication may arise from rapid IV administration of N-acetylcysteine?**

Anaphylactoid reaction.

○ **With what laboratory test may N-acetylcysteine interfere?**

It may cause a false positive for urine ketones.

○ **T/F: Intravenous N-acetylcysteine is FDA approved for use in the US.**

False.

○ **What is the toxic metabolite of acetaminophen produced via the cytochrome oxidase P450 isoenzymes?**

N-acetyl-p-benzoquinoneimine (NAPQI).

○ **Why is excess NAPQI produced in acetaminophen overdose?**

The normal sulfation and glucuronidation pathways are saturated; so more acetaminophen is metabolized to NAPQI by the cytochrome P450 isoenzymes.

○ **Why does NAPQI accumulate after acetaminophen overdose?**

Hepatic glutathione stores are depleted.

○ **T/F: Acetaminophen overdose may cause early metabolic acidosis**

True, in severe overdoses.

○ **What is the most sensitive indicator of liver injury after acetaminophen overdose?**

Aspartate aminotransferase (AST) level.

○ **How early are elevations of the AST are seen after acetaminophen overdose?**

After 8 to 12 hours in severe toxicity.

○ **When is the period of maximal liver injury after acetaminophen overdose?**

3 to 4 days post-ingestion – stage III.

○ **What is phase IV of acetaminophen overdose?**

The recovery phase in those who survive phase III.

○ **Is a 2 hour acetaminophen useful?**

Since the nomogram starts at four hours, a two hour level is difficult to interpret. However, a very low level at two hours probably rules out a significant ingestion, except potentially in cases where an extended release product was ingested or gut motility is decreased.

○ **Are children at more or less risk of acetaminophen toxicity?**

Children seem to be at less risk, except in the case of chronic ingestions in febrile infants.

○   **What groups of patients may be at increased risk of acetaminophen toxicity?**

Febrile infants, patients taking medicines which induce cytochrome P450 isoenzymes, the malnourished, HIV patients.

○   **How does acetaminophen metabolism in children and adults differ?**

In adults, significantly more acetaminophen undergoes glucuronidation than sulfation, while in children the opposite is true.

○   **When should NAC therapy be instituted empirically?**

If an acetaminophen level is not available within 8 hours of the ingestion.

○   **Does activated charcoal administration decrease the half-life of acetaminophen?**

No.

○   **How may NAC decrease the amount of NAPQI that is generated?**

By enhancing the sulfation pathway of metabolism.

○   **What is the primary indication for the use of ethosuximide?**

Petit mal seizures.

○   **What are the anti-convulsant mechanisms of action of valproic acid?**

$Na^+$ channel inactivation and inhibition of GABA breakdown by GABA transaminase.

○   **What fatal CNS effect may occur after valproic acid overdose?**

Cerebral edema.

○   **What patients are at higher risk of valproic acid induced liver failure?**

Children under two and those on multiple anticonvulsants.

○   **Narcan has been used to reverse the sedation after overdose of which anticonvulsant?**

Valproic acid.

○   **What is the clinical implication of QRS duration greater than 100 milli seconds in cyclic antidepressant overdose?**

Approximately 1/3 of patients will seize.

○   **What is the treatment of dystonic reactions?**

Anticholinergic agents, such as diphenhydramine (1-2 mg/kg IV) or benztropine mesylate (1-2mg IV).

○   **What is the treatment of dystonic reactions if anticholinergic agents are not effective?**

If anticholinergic agents are ineffective, reconsider the diagnosis and treat with benzodiazepines.

○ **What is the pathophysiology of tardive dyskinesia?**

Chronic blockade of dopamine receptors causes an increase in release of dopamine, particularly in the nigrostriatal neurons.

○ **Why do tricyclic antidepressants cause seizures in overdose?**

The tricyclic antidepressants bind to the picrotoxin site on the GABA channel and inhibit chloride flow.

○ **T/F: Patients who ingest large amounts of tricyclic antidepressants and arrive in the emergency department with minimal symptoms usually do not worsen.**

False. In one study, 50% of all patients with mild toxicity rapidly worsened within the first hour.

○ **What percent of patients with tricyclic antidepressant toxicity and a QRS > 100 msec will develop seizures?**

30%.

○ **What percent of patients with tricyclic antidepressant toxicity and a QRS > 160 msec will develop dysrhythmias?**

50%.

○ **What morphologic change in the AVR lead is predictive of tricyclic antidepressant toxicity?**

Rightward axis shift in the terminal 40 msec.

○ **What is the first-line treatment of wide complex tachycardia from tricyclic antidepressant toxicity?**

Sodium bicarbonate.

○ **What is the second-line treatment of wide complex tachycardia from tricyclic antidepressant toxicity?**

Hypertonic saline.

○ **What antidotes are contraindicated in tricyclic antidepressant toxicity?**

Physostigmine and flumazenil.

○ **What is the first-line therapy for hypotension from tricyclic antidepressant toxicity?**

After adequate fluid resuscitation, an alpha agonist such as norepinephrine is most appropriate.

○ **What are the side effects of SSRIs in therapeutic use?**

Lightheadedness, anorexia and blurred vision. The SSRIs may also cause increases in serum glucose, cortisol, ACTH and vasopressin leading to an SIADH-like syndrome. Platelet dysfunction may also occur.

○ **What are the clinical signs of serotonin syndrome?**

Mental status changes (agitation, sedation, coma), musculoskeletal irritability (tremor, rigidity, myoclonus or hyperreflexia), autonomic instability and fever.

○ **What is the cause of serotonin syndrome?**

Excessive stimulation of the 5HT 1A receptor. This may occur particularly when two serotonergic medications are used concurrently, but has been reported with single medications.

○ **What is the time of onset of serotonin syndrome?**

Minutes to hours after ingestion.

○ **What is the time of onset of the neuroleptic malignant syndrome?**

Generally 3 to 9 days after the neuroleptic dose.

○ **What is the antidote used to treat acetaminophen toxicity?**

N-acetylcysteine.

○ **What is the oral dose of N-acetylcysteine?**

First dose is 140 mg/kg, then 70 mg/kg q4 hours for 17 doses.

○ **What are the two primary active constituents of syrup of ipecac?**

Emetine and cephaline.

○ **What is the antidote used to treat iron toxicity?**

Deferoxamine.

○ **What is the dose for deferoxamine?**

15 mg/kg/hr.

○ **What is the antidote currently used to treat cyanide toxicity in the United States?**

Pasadena Cyanide Kit. This kit includes amyl nitrate, sodium nitrate and sodium thiosulfate.

○ **Why should the "extract" of ipecac never be used to induce emesis?**

The extract is much more potent than the syrup (14X) and deaths have occurred following its use.

○ **What is the antidote used to treat organophosphate toxicity?**

Atropine for muscarinic effects and 2-PAM for nicotinic effects.

○ **What is the antidote that may be used to treat black widow spider bite related toxicity?**

Latrodectus antivenom.

○ **What is the dose of black widow antivenom?**

1-2 vials.

○ **Black widow antivenom is derived from what animal?**

Horse serum.

○ **What is the antidote that may be used to treat scorpion sting related toxicity?**

Species specific scorpion antivenom.

○ **What is the antidote that may be used to treat ethylene glycol toxicity?**

Ethanol or 4 methyl pyrazole (fomepizole).

○ **What is the antidote that may be used to treat methanol toxicity?**

Ethanol or 4 methyl pyrazole (fomepizole).

○ **What is the elimination half life of naloxone?**

Approximately one hour.

○ **What is the antidote that may be used to treat lead toxicity?**

EDTA, BAL, DMSA.

○ **What is the antidote that may be used to treat anticholinergic syndrome related toxicity?**

Physostigmine.

○ **What is the antidote that may be used to treat INH related toxicity?**

Pyridoxine.

○ **What is the drug that may be used to treat methemoglobinemia?**

Methylene blue.

○ **What is the antidote that may be used to treat carbon monoxide related toxicity?**

Oxygen.

○ **What is the antidote that may be used to treat opioid related toxicity?**

Naloxone.

○ **What is the antidote that may be used to treat beta-blocker related toxicity?**

Glucagon.

○ **What is the action of flumazenil?**

Highly selective competitive inhibitor of CNS benzodiazepine receptors.

○ **Which route for the administration of N-acetylcysteine is more efficacious; IV or PO?**

They are equally efficacious.

○ **What are the indications for whole bowel irrigation?**

Sustained release products or slowly dissolving tablets (paint chips, concretions), foreign bodies (crack vials, etc), body packers, and drugs not adsorbed by charcoal (lithium, iron, metals).

○ **If pralidoxime chloride is administered intravenously too quickly, what complication may occur?**

Hypertension.

○ **What adverse reaction to NAC is found following IV use but not oral use?**

Anaphylactoid reactions.

○ **What carbamate-like drug can be used as a "protectant" against organophosphate or nerve agent toxicity?**

Pyridostigmine bromide.

○ **For which substances would urinary alkalinization be indicated?**

Aspirin, Chlorpropamide, Phenobarbital.

○ **What is the mechanism of warfarin's anticoagulant action?**

Warfarin inhibits the reduction of vitamin K and decreases the concentration of the active form of vitamin K.

○ **What will reverse the action of warfarin?**

Vitamin K.

○ **How does vitamin K reverse warfarin-induced coagulopathy?**

Vitamin K provides functional coagulation factors and bypasses the metabolic block that results in the synthesis of defective coagulation factors.

○ **How long does it take vitamin K to reverse the effects of warfarin?**

Effects begin at 6-8 hours, but do not peak for 1-2 days.

○ **What can you do for immediate restoration of hemostasis in the case of warfarin overdose?**

Transfusion of fresh frozen plasma.

○ **What is the major toxicity of warfarin?**

Bleeding.

○ **What are the effects of angiotensin converting enzyme inhibitor (ACEI) overdose?**

Symptoms after ACEI overdose are unusual and are limited to hypotension.

○ **What may reverse the hypotension in ACEI overdose?**

Naloxone has been reported to reverse hypotension. ACEIs may inhibit the metabolism of enkephalins leading to opiate-induced hypotension. Hypotension should, of course, be treated with fluids.

○ **What is the difference between a bacteriostatic and bactericidal antibiotic?**

A bacteriostatic drug inhibits bacterial growth while a bactericidal agent will kill the bacteria.

○ **What is the mechanism of action of the sulfonamides?**

Inhibition of folic acid synthesis mainly by competitive inhibition of the enzyme dihydropteroate synthetase.

○ **What is the natural metabolite that the sulfonamides compete with?**

PABA (p-aminobenzoic acid).

○ **Which is the most common adverse effect associated with the use of sulfonamides?**

Allergic reactions especially skin rashes.

○ **What are the advantages of combining sulfamethoxazole with trimethoprim?**

Bactericidal effect; decreased resistance; less toxicity and an extended spectrum of activity.

○ **What is the major adverse effect associated with penicillin use?**

Hypersensitivity reactions.

○ **What toxicities are associated with ampicillin?**

The incidence of rash is high in some patients. Also pseudomembranous colitis may occur.

○ **What is the purpose of combining clavulanic acid with penicillin?**

This combination provides a synergistic effect. Clavulanic acid is a beta lactamase inhibitor and thus extends the action of the penicillin.

○ **What additional toxicity may be associated with the combinations of beta lactamase inhibitors with beta lactam antibiotics?**

GI effects such as diarrhea.

○ **What is the advantage of amoxicillin over ampicillin?**

Amoxicillin has better oral bioavailability.

○ **Are amoxicillin and ampicillin inactivated by penicillinase?**

Yes.

○ **Which group of cephalosporins has the best penetration into the CNS?**

Third generation.

○ **What is the major adverse effect associated with cephalosporin use?**

Rashes and other hypersensitivity reactions.

○ **What ribosomal subunit do the macrolide antibiotics bind to?**

50S.

○ **What other antibiotics bind to this subunit?**

Clindamycin and chloramphenicol.

○ **What are the advantages of the newer macrolide antibiotics over erythromycin?**

Less GI irritation and better absorption.

○ **What is the most serious toxicity associated with the use of erythromycin?**

Cholestatic hepatitis.

○ **Which erythromycin preparation is cholestatic hepatitis most commonly associated with?**

Erythromycin estolate (Ilosone).

○ **What is the major type of antibacterial activity associated with clindamycin?**

Anaerobic organisms especially *Bacteroides fragilis*.

○ **What is the most serious toxicity associated with the use of clindamycin?**

Pseudomembranous colitis (AAPC).

○ **How is AAPC (Antibiotic-Associated Pseudomembranous Colitis) caused?**

By a toxin secreted by clindamycin resistant strains of *C. difficile*.

○ **What drugs are used to treat AAPC?**

Vancomycin and metronidazole.

○ **What is the common toxicity associated with the use of vancomycin?**

Red neck or red man syndrome.

○ **What are the two most serious toxicities associated with the use of vancomycin?**

Ototoxicity and nephrotoxicity.

○ **Describe the mechanism of action of metronidazole?**

The anaerobic environment produces certain chemically active reduction products, which can disrupt DNA and inhibit nucleic acid synthesis.

❍ **What are the common adverse effects of metronidazole?**

GI upset and some neurological toxicity (CNS effects and peripheral neuropathy).

❍ **What is the gray baby syndrome?**

Infants with their limited ability to metabolize chloramphenicol experience a syndrome, which includes as ashen gray cyanosis, which may be fatal.

❍ **Why are the tetracyclines contraindicated in young children.**

They can cause discoloration of the teeth and can inhibit bone growth.

❍ **What is the mechanism of the tetracyclines effect in bones and teeth?**

Tetracyclines bind to calcium and then become deposited in the bones and teeth. Discoloration of the teeth is sometimes due to oxidation of the tetracycline-calcium complex.

❍ **What are the clinical uses of ketoconazole?**

A few systemic fungal infections and dermatophyte infections that are resistant to griseofulvin.

❍ **What adverse reactions are associated with the use of ketoconazole?**

GI intolerance, endocrine effects (decreased libido, oligospermia etc.) and hepatic toxicity.

❍ **Why does pyridoxine prevent the neurotoxicity associated with the use of INH?**

INH causes pyridoxine deficiency by forming hydrazones that inhibit the conversion of pyridoxine to the active form pyridoxal phosphate.

❍ **What is the mechanism of action of rifampin?**

It inhibits mycobacterial DNA-dependent RNA polymerase.

❍ **How does the body excrete rifampin?**

It is rapidly eliminated in the bile, followed by an enterohepatic recirculation. Eventually about 60% is excreted via the intestine.

❍ **How is rifampin metabolized?**

It is progressively diacetylated in the liver with the metabolite retaining full activity. It induces its own metabolism.

❍ **What adverse effects are associated with the use of rifampin?**

Gastrointestinal disturbances and hepatotoxicity.

❍ **What additional toxicity is sometimes seen when rifampin is used in high dose intermittent therapy?**

It produces several effects thought to have an immunological basis, including thrombocytopenia, hemolytic anemia, acute renal failure and the respiratory flu syndrome.

○ **What type of drug-drug interactions are associated with rifampin use?**

Rifampin is a potent inducer of liver microsomal enzymes and may affect the metabolism of a variety of other drugs.

○ **Structurally what is acyclovir?**

An analog of guanosine or deoxyguanosine with an acyclic side chain.

○ **What is the mechanism of action of acyclovir?**

It is phosphorylated to mono, di- and tri- phosphates. As the nucleotide it is an inhibitor of viral DNA polymerase and is incorporated into the growing DNA chain where it can act as a chain terminator due to the lack of the 3'- hydroxyl group.

○ **What is the most common adverse effect associated with the use of acyclovir?**

Renal toxicity.

○ **What causes the renal toxicity associated with acyclovir?**

High urine levels of the drug cause crystalline nephropathy.

○ **What other adverse effects are associated with the use of acyclovir?**

Neurotoxicity is uncommon and GI upset, headache and rash occur when it is given orally. There may also be lacrimation, itching, burning and pain when it is used in the eye.

○ **What is valacyclovir?**

A prodrug of acyclovir that is rapidly converted to acyclovir after absorption. It has a mechanism of action identical to that of acyclovir.

○ **What adverse effects are associated with the use of valacyclovir?**

It is generally well tolerated, but a thrombotic thrombocytopenic purpura/hemolytic anemia syndrome has been reported in some severely immunocompromised patients treated with high doses for prolonged periods. Hallucinations and confusion also may occur. Other adverse effects are similar to acyclovir.

○ **What are the toxic effects of quinine and quinidine?**

Cinchonism (tinnitus, headache, nausea, hearing and visual disturbances); hyperinsulinemia and severe hypoglycemia; severe hypotension when given too rapidly by i.v.; overdoses produce more severe symptoms including GI and C.V. disturbances. There may also be hemolysis in glucose-6-phosphate dehydrogenase deficient patients.

○ **What odor may emanate from an arsenic toxic patient?**

Garlic.

○ **What is generally thought to be the drug of choice in a patient with a beta-blocker overdose who is bradycardic and hypotensive without response to intravenous fluids and atropine?**

Glucagon.

○ **Stimulating what other receptor can increase decreased intracellular cAMP from beta-receptor blockade?**

Glucagon.

○ **What symptom is commonly seen when glucagon is administered rapidly intravenously?**

Vomiting.

○ **In which of the beta-blocker overdoses should hemodialysis be considered?**

Acebutolol, nadolol, atenolol, sotalol.

○ **How long should patients with sustained release beta-blocker overdose be observed?**

24 hours.

○ **What two abnormalities on the chemistry panel may be seen with beta-blocker overdose?**

Hyperkalemia and hypoglycemia.

○ **Which group of beta-blocker overdosed patients has a higher incidence of hypoglycemia?**

Children.

○ **What toxin related disease in infants is related to the ingestion of raw honey?**

Infantile botulism.

○ **What is the *sine quo non* of botulism poisoning presentation?**

Bulbar palsy.

○ **Name four sources of botulism.**

Botulism occurs with the ingestion of a preformed toxin in improperly preserved, canned, smoked, or fermented foods, improperly stored fried onions, baked potatoes, potato yogurt sweetened with aspartame, and turkey stuffing.

○ **Name the bacteria that produces the botulinum neurotoxin.**

*Clostridium botulinum*.

○ **How does the *Clostridium botulinum* cause toxicity?**

The neurotoxin causes motor weakness by binding to the cholinergic nerve terminals of the axon and inhibiting acetylcholine release.

○ **How does death normally occur from botulism?**

Respiratory muscle failure.

○ **What is the order of progressive muscle involvement in a patient with botulism?**

Muscles served by cranial nerves, followed by extremity muscles and finally respiratory muscles.

○ **In what kind of patient should botulism be considered?**

Any patient with a history of gastrointestinal symptoms, dry mouth, difficulty swallowing and visual symptoms has botulism until proven otherwise.

○ **What samples should be collected from a child suspected to have botulism?**

Serum, stool, gastric contents and suspect foods should be tested for botulinum toxin and *Clostridium botulinum*.

○ **What type of monitoring does a child suspected of having botulism need?**

Respiratory status must be followed using measurements of vital capacity, peak expiratory flow rate, negative inspiratory force, pulse oximetry, and gag reflex.

○ **When should a child with botulism be intubated?**

Some sources suggest that intubation should be considered in a child suspected of having botulism when the vital capacity falls to less than 30% of predicted.

○ **What are the common manifestations of infant botulism?**

Constipation, feeding difficulty, weak cry, decreased muscle tone, ophthalmoplegia, and loss of facial grimacing can occur.

○ **How is infant botulism different from that observed in adults?**

In the adult form, the preformed toxin is ingested. The toxin is produced in vivo in cases of infant botulism.

○ **Why is the bacteria able to produce toxin in infants?**

The infant gut lacks the intestinal flora, gastric acids and bile acids that inhibit bacterial growth in adults.

○ **At what age is botulism most commonly observed in infants?**

1-13 months.

○ **What is the most common food associated with infant botulism?**

Honey.

○ **What is the least common cause of botulism?**

Wound botulism.

○ **How many strains (serotypes) of *Clostridium botulinum* exist?**

Seven; A, B, C, D, E, and F.

○ **What strains of *Clostridium botulinum* are most frequently implicated in human disease?**

A, B, and E.

○  **What conditions must exist for botulinum spores to germinate?**

They require an anaerobic environment with a pH greater than 4.6.

○  **How can botulinum spores be destroyed?**

Pressure cooking for 30 minutes at 120° C will destroy the spores.

○  **Is the toxin more difficult or less difficult to destroy than the spores?**

The toxin is much more heat labile than the spores. Boiling at 100°C for minute will destroy the toxin.

○  **What can be added to foods to inhibit *Clostridium* growth?**

Nitrites.

○  **How long after ingestion of botulinum do symptoms occur?**

The incubation period is usually 12-36 hours, but can take as long as 8 days.

○  **Does breastfeeding help protect infants from botulism?**

No, breast fed infants are more likely to develop botulism.

○  **What subset of patients are at highest risk for developing wound botulism?**

Drug abusers who inject subcutaneously with infected needles, forming abscesses in which the bacterium can produce toxin.

○  **What types of botulin antitoxins are available?**

There are bivalent and trivalent vaccines. The USAMRIID has an investigational heptavalent vaccine.

○  **How do the antitoxins work?**

They bind circulating free toxin and prevent the progression of illness.

○  **When is the antitoxin most effective?**

It should be given within 24 hours of the onset of symptoms.

○  **What test should be performed prior to administering the antitoxin?**

A skin test to rule out hypersensitivity should be performed. Serum sickness is a potential complication because the antitoxin is derived from horse serum.

○  **Is botulism a reportable disease?**

Yes, botulism should be reported to local or state health departments or the Centers for Disease Control.

○  **What is the most common form of botulism?**

Infant botulism accounts for two thirds of reported cases.

○ **Where is botulism most commonly found in North America?**

Alaska, California, Oregon, and Washington have the highest incidences of botulism.

○ **Where are the different toxin types most often found?**

Type A and B are ubiquitous in soil, type E is found in mud and sand in oceans. Type A occurs more commonly west of the Mississippi, type B more often east of the Mississippi.

○ **Should antibiotics be used in the treatment of botulism?**

Antibiotics should be used only to treat secondary infections.

○ **What is guanidine's effect in patients with botulism?**

It increases the release of acetylcholine at the nerve terminal but has not been shown to be clinically useful.

○ **What is the dose of antitoxin in suspected botulism cases?**

1-2 vials.

○ **Should antitoxin be used in cases of infant botulism?**

No.

○ **Should cathartics be used after botulism ingestion?**

Cathartics should not be used, especially those containing magnesium because they may exacerbate muscle weakness.

○ **Which adults are susceptible to an adult-form of infant botulism?**

Adults with bowel pathology such as Cohn's disease or achlorhydria that allows the bacteria to produce toxin.

○ **What kind of organism is *Clostridium botulinum*?**

It is a gram-positive, anaerobic organism.

○ **What pupil findings are suggestive of botulism?**

Fixed or dilated pupils in an alert patient.

○ **How long do the symptoms of botulism persist?**

Hospitalizations last 1-10 days, but symptoms such as fatigue can last 1-2 years.

○ **What drug may mildly and transiently improve the symptoms of botulism.**

Edrophonium may improve symptoms slightly, although too much less an extent than in a patient with myasthenia gravis.

○ **Honey should not be given to children younger than what age?**

1 year.

○   **How are deep tendon reflexes affected in botulism?**

Reflexes are either normal or hypoactive.

○   **What are the CSF findings in botulism?**

Lumbar puncture usually reveals normal CSF, although occasionally slightly elevated protein may be present.

○   **What are the indications for hyperbaric oxygen therapy in carbon monoxide poisoning if there is easy access to a hyperbaric chamber?**

COHbg level > 25%, syncope, coma, seizures, altered mental status, myocardial ischemia, focal neurologic deficit, ventricular dysrhythmias, pregnancy with a COHb > 15% or persistent neurologic symptoms after oxygen therapy.

○   **What percentage of patients with carbon monoxide intoxication will develop delayed neurologic sequelae?**

14-43%.

○   **When is the onset of delayed neurologic sequelae after carbon monoxide poisoning?**

2-40 days after exposure.

○   **Carbon monoxide has an affinity for hemoglobin that is greater than oxygen's. How much larger?**

Two hundred and fifty times.

○   **How many deaths are caused by carbon monoxide poisoning per year?**

CO causes approximately 3000-5000 deaths per year in the US.

○   **What are the most common symptoms of carbon monoxide toxicity?**

Headache (91%), nausea and vomiting (47%), dizziness and weakness (53%) and dyspnea (40%).

○   **In which time frame do the delayed neurologic sequelae of carbon monoxide occur: first hour after exposure, one to six hours, six to twenty-four hours or two to forty days?**

The delayed neurologic sequelae after carbon monoxide exposure typically develop between two and forty days after the exposure.

○   **What odor is consistent with ambient levels of carbon monoxide?**

None, it is an odorless gas.

○   **T/F: Carbon monoxide casualties have resulted from the generation of carbon monoxide as the result of blasting operations?**

True.

○ **What is the level of CO that is considered immediately dangerous to life and health (IDLH)?**

1200 ppm.

○ **What is a "normal" serum level of carboxyhemoglobin (COHgb) in a child not exposed to exogenous carbon monoxide?**

Generally below 3%.

○ **What is the source of the baseline carboxyhemoglobin level in non-exposed patients?**

Carbon monoxide is a byproduct of heme degradation.

○ **Name four sources of carbon monoxide.**

Incomplete combustion of fossil fuels (propane heaters, boat engines, tractor engines, car engines, etc), fire/smoke inhalation, cigarette smoke, and methylene chloride.

○ **How does methylene chloride produce carbon monoxide?**

Methylene chloride is a paint stripper that is easily absorbed from the skin or inhaled. It is metabolized to carbon monoxide in the liver.

○ **How does carbon monoxide affect hemoglobin oxygen binding?**

CO has an affinity for hemoglobin that is 250 times greater than oxygen. This leads to decreased arterial oxygen content despite a normal $pO_2$.

○ **How does carbon monoxide affect the oxygen-hemoglobin dissociation curve?**

Carbon monoxide causes a conformational change in hemoglobin that allows the three remaining oxygen molecules to be held more tightly. This leads to a left shift in the oxygen-hemoglobin dissociation curve.

○ **What is carbon monoxide's effect on mitochondrial cytochrome oxidase?**

CO binds to cytochromes A3 and P450 and inhibits cellular respiration and ATP production.

○ **What is carbon monoxide's effect on myoglobin?**

CO binds to myoglobin leading to myocardial impairment. This binding is increased in hypoxic conditions.

○ **What is carbon monoxide's effect on platelets?**

CO causes displacement of NO from platelets leading to smooth muscle relaxation and vasodilation.

○ **What clinical signs/symptoms are expected with a COHgb level of 10-20%?**

Headache, nausea, vomiting and dizziness.

○ **What are the ophthalmologic signs of severe carbon monoxide poisoning?**

Flame hemorrhages, papilledema and bright red retinal veins (equilibration of the color of arteries and veins).

○ **T/F: Fetal COHgb levels are lower than maternal levels.**

False. Fetal COHgb levels are 10-15% higher than maternal levels.

○ **T/F: Fetal COHgb levels do not equilibrate with maternal levels for up to 24 hours.**

True. Fetal levels lag behind maternal levels and equilibrate after 14-24 hours of exposure.

○ **What percentage of children born to women with CO toxicity will have neurologic sequelae?**

Up to 60%.

○ **What is the complication rate of hyperbaric oxygen therapy?**

Approximately 5%.

○ **What is the severe complication rate of hyperbaric oxygen therapy?**

Approximately 3%. 1% develop dysrhythmias, 1% develop tension pneumothorax, 1% arrest, 2% develop hypotension and 3% have a seizure. Many of these complications may be related to underlying diseases.

○ **Can just a small increase in calcium channel blocker dose be potentially lethal?**

Yes.

○ **What rhythm abnormality results when a calcium antagonist binds the calcium channel receptors in the sinoatrial node?**

Sinus bradycardia, pause, or arrest.

○ **Is hyperglycemia a common finding in calcium channel blocker overdose?**

Yes. Probably because there is calcium mediated release of insulin from the beta cells of the pancreas that may be blocked by high concentrations of calcium channel blockers.

○ **Can nausea/vomiting be seen in calcium channel blocker overdose?**

Yes.

○ **Are CNS changes a prominent feature of calcium channel blocker poisoning independent of blood pressure and cardiac output changes?**

No.

○ **What is the initial treatment (other than intravenous saline and atropine) for patients that have taken a calcium channel blocker overdose and are bradycardic and hypotensive?**

Intravenous calcium.

○ **What is the difference between calcium chloride and calcium gluconate?**

Calcium chloride is 3 times as concentrated as calcium gluconate.

○   **What is the decontamination method of choice for an overdose of a sustained release calcium channel blocker presenting greater than 1 hour post-ingestion.**

Polyethylene glycol (Go-lytely).

○   **If there is no effect in treating a patient with calcium channel blocker toxicity that is bradycardic and hypotensive with calcium, atropine, and catecholamines, which drug should be considered?**

Glucagon.

○   **Can catecholamines be used to treat bradycardia and hypotension?**

Yes.

○   **In biochemical terms, why may glucagon work to reverse the effects of calcium channel blockade?**

It increases calcium entry into the heart cells via increased cAMP and protein kinase activity.

○   **What treatment that increases "substrate" delivery to the myocardium is very promising.**

Insulin and glucose (hyperinsulinemic euglycemia treatment).

○   **If insulin and glucose are administered, what electrolyte must be closely observed?**

Potassium.

○   **Is hemodialysis or hemoperfusion likely to enhance the elimination of calcium channel blockers?**

No.

○   **Is it true that sustained release calcium channel blockers (e.g. verapamil SR, diltiazem CD, nifedipine XL) are "long acting" because the medication remains in the gut and slowly releases the medication**

Yes.

○   **What implications does this have in these overdoses regarding GI decontamination?**

Further absorption can theoretically be decreased by GI decontamination even 1-2 hours after ingestion with repeated dose activated charcoal or whole bowel irrigation.

○   **Are symptoms from sustained release calcium channel blocker overdose, e.g. verapamil SR, generally more delayed than regular verapamil?**

Yes.

○   **What is the initial dose of glucagon in calcium channel antagonist toxicity?**

2-5 mg over 1-3 minutes in adults and 50 mcg/kg in children.

○ **Can ingestion of small amounts of household bleach (2 teaspoons) cause severe gastrointestinal irritation?**

No.

○ **What sort of damage is seen on endoscopy with bleach ingestion?**

Endoscopy is indicated if there are severe symptoms such as pain, vomiting, hematemesis. Usually there is mucosal irritation, which appears as a white film on the esophageal and gastric mucosa. There is rarely an ulcer.

○ **How about the patient that drinks "Drano"? Is this a serious ingestion?**

Yes.

○ **What type of necrosis does "Drano" cause?**

Liquefactive necrosis.

○ **What is the significance of this type of necrosis?**

Liquefactive necrosis allows the material, in this case a strong base, to penetrate deeply into the tissue, such as the esophageal wall, resulting in a thick layer of injury. Thus there is a larger chance of perforation, and if perforation does not occur immediately, there is a high chance of stricture formation.

○ **Should a child that drank "Drano" undergo gastric lavage, or induction of vomiting?**

No. There is more danger when the strong base comes back up the esophagus.

○ **Should the child that drinks "Drano" be given charcoal?**

No. Charcoal may also cause vomiting, and there is nothing to be gained by preventing the absorption of lye as its toxicity from local contact. It will also obscure the endoscopist's view.

○ **What should be done if a child drinks "Drano"?**

You can try to dilute the ingested material in the stomach by asking the patient to drink water or milk. If the ingestion was immediate, there is a report of immediately drinking a mild acid such as Coca-Cola (Phosphoric acid), which resulted in a better outcome than drinking water.

○ **What type of chemical (acid or base) is found in most toilet bowl cleaners?**

Acid.

○ **What type of "burn" does this type of material cause if exposed in high concentration?**

Coagulative necrosis.

○ **What is the significance of this type of necrosis on long term sequelae?**

Because the coagulation of tissue proteins occurs by contact, the acid is prevented from reaching the deeper layers of the tissue, so injury, which can appear horrible, is limited to the more superficial layers, and therefore there are fewer long term effects than one would see with burns by a strong base.

○ **Which is the more dangerous inhalation household bleach or swimming pool disinfectants?**

Swimming pool disinfectants, as these may be up a 20% concentration while household bleach is usually a 3-5% concentration.

○ **What are soaps?**

Salts of fatty acid.

○ **What symptoms do they produce when acutely ingested?**

Nausea, vomiting.

○ **What symptom may develop the next day after soap ingestion?**

Diarrhea.

○ **What is the difference between soap and a detergent?**

A detergent contains surfactant.

○ **What does the class of material in detergents allow?**

Reduction of surface tension, allowing easier wetting of surfaces.

○ **What is the main toxicity of detergents?**

Mucous membrane irritation, skin irritation, possibly superficial mucosal erosion.

○ **Is the dishwasher detergent sludge remaining in the dispenser toxic?**

Yes, because it is very concentrated.

○ **Is inhaling detergent toxic?**

Yes, Inhaling powdered detergent can result in respiratory problems the most severe of which is upper airway obstruction (drooling, stridor) which may require intubation.

○ **What is additional toxicity of "enzyme-containing" detergents?**

As these "enzymes" are proteins, they can cause skin sensitization and allergic reactions, which is some patients may even results in bronchospasm.

○ **Can there be tetany and hypocalcemia resulting from ingestion of large amounts of phosphate containing detergents?**

Yes, theoretically.

○ **Has there ever been a death from detergent ingestion?**

Yes, one known in 1994 data, maybe others, but these are exceedingly rare.

○ **"Pine sol" disinfectant contains an anionic detergent, isopropyl alcohol, and pine oil. Should vomiting or gastric lavage be performed?**

No. Anionic detergents are not seriously toxic. Isopropyl alcohol in the amount that is most likely going to be ingested is not seriously toxic. The pine oil can cause chemical pneumonitis as it is low viscosity and all attempts should be made to prevent aspiration.

○ **Phenol was originally used in many households (and hospitals) as a potent germicidal agent, but now found mostly in topical skin preparations such as _____.**

Campho-Phenique, and commercial skin pealing agents.

○ **Creosote, creosol, phenylphenol, hydroquinone, eugenol are derivative of what chemical?**

Phenol.

○ **Is "Lysol," a common household disinfectant a phenolic compound?**

Yes. It is bisphenol. It denatures proteins and in the case of bacterial disrupts their cell walls, killing them. In humans it produces a coagulation necrosis and thus corrosive injury.

○ **What skin exposure characteristically caused painless white "burns".**

Phenol exposure. It then turns red and brown.

○ **By what two mechanisms do mercuric chloride button batteries lodged in the esophagus produce injury? What is the worst that could happen?**

1. Leakage of the corrosive metallic salt.
2. Local discharge of electrical current at the site of impaction.

The worst complication is perforation, which on plain x-ray may appear as free air in the mediastinum.

○ **Is it necessary to remove the button battery if it is seen in the esophagus? How about if it is under the diaphragm? How is removal accomplished?**

Yes if it is in the esophagus, no if it is past the lower esophageal sphincter. Removal is accomplished by endoscopy.

○ **Naphthalene used to be the active ingredient in mothball. What is it now?**

Paradichlorobenzene.

○ **What was the toxicity of naphthalene?**

Nausea, vomiting with ingestion; mucous membrane irritation with inhalation. CNS effects ranging from agitation, lethargy, and seizures. In patients with G6PD deficiency, severe hemolysis can result.

○ **Is paradichlorobenzene toxic?**

Yes, but not nearly as toxic as naphthalene. Has produced liver necrosis and tremors in animals.

○ **Is there any way to distinguish naphthalene and paradichlorobenzene?**

Physically there are very difficult to distinguish. Paradichlorobenzene is radiopaque which naphthalene is not.

○ **Should you administer milk, or other fatty substances, to a patient who acutely ingested naphthalene or paradichlorobenzene in an effort to dilute it.**

No. These substances may enhance absorption.

○ **What are the active ingredients in deodorants? Are they toxic?**

Aluminum and Zinc, low toxicity.

○ **What is the active ingredient in fingernail polish or fingernail polish remover?**

These are generally hydrocarbon solvents such as acetone, acetates, toluene, and aromatic hydrocarbons.

○ **What toxic chemical may artificial-fingernail remover contains?**

Acetonitrile (vinyl cyanide). This breaks down in vivo to form cyanide. Some artificial-fingernail removers contain nitromethane.

○ **What is the active ingredient in "nail primer" or artificial nail "extender"?**

Methacrylic acid (2-methypropanenoic acid). Has a bad odor and is a caustic. It is also used in bone cements. inhalation can result in respiratory distress. It is non-toxic once polymerized.

○ **How long should a patient with a skeletal muscle relaxant overdose be observed?**

At least 6 hours because of the possibility of delayed absorption.

○ **Is Flumazenil useful in "reviving" patients with skeletal muscle relaxant overdose?**

No.

○ **Should ipecac be used in patients with skeletal muscle relaxant overdose?**

No. The mental status can deteriorate and seizures can develop suddenly, thus the risk of aspiration is too great.

○ **Is charcoal useful?**

Yes.

○ **Is hemodialysis or hemoperfusion useful?**

No, because there is extensive tissue distribution.

○ **What is the onset of action of Dig-specific antibodies?**

Onset averages 19 minutes after infusion, however peak effect is approximately 4 hours.

○ **How is the dose of digoxin-specific antibodies calculated?**

# of vials of Digoxin-Fab = [ serum digoxin (mg/dL) x Body weight (kg) ] / 100.

○ **What is the volume of distribution for digoxin?**

5-6 L/kg.

○ **What is the effect of toxic levels of digitalis?**

The sodium/potassium ATPase pump is inhibited, allowing no potassium to be transported into the cells.

○ **What is the most common rhythm disturbance seen in digitalis toxicity?**

Premature ventricular contractions.

○ **Toxic levels of digitalis acting at what anatomic site in the heart cause premature ventricular contractions (PVC s)?**

The Purkinje fibers.

○ **How do toxic levels of digitalis affect the Purkinje fibers?**

Toxic levels of digitalis decrease resting potential and conduction velocity, increase muscle fiber sensitivity to electrical stimuli, and increase automaticity.

○ **Name four plants in which cardiac glycosides can be found?**

Oleander, foxglove, lily of the valley, red squill, and rhododendron.

○ **What constitutes a toxic dose of digitalis?**

Acute ingestions of 1mg of digitalis in children and 3mg of digitalis can produce elevated serum levels.

○ **Are children or adults more resistant to digitalis overdose?**

Children appear to have less cardiotoxicity from digitalis overdose than adults do.

○ **How does the volume of distribution of digoxin compare to digitoxin?**

The volume of distribution of digoxin is large (5-10 L/kg) compared to digitoxin (0.5 L/kg).

○ **What is the elimination half-life of digoxin?**

30-50 hours.

○ **Why is the elimination half-life of digitoxin 5-8 days compared to 30-50 hours for digoxin?**

Digitoxin undergoes more extensive enterohepatic circulation than digoxin.

○ **How much foxglove or oleander must be ingested to reach toxic levels of digitalis?**

Even a few leaves of either foxglove or oleander are enough to cause toxicity.

○ **How does the use of digitalis specific antibodies affect the measurement of serum digoxin levels?**

The use of Fab fragments of digoxin cause a falsely elevated serum digoxin level.

○ **When do peak levels occur after digoxin ingestion?**

About 1.5 to 2 hours.

○ **When does digoxin reach steady state after ingestion?**

6 to 8 hours.

○ **Is it the peak or steady state level that correlates with toxicity in digoxin overdose?**

The steady state level should be used to determine toxicity and dosages of Fab fragments.

○ **What are the most common symptoms in digitalis intoxication?**

Fatigue, nausea, visual disturbances and anorexia occur in 80% of cases.

○ **Above what potassium level is the administration of digitalis specific antibodies recommended?**

Greater than 5 mEq/L.

○ **How are digitalis antibodies produced?**

It is derived from sheep immunized with digitalis and the IgG is split with papain.

○ **What classic visual disturbance occurs in patients with digitalis toxicity?**

Patients report seeing a yellow-green halo around objects.

○ **Which medications should NOT be used to treat ventricular arrhythmias thought to be due to digitalis toxicity?**

Quinidine, procainamide, and bretylium may worsen the dysrhythmia.

○ **Ventricular dysrhythmias due to digitalis toxicity may respond to what medications?**

Lidocaine and phenytoin.

○ **Why are phenytoin and lidocaine indicated for the treatment of dysrhythmias secondary to digitalis intoxication?**

They depress ventricular automaticity without slowing AV nodal conduction.

○ **Why should cardiac pacing be used with extreme caution in patients with digitalis toxicity?**

Pacing induced dysrhythmias are common, occurring in one study in 36% of patients with 13% morality in one study.

○ **Should cardioversion be used in life-threatening dysrhythmias caused by digitalis toxicity?**

Cardioversion should only be used when all other methods fail to control the dysrhythmia because malignant ventricular dysrhythmia may occur.

○ **What are possible side effects of digoxin-specific antibody therapy?**

Hypokalemia, worsening congestive heart failure, and rash have been reported in treated patients.

○ **Why is the measurement of digoxin levels after digoxin specific antibodies not clinically useful?**

Most laboratories cannot measure free digoxin levels. Therefore the level obtained after antibody administration will represent free plus bound digoxin.

○ **How is digitalis eliminated?**

It is filtered by the glomeruli and secreted by the renal tubules.

○ **What are the indications for Digoxin-specific antibodies in acute digoxin toxicity?**

Hyperkalemia (>5.0 mg/dL), potentially lethal arrhythmias, progressive refractory bradydysrhythmia, or highly elevated digoxin levels (>10 ng/mL at steady state or >15 ng/mL at any time).

○ **Which subunit of the Na/K ATPase does digoxin bind?**

Alpha.

○ **What is the mortality rate of patients with acute digoxin toxicity and a serum potassium between 5.0 mEq/L and 5.5 mEq/L?**

50%.

○ **What is the mortality rate of patients with acute digoxin toxicity and a serum potassium above 6.5 mEq/L?**

Approaching 100%.

○ **What is the volume of distribution of digoxin?**

16 L/kg in children.

○ **Is hemodialysis effective in eliminating digoxin?**

No.

○ **What medication should be avoided in the treatment of digoxin-related bradycardia?**

Isoproterenol may increase ventricular ectopy and is therefore contraindicated.

○ **What enzyme catalyzes the synthesis of acetylcholine?**

Choline acetyltransferase.

○ **Where is acetylcholine stored?**

In the pre-synaptic nerve terminals.

○ **Acetylcholine (Ach) is the transmitter at what sites?**

At preganglionic fibers to all ganglia; postganglionic parasympathetic fibers to smooth muscle, heart and glands; postganglionic sympathetic fibers to sweat glands; motor fibers to skeletal muscle and in the CNS.

○ **How do autonomic drugs influence neurotransmission?**

They can alter synthesis of the transmitter, modify the storage mechanism for neurotransmitters, change transmitter release, modify the inactivation mechanism of the transmitter and activate or block receptors. The latter is the most common mechanism.

○ **What are the steps in synaptic transmission?**

Depolarization of presynaptic terminals, calcium influx and transmitter release. Combination of the transmitter with the postsynaptic receptor, receptor response, destruction or dissipation of the transmitter and repolarization of the postsynaptic membrane.

○ **How is acetylcholine released from terminal vesicles?**

An action potential induces an influx of calcium and initiates of exocytosis.

○ **How does botulinum toxin work?**

It inhibits the release of acetylcholine.

○ **What is meant by the term cholinergic crisis?**

This is an effect caused by excessive doses of AchE inhibitors. Symptoms include miosis, sweating, salivation, lacrimation, a hyperactive bowel, muscle weakness and paralysis.

○ **What determines the duration of cholinesterase inhibition?**

The type of bond formed between the drug and the enzyme.

○ **What are the therapeutic uses of physostigmine?**

It is used in the treatment of wide-angle glaucoma and for the reversal of anti-cholinergic toxicity.

○ **Name some insecticides that are anticholinesterase agents?**

Parathion, Malathion, diazinon, Fenton and chlorpyrifos.

○ **What is the toxicological significance of parathion?**

It may be involved in accidental poisoning, suicide and homicide.

○ **What are the symptoms of parathion toxicity?**

There are nicotinic signs (muscle weakness and fatigability) and muscarinic signs (salivation, GI hyperactivity, bronchoconstriction etc.) as well as CNS effects such as confusion, ataxia, slurred speech, loss of reflexes, generalized convulsions and respiratory paralysis.

○ **How is parathion poisoning as well as poisoning with other irreversible cholinesterases treated?**

It depends on how soon after the patient is seen. The area should be decontaminated then respiration supported and then atropine and pralidoxime can be used as antidotes.

○ **What is pralidoxime?**

A cholinesterase reactivator.

○ **What is the rationale for the use of pralidoxime?**

It is very reactive with phosphorylated enzymes. It is causes reactivation of phosphorylated acetylcholinesterase.

○ **How does pyridostigmine compare to other cholinesterase inhibitors?**

It has a longer duration of action than neostigmine.

○ **What are the signs of mushroom poisoning due to muscarine containing mushrooms?**

The usual signs of muscarine excess including nausea, vomiting, diarrhea, vasodilatation, reflex tachycardia, sweating, salivation and possible bronchoconstriction.

○ **How is mushroom poisoning due to muscarine containing mushrooms treated?**

It is treated with atropine.

○ **What are the belladonna alkaloids?**

A group of alkaloids isolated from plants related to deadly nightshade. They have antimuscarinic effects.

○ **Name the belladonna alkaloids?**

Atropine and scopolamine.

○ **What are the sites of action of atropine?**

It acts at muscarinic receptors, including those in blood vessels, sweat glands and the CNS.

○ **What is the mechanism of action of atropine and other belladonna alkaloids?**

They antagonize the action of Ach at muscarinic cholinergic receptors. Only at large doses do they act at nicotinic cholinergic receptors.

○ **What is the order in which different tissues are effected by increasing doses of atropine?**

Receptor blockade depends on the dose of atropine. Salivary and bronchial secretions and sweating are depressed first. Then mydriasis, cycloplegia and vagal blockade of the heart occur, then tone and motility of the GI tract and urinary bladder are affected and finally gastric secretion is partially inhibited.

○ **How does atropine effect the CNS?**

At a low doses it causes mild vagal stimulation and at larger doses it causes restlessness, excitement, irritability and hallucinations.

○ **What are the ocular effects of atropine?**

Mydriasis, cycloplegia and photophobia.

○   **Why does atropine cause tachycardia?**

It occurs as a result of vagal blockade.

○   **What is the effect of atropine on the respiratory system?**

It decreases bronchial secretions and relaxes bronchial smooth muscle.

○   **What are the GI effects of atropine?**

It inhibits salivary secretions and reduces the tone and motility of the GI tract. There is also a partial reduction of gastric secretion.

○   **What are the therapeutic uses of atropine?**

It is used in preoperative medication, in bradycardia, in ophthalmology to produce mydriasis, to reduce cholinergic hyperactivity. It is also used to treat Parkinsonism, as an antispasmodic, and in some OTC preparations for rhinitis and hay fever.

○   **What are the adverse effects of atropine?**

Dry mouth, blurred vision, photophobia, tachycardia, GI distress and hot and dry skin.

○   **What groups of patients are very susceptible to atropine toxicity?**

Children, especially infants, are very sensitive to the hyperthermic effects of atropine. Deaths have followed doses as small as 2 mg.

○   **What is another name for adrenergic agonists?**

Sympathomimetics.

○   **What types of sympathomimetics are there?**

Direct agents, indirectly acting agents, mixed agents and those that act reflexly by stimulation of alpha or beta adrenergic receptors in the circulation.

○   **What is meant by the term indirect acting agent?**

A drug that acts as a result of releasing norepinephrine from the nerve ending.

○   **Name two indirect acting adrenergic agonists?**

Tyramine and amphetamine.

○   **What organ systems does epinephrine exert its prominent effects on?**

The cardiovascular system (vasoconstriction of arterioles in the skin; viscera and mucus membranes) and the respiratory system. In addition it has certain metabolic effects such as increased glycogenolysis and release of glucagon and decreased release of insulin which results in hyperglycemia.

○   **What are the cardiac effects of epinephrine?**

There is an increased heart rate and contractility.

○ **What are the vascular effects of epinephrine?**

Cutaneous blood flow is reduced, renal blood flow is reduced, skeletal blood flow can be increased or decreased, and coronary blood flow is increased.

○ **How is blood pressure effected by epinephrine?**

There is increased systolic pressure, decreased diastolic pressure and no change in mean pressure.

○ **How is blood pressure effected by norepinephrine?**

There is increased systolic, diastolic and mean blood pressure.

○ **What are the effects of epinephrine on the respiratory tract?**

There is bronchodilation.

○ **What are the metabolic effects of epinephrine?**

There is increased glycogenolysis and release of glucagon and decreased release of insulin resulting in hyperglycemia.

○ **What are the adverse effects of epinephrine?**

Cardiac arrhythmias, hypertension, palpitations, dizziness, anxiety, headache, tremor, myocardial infarction due to increased cardiac work and pulmonary edema.

○ **What are the toxic effects of amphetamine?**

Psychological and physical dependence, psychosis, confusion, insomnia, headache, restlessness, heart palpitations, tachycardia and impotence.

○ **What effects of amphetamine show tolerance?**

The anorexigenic and mood improvement effects.

○ **Name two uses of amphetamine?**

Attention deficit hyperactivity syndrome and narcolepsy.

○ **What are the pharmacological effects of phenylpropanolamine?**

It causes vasoconstriction and stimulation of the hypothalamic satiety center.

○ **What are the therapeutic uses of phenylpropanolamine?**

It is used as a nasal decongestant and an appetite suppressant.

○ **What is the therapeutic use of terbutaline?**

It is a bronchodilator used to treat asthma.

○ **What is propranolol?**

A nonselective beta adrenergic blocker.

○ **The olol suffix on a drug means the drug is what?**

The drug is a beta blocker.

○ **Describe the C.V. effects of propranolol?**

The heart rate decreases, cardiac output decreases, oxygen consumption decreases, there is a slowly developing reduction in blood pressure and sinus rate is decreased as well as conduction is slowed.

○ **What are the metabolic effects of propranolol?**

The normal rise in plasma free fatty acids associated with the beta response is inhibited and the hyperglycemic response to epinephrine is reduced.

○ **Does propranolol effect bronchial smooth muscle?**

It increases the tone of bronchial smooth muscle and airway resistance is increased.

○ **What are the side effects of propranolol?**

There is fatigue, lethargy, GI upset, wheezing and coldness in the extremities.

○ **What adverse effects are associated with the use of nonselective beta blockers?**

Bradycardia, bronchoconstriction, they may hide the warning signs of hypoglycemia, fatigue, depression and sexual dysfunction.

○ **What is the mechanism of action of metoprolol?**

It is a competitive blocker of $beta_1$ receptors with no agonist properties.

○ **What are the C.V. effects of metoprolol?**

It inhibits the inotropic and chronotropic actions of the $beta_2$-adrenergic agonists and it reduces blood pressure.

○ **How is phenoxybenzamine used clinically?**

It is used for pheochromocytoma and benign prostatic hypertrophy.

○ **What are the toxicities associated with the use of phenoxybenzamine?**

Postural hypotension, reflex tachycardia and nasal stuffiness.

○ **What is methylphenidate?**

An amphetamine variant whose major pharmacologic effects and abuse potential are similar to those of amphetamine. It is a mild CNS stimulant with more prominent effects on mental than motor activities.

○ **What is the therapeutic use of methylphenidate?**

It is effective in treating attention deficit hyperactivity disorder and narcolepsy.

○ **What is the toxicity of methylphenidate?**

Large doses produce signs of generalized CNS stimulation that may lead to convulsions. It shares the abuse potential of the amphetamines.

○ **What is an LD50?**

The dose lethal to 50% of the population. It is analogous to the ED50.

○ **What is meant by NOAEL and NOEL?**

No observed adverse effect level or no observed effect level.

○ **What is the appropriate dose of polyethylene glycol for whole bowel irrigation in a child?**

0.5-1.0 L/hour.

○ **What substance is the most common cause of toxin related death?**

Carbon monoxide.

○ **What toxin causes more deaths in the US than any other?**

Carbon monoxide – over 5000 deaths per year in the US.

○ **What factors influence the ability to remove a substance from the body by the use of hemodialysis?**

Molecular size, volume of distribution, degree of protein binding.

○ **What are the most common exposures in children below the age of six?**

According to the AAPCC data from 1991-1995, the most common exposures are the following (yearly average in parenthesis):

1. Cosmetics/personal care items (123,505)
2. Cleaning substances (115,632)
3. Analgesic agents (82,542)
4. Plants (80,250)
5. Cough/cold preparations (73,560)
6. Topical agents (53,335)

○ **What is the most common etiology of toxin induced death in all age groups ?**

Carbon monoxide.

○ **When is peritoneal dialysis indicated in the treatment of the poisoned patient?**

Virtually never.

○ **What are the causes of high anion gap metabolic acidosis?**

Methanol, metformin.
Uremia.
DKA, AKA.
Paraldehyde, Phenformin.
Iron, INH.
Lactic acidosis.

Ethylene glycol.
Salicylates.
Caffeine, CO, CN.
Acetaminophen (massive), Acids (propionic acid – ibuprofen, valproic acid).
Theophylline.

○ **What is osmolality?**

Osmolality is the molal concentration of solutes. This is the number of particles in one kilogram of solution.

○ **How is osmolality measured?**

Generally by freezing point depression. Vapor pressure method is associated with more falsely low measurements.

○ **What is osmolarity?**

Osmolarity is the molar concentration of solutes. This is the number of particles in a liter of solution. This value is generally calculated: $2*Na + BUN/2.8 + Glucose/18 + Etoh/4.6$

○ **What is the surface area of activated charcoal? Super-activated charcoal?**

Activated charcoal has a surface area of 950 m2/g and super-activated charcoal has a surface area of 2000 m2/g.

○ **How should the elevated temperature associated with toxic (agitated delirium) be treated?**

Pack the patient in ice as quickly as possible.

○ **What is an anaphylactoid reaction?**

An anaphylactoid reaction is very similar to anaphylaxis; however, it does not require prior exposure to the reaction product. Cases may occur from a radiopaque contrast media or from medications, such as NSAIDs.

○ **Which drugs commonly cause bradycardia?**

ß-blockers, cardiac glycosides, pilocarpine, and cholinesterase inhibitors (such as organophosphates) are responsible for bradycardia. Sympathomimetics, such as amphetamines and cocaine, and anticholinergics, such as atropine and cyclic antidepressants, commonly cause tachycardia.

○ **What drug commonly causes both horizontal and vertical nystagmus?**

Phencyclidine (PCP).

○ **Name 5 drugs or conditions that cause hypertension and/or tachycardia.**

Sympathomimetics.
Withdrawal.
Anticholinergics.
MAO Inhibitors.
Phencyclidine (PCP).

A mnemonic for this is SWAMP.

○ **Name six common drugs that can cause hyperthermia.**

<u>S</u>alicylates.
<u>A</u>nticholinergics.
<u>N</u>euroleptics.
<u>D</u>initrophenols.
<u>S</u>ympathomimetics and <u>PCP</u>.

The mnemonic for this one is SANDS-PCP.

○ **Which drugs or environmental exposures can induce bullous lesion formation?**

Sedative hypnotics, carbon monoxide, snake bite, spider bite, caustic agents, and hydrocarbons.

○ **What is a mnemonic for remembering the drugs that cause nystagmus?**

MALES TIP:
M = methanol.
A = alcohol.
L = lithium.
E = ethylene glycol.
S = sedative hypnotics and solvents.
T = thiamine depletion and Tegretol (carbamazepine).
I = isopropanol.
P = PCP and phenytoin.

○ **What is a mnemonic for remembering drugs that are radiopaque?**

BAT CHIPS
B = barium.
A = antihistamines.
T = tricyclic antidepressants.
C = chloral hydrate, calcium, cocaine.
H = heavy metals.
I = iodine.
P = phenothiazine, potassium.
S = slow-release (enteric coated).

○ **Name some side-effects of alkalization of the urine.**

Hypernatremia and hyperosmolality.

○ **What is the mechanism of action of syrup of ipecac?**

Induces vomiting by stimulation of the chemotactic trigger zone in the brain and causes local stomach irritation.

○ **Which is more toxic, syrup of ipecac or fluid extract of ipecac?**

The fluid extract is much more potent (>10x).

○ **What are the main active compounds in syrup of ipecac?**

Emetine and cephaline.

○ **What are the components of Lomotil?**

Atropine and diphenoxylate.

○ **Which anti-diarrheal contains difenoxin and atropine?**

Motofen.

○ **What is loperamide?**

A meperidine analogue sold over the counter as Imodium, an anti-diarrheal.

○ **Why may the toxic effects of Lomotil be delayed several hours or more?**

Since Lomotil slows gastrointestinal transit time, its absorption may be delayed. Also, the more-potent opioid metabolite difenoxin may accumulate as it has a longer serum half-life.

○ **What are the indications for deferoxamine therapy in iron poisoning?**

Serum iron greater than 400-500 mcg/dL or serious clinical signs of toxicity (shock, acidosis, severe gastroenteritis).

○ **What blood tube causes false depression of iron levels?**

Lavender tubes contain EDTA and falsely decrease the iron levels.

○ **What percent of ferrous sulfate tablets are elemental iron?**

20%.

○ **Infection with what organism is likely in patients who are iron overloaded?**

*Yersinia enterocolitica*.

○ **How much iron will be bound by 100 mg of deferoxamine?**

9.3 mg.

○ **What is the toxic dose of iron?**

Severe toxicity is rare with ingestions of less than 40 mg/Kg however mild symptoms such as nausea may occur at lower doses.

○ **How much elemental iron is present in ferrous gluconate containing preparations?**

12%.

○ **How much elemental iron is present in ferrous fumarate containing preparations?**

33%.

○ **The red tinted urine that results from treatment of iron overdose with deferoxamine is known as?**

Vin rose.

○ **What is the acid-base disturbance that occurs with iron toxicity?**

Metabolic acidosis.

○ **What is the etiology of acidosis in iron toxicity?**

Iron is converted from ferrous to ferric ($Fe^{2+}$ to $Fe^{3+}$) and a hydrogen ion is released. Iron also causes lactic acidosis by inhibiting oxidative phosphorylation and increasing anaerobic metabolism by causing hypotension.

○ **What is iron's effect on coagulation?**

Iron inhibits thrombin formation and activity.

○ **What x-ray may be helpful in suspected iron toxicity?**

Abdominal x-ray may show radiopaque pills.

○ **What pattern of liver injury occurs with iron toxicity?**

Periportal hemorrhagic necrosis.

○ **Why may oral deferoxamine administration after iron overdose worsen the toxicity?**

Deferoxamine combines with iron to form ferrioxamine, which is better absorbed than elemental iron, thus increasing total iron absorption.

○ **What is the first stage of iron toxicity?**

Iron overdose causes acute GI irritation resulting in abdominal pain, nausea, vomiting, and diarrhea. Iron is corrosive to the GI mucosa and may cause significant gastrointestinal ulceration, hemorrhage and necrosis.

○ **What is the second stage of iron toxicity?**

The patient may experience a "latent" period after the initial gastrointestinal effect resolve.

○ **What is the third stage of iron toxicity?**

Patients with severe toxicity will develop shock and worsening metabolic acidosis.

○ **What is the fourth stage of iron toxicity?**

Hepatic failure.

○ **What is the fifth stage of iron toxicity?**

The corrosive effects of the iron on the gastrointestinal system may result in strictures.

○ **T/F: Measurement of TIBC is useful in predicting iron toxicity after overdose.**

False.

○ **What is the major side effect of IV deferoxamine administration?**

Hypotension.

○ **What are the indications for deferoxamine therapy after iron overdose?**

Serum iron level above 500 µg/dL or significant signs of toxicity (shock, acidosis).

○ **How long should an asymptomatic patient be observed after suspected iron overdose?**

6 hours.

○ **How long after acute overdose does the peak blood level occur?**

Approximately 4.5 hours.

○ **What change in the urine may be seen after deferoxamine treatment?**

A "vin rose" color caused by elimination of deferoxamine.

○ **At what rate is deferoxamine infused?**

15 mg/hg/hr.

○ **What toxicity may occur after greater than 24 hours of deferoxamine therapy?**

ARDS.

○ **T/F: Any patient with significant iron toxicity will manifest a WBC count greater than 15,000 and/or blood glucose greater than 150 mg/dL.**

False. These parameters have been associated with elevated iron levels but are not accurate predictors.

○ **T/F: Iron is not significantly adsorbed by activated charcoal.**

True.

○ **What dose of ingested iron will generally cause severe toxicity?**

60 mg/kg or more.

○ **What compound is formed by the binding of iron to deferoxamine?**

Ferrioxamine.

○ **Which types of iron preparations are least likely to be seen on abdominal x-ray after ingestion?**

Chewable and liquid formulations.

○ **T/F: The deferoxamine challenge test is useful after iron overdose.**

False. The deferoxamine challenge involves administration of an IM deferoxamine dose. A positive test occurs if the urine changes color, indicating the presence of ferrioxamine. This test is considered unreliable.

○ **T/F: Deferoxamine can chelate iron which is bound to ferritin and transferrin.**

False.

○ **How do most children with acute, severe lead intoxication present to the ED?**

They are encephalopathic and often seizing.

○ **What age group of patients are at greatest risk for lead toxicity?**

Children less than 36 months of age.

○ **Is more ingested lead absorbed by the intestines in this population?**

Yes.

○ **How is iron deficiency related to the possibility of lead toxicity?**

Iron deficiency for unknown reasons increases the intestinal absorption of lead.

○ **Why may the brain of these patients be exposed to relatively more lead?**

They have an incomplete blood-brain barrier.

○ **In addition to the above, why is childhood lead poisoning of greater concern than adult?**

More susceptible to lead's neurotoxic effects. Exposure of the developing brain can lead to permanent deficits in intelligence and behavior.

○ **At what blood lead level is a child considered to be lead poisoned?**

10 mcg/dL.

○ **Do children at this level need chelation therapy?**

No, but an investigation into possible lead sources and an emphasis on lead healthy lifestyle should ensue.

○ **Is the number of lead poisoned children in the U.S. closer to 8% or 2%?**

8%.

○ **Does lead (e.g. lead paint) have a noxious taste?**

No, it tastes sweet.

○ **What are the principle sources of lead exposure?**

Lead in paint, soil, and dust.

○ **Children of what racial group seems to be disproportionately affected?**

African American.

○ **Can lead be inhaled?**

Yes, lead dust and lead oxide fumes are very efficiently absorbed by this route.

○   **Is the unborn fetus at risk?**

Yes, lead readily crosses the placenta.

○   **When did the lead content of paint begin to be regulated?**

1977.

○   **What tests can be used in home inspections for lead?**

Sodium sulfide (produces lead sulfide, which is grayish black), and X-ray fluorescence.

○   **Do folk, alternative, or herbal medications ever contain lead?**

Yes.

○   **Which body compartment has the greatest lead content?**

Bone.

○   **What X-ray finding is seen in growing children?**

Lead lines.

○   **Is it actual lead that is being imaged on these X-rays?**

No, they are growth arrest lines.

○   **Which type of nerve is affected more by lead, sensory or motor?**

Motor. It is thought that lead neuropathy is an anterior horn cell disease with dying back of the motor neuron.

○   **What characteristic finding is frequently seen on microscopic examination of the RBC in patients with prolonged lead poisoning?**

Basophilic stippling.

○   **What 2 enzymes in the heme synthesis pathway are inhibited by Pb?**

Delta aminolevulinic acid dehydratase and ferrochelatase.

○   **What are two substances that accumulate due to this inhibition?**

Delta aminolevulinic acid (possibly neurotoxic), and erythrocyte protoporphyrin.

○   **What is the utility of measure erythrocyte protoporphyrin in the blood?**

The effect on erythrocyte protoporphyrin lasts longer than elevated blood lead level, thus the effect of large exposure weeks earlier can be gauzed. It is not affected by "lead rebound," only by re-exposure.

○   **Is the blood lead level a good indicator of total body burden of lead?**

No.

○ **What are the two parenteral chelators available for severe lead poisoning?**

British Anti-Lewisite (BAL) and EDTA.

○ **BAL cannot be given to patients allergic to what substance?**

Peanut oil, as this is its carrier.

○ **In what group of patients must BAL be given cautiously?**

G6PD deficiency.

○ **What substance should not be given orally to patients on BAL?**

Iron.

○ **Should someone with encephalopathy and a blood level greater than 100 mcg/dL (70 mcg/L in children) be chelated parenterally?**

Yes.

○ **Can EDTA be given orally?**

No. It is not well absorbed, and it may increase the absorption of lead.

○ **What trace element deficiency can develop with EDTA chelation for lead?**

Zinc.

○ **If a patient on EDTA has developed proteinuria, glycosuria, or hematuria, what has happened?**

Renal toxicity from the EDTA.

○ **Does EDTA effectively decrease further a lead level 40 mcg/dL?**

No, probably not.

○ **What are the oral chelators that are available for lead chelation?**

Dimercaptosuccinic acid (DMSA, Succimer), D-penicillamine.

○ **What organs develop side effects of D-penicillamine?**

Gastrointestinal, dermatologic, bone marrow, renal.

○ **What are the side effects of DMSA?**

Rash, WBC depression, LFT abnormalities. There will frequently be a rebound phenomena as lead from non-blood stores mobilize into the blood. EP is not affected by this rebound, but would be if there were re-exposure.

○ **LSD is derived from what alkaloids?**

Ergots.

○ **What is the onset of action and half-life of LSD?**

Onset of action is approximately 30 minutes after ingestion and peak effect is 3-5 hours. Elimination half-life is 2.5 hours.

○ **What hallucinogenic alkaloid is found in *Lophophora williamsii* (peyote)?**

Mescaline.

○ **What neurotransmitter is responsible for the hallucinogenic action of LSD and the other hallucinogens?**

Hallucinogens are 5-HT2 receptor agonists.

○ **What are the effects of LSD on the physical examination?**

Sympathomimetic symptoms predominate; tachycardia, tachypnea, mydriasis and diaphoresis.

○ **What mushroom has hallucinogenic properties?**

*Amanita muscaria.*

○ **What popular hallucinogenic drugs belong to the phenylethylamine class?**

Mescaline, MDMA (Ecstasy, 3,4 methylenedioxymethamphetamine), PMA (para-methoxyamphetamine), MDA (3,4-methylenedioxyamphetamine), methamphetamine and DOB (4-bromo-2,5-dimethoxyamphetamine).

○ **Is the patient on a bad Lysergic Acid Diethylamide (LSD) "trip" oriented?**

Yes, even though they are fearful, and display bizarre reasoning.

○ **Can the patient on LSD have dilated pupils and hyperthermia?**

Yes, dilated pupils are often seen, hyperthermia is very high overdoses, presumable from the stimulation of $5-HT_2$ receptors.

○ **Can the patient taking LSD have bruxism?**

Yes. Bruxism refers to constant chewing or biting motions characteristic of MDMA (Ecstasy) and LSD use/abuse, not often seen in other psychoactive medication use.

○ **Is there an antidote for LSD?**

No, but benzodiazepines may be useful, often in large amounts.

○ **What chemical is detected in the urine immunoassay for marijuana?**

11nor-9-carboxy-delta 9-THC.

○ **What form of tetrahydrocannabinol is found in marijuana plant?**

The acid form, mostly acid A, of THC (delta 9 tetrahydrocannabinol) is found in the plant product. The THC acid A (and the acid B) must be heated to form THC.

○ **How are cannabinoids excreted?**

2/3 is excreted in the feces and 1/3 is excreted into the urine.

○ **How long will a urine drug screen testing for 11nor-9-carboxy-delta 9-THC be positive after one exposure to marijuana?**

2-10 days.

○ **How long will a urine drug screen testing for 11nor-9-carboxy-delta 9-THC be positive after chronic use of marijuana?**

Up to four weeks.

○ **What is the main psychoactive chemical in marijuana?**

Delta-9-tetrahydrocannabinol (THC).

○ **Is this chemical available legally?**

Yes, it is marketed as dronabinol (Marinol).

○ **What is the mechanism of action of marijuana?**

It binds anandamide receptors in the brain. "Anandia" is translated from the Sanskrit as the word: "bliss".

○ **What are the clinical symptoms of marijuana ingestion/overdose?**

It may have a variety of effects depending on a multitude of concurrent psychosocial or pharmacologic stimulation, but generally there is euphoria, a stimulant effect, and with higher doses a hallucinogenic and paranoid effect. There can also be a sedative effect and an orthostatic hypotensive effect after the initial stimulatory effect.

○ **What are some signs of marijuana ingestion/overdose?**

Tachycardia, orthostatic hypotension, conjunctival injection, slurred sleep, incoordination, and stupor in excessive overdose.

○ **Is there an antidote for a paranoid, psychotic patient overdosed on marijuana?**

There is no direct antidote; however, benzodiazepines would be effective. Orthostatic hypotension responds to fluids.

○ **What is considered to be a lethal level of methemoglobin?**

70%.

○ **Pulse oximetry readings (oxygen saturation) approximate what value in the face of methemoglobinemia?**

85%.

○ **At what level of methemoglobin can cyanosis be expected to be seen?**

15-20%.

○ **What is the Valence State of iron in methemoglobinemia?**

+3 (ferric).

○ **What mutated form of hemoglobin allows easier oxidation to methemoglobin?**

Hemoglobin M.

○ **What is the reduced form of iron capable of oxygen transport?**

$Fe^{2+}$ (ferrous).

○ **What is methemoglobin?**

Hemoglobin in which the iron molecule has been oxidized to $Fe^{3+}$ (ferric).

○ **Why is there a baseline level of methemoglobin in the body?**

Oxygen transport occasionally results in a loss of an electron from the iron to the leaving oxygen molecule.

○ **What concentration of methemoglobin is necessary to observe cyanosis in a patient?**

1.5 g/dL.

○ **What concentration of sulfhemoglobin is necessary to observe cyanosis in a patient?**

0.5 g/dL.

○ **What characteristic may one observes when drawing a blood sample from a patient with significant methemoglobinemia?**

"Chocolate brown" color of the blood.

○ **Why is pulse oximetry abnormal in the patient with methemoglobinemia?**

The pulse oximetry device is designed to measure the absorption characteristics of oxyhemoglobin and deoxyhemoglobin. Methemoglobin has different absorption characteristics and will interfere with the readings.

○ **What pulse ox readings may one see in a patient with methemoglobinemia?**

As methemoglobin level rises, the pulse ox will drop until leveling off at 85% with methemoglobin concentrations of 30% or higher.

○ **What type of device is needed to measure a methemoglobin level?**

A co-oximeter.

○ **What is the significance of the "saturation gap" in a patient with methemoglobinemia?**

The patient's oxygen saturation measured by pulse oximetry will be lower than the calculated oxygen saturation on the arterial blood gas analysis. This is due to methemoglobin's interference with accurate pulse oximetry.

○ **What substances may cause a falsely elevated methemoglobin level?**

Serum triglycerides, sulfhemoglobin and methylene blue.

○ **What cause of methemoglobin has been associated with fatal cases in infants?**

Nitrates in well water.

○ **What are the major classes of compounds that cause methemoglobinemia?**

Nitrites, nitrates, sulfonamides, quinines, bromates.

○ **What is the baseline level of methemoglobin in a healthy child?**

Less than 1%.

○ **What are the two enzymes that are responsible for reducing methemoglobin?**

NADH methemoglobin reductase and NADPH methemoglobin reductase.

○ **What enzyme is responsible for the majority of methemoglobin reduction?**

NADH methemoglobin reductase.

○ **Why may infants less than four months of age be more susceptible to methemoglobinemia?**

The enzyme NADH methemoglobin reductase does not reach full activity level until around this age.

○ **What genetic defect may give patients a baseline elevation of methemoglobin up to 50%?**

NADH methemoglobin reductase deficiency.

○ **What vitamin may act to reduce methemoglobin?**

Ascorbic acid (vitamin C).

○ **What is the antidote for methemoglobinemia?**

Methylene blue.

○ **How does methylene blue help to reduce methemoglobin?**

Methylene blue is converted to leukomethylene blue by the NADPH methemoglobin reductase. The leukomethylene blue then reduces the methemoglobin.

○ **At what level of methemoglobinemia may symptoms first appear?**

15%.

○ **What are the first symptoms of significant methemoglobinemia?**

Dyspnea, fatigue, headache, dizziness.

○ **What substances are associated with both methemoglobinemia and hemolysis?**

Amyl nitrite, aniline, dapsone, phenazopyridine.

○ **What is the normal rate of reduction of methemoglobin?**

15% per hour.

○ **How is methylene blue administered in cases of methemoglobinemia?**

1-2 mg/kg of 1% solution IV over 5 minutes. A repeat dose of 1 mg/kg may be given.

○ **What is the chemical name for methylene blue?**

Tetramethyl thionine chloride.

○ **What is the major toxicity of dapsone overdose?**

Prolonged methemoglobinemia.

○ **Why is methylene blue ineffective in patients with no G-6-PD activity?**

Patients with no G-6-PD are unable to generate NADPH in the red cell which is necessary for NADPH methemoglobin reductase to convert methylene blue to leukomethylene blue.

○ **What are the indications for methylene blue therapy?**

It is indicated in any patient with symptomatic methemoglobinemia.

○ **What are possible side effects of large doses of methylene blue?**

Paradoxical methemoglobinemia and hemolysis.

○ **Which local anesthetic agents may cause methemoglobinemia?**

Benzocaine and lidocaine.

○ **What two analgesics may cause methemoglobinemia?**

Phenacetin and phenazopyridine.

○ **Ingestions of which two types of mushrooms has been associated with renal failure?**

*Cortinarius* and *Amanita*.

○ **Which group of mushrooms contains a chemical which can be hydrolyzed to monomethylhydrazine?**

*Gyromitra* species.

○ **What percentage of mushroom-related deaths are caused by *Amanita* species?**

Approximately 90%.

○ **What three types (genus) of mushroom contain cyclopeptides?**

*Amanita*, *Galleria*, and *Lepiota*.

❍ **When can Aminotransferase levels be expected to rise after *Amanita* poisoning?**

Within 2-3 days.

❍ **What endocrine abnormalities may be related to *Amanita* poisoning?**

Elevated insulin and calcitonin levels and depressed triiodothyronine levels.

❍ **Which cyclopeptide-containing mushroom produces a mixed polyneuropathy in 50% of cases?**

*Lepiota* species.

❍ **What toxins do *Amanita phalloides* contain?**

Amatoxins, phallotoxins and virotoxins.

❍ **What is the mechanism of action of alpha-amanita?**

Inhibits RNA polymerase II, thereby preventing DNA transcription.

❍ **Is there any therapy for *Amanita* mushroom toxicity?**

Thioctic acid, penicillin, silibinin, cimetidine and multiple doses of activated charcoal have been suggested, but none have been definitively determined to be advantageous.

❍ **A patient has status epilepticus 6-10 hours after eating a mushroom that looked like a brain. Which mushroom did they eat?**

Monomethylhydrazine-containing mushrooms (*Gyromitra*).

❍ **What is the antidote for *Gyromitra* mushroom poisoning?**

Pyridoxine. Gyromitrin is metabolized to monomethylhydrazine which reacts with pyridoxine and inhibits GABA function leading to status epilepticus. Pyridoxine may limit this toxicity.

❍ **Which mushrooms cause a cholinergic toxidrome?**

*Clitocybe* and *Inocybe*.

❍ **What symptoms would you expect after a meal of *Coprinus* mushrooms and a glass of wine?**

Coprinus mushrooms contain the toxin coprine that can cause a disulfiram-like effect (hypotension, tachycardia, flushing, nausea and vomiting).

❍ **What is the toxicity of *Amanita gemmate* and *Amanita muscaria*?**

These mushrooms contain ibotenic acid and muscimol which produce a GABAergic syndrome of somnolence, hallucinations, myoclonus and can cause seizures.

❍ **What chemical toxin is contained in *Conocybe cyanopus*, *Panaelus foenisecii*, *Gymnopilus spectabilis*, *Psilocybe caerulescens*, and *Psathyrella foenisecii*?**

Psilocybin, a hallucinogenic compound.

○ **Which class of mushroom causes delayed renal failure?**

*Cortinarius* species contain orellanine that can produce renal failure up to weeks after ingestion.

○ **What is lycoperdonosis?**

Lycoperdonosis is a syndrome of nasopharyngitis; vomiting, pneumonitis, shortness of breath; myalgias and fever caused by the inhalation of puffball mushrooms of the *Lycoperdon* species. Inhalation of spores is used as a treatment for epistaxis.

○ **What is the toxic dose of amanitin?**

0.1 mg/kg.

○ **How much Amanitin is contained in one *Amanita* species cap?**

10-15mg.

○ **What is the theoretical mechanism of action for penicillin therapy for *Amanita* species toxicity?**

Penicillin prevents alpha-amanitin from entering the hepatocyte.

○ **What is the mortality rate of patients who develop liver failure secondary to *Amanita* toxicity?**

20-30%.

○ **What percentage of patients who call their Poison Center after ingesting a mushroom eventually develops symptoms?**

50%.

○ **What percentage of patients who call their Poison Center after ingesting a mushroom eventually develop severe symptoms?**

0.2%.

○ **If vomiting begins 30 minutes after ingestion, is that patient at increased risk of severe toxicity or decreased risk?**

If vomiting occurs prior to 3-4 hours after ingestion, the mushroom was most likely not toxic. However, many patients eat several mushrooms and may have eaten a mixture of toxic and non-toxic mushrooms.

○ **What is the neonatal toxicity of Blue Cohosh?**

Myocardial depression and shock has occurred in neonates born to mothers who take Blue Cohosh.

○ **Chronic ingestion of licorice can result in what electrolyte abnormality?**

Hypokalemia.

○ **Squill, oleander, foxglove and Ch'an Su result in toxicity identical to what medication?**

Digoxin. All of the above are cardiac glycosides.

○ **Ingestion of jimson weed results in what toxidrome?**

Anticholinergic.

○ **What is the active ingredient in St. John's Wort?**

Hypericin – it most likely acts as a serotonin reuptake inhibitor.

○ **Which NSAID has been associated with agranulocytosis?**

Phenylbutazone.

○ **NSAIDs inhibit what enzyme to produce their therapeutic effect?**

Cyclo-oxygenase.

○ **What is the toxicity of massive ibuprofen overdose?**

Seizures, coma, metabolic acidosis, renal and liver failure.

○ **What percentage of adverse drug reactions are related to NSAIDs?**

About 25%.

○ **Which NSAID may cause a false-positive salicylate assay?**

Diflunisal.

○ **Which veterinary NSAID has caused aplastic anemia and agranulocytosis?**

Phenylbutazone, formerly used in humans, can be highly toxic a relatively low dose (2g in a child; 4-40g in an adult) is now only available for veterinary medicine.

○ **What is the unique aspect of NSAID toxicity secondary to the anthranilic acids (mefenamic acid and meclofenamate)?**

Reported rate of seizures in 20% of patients.

○ **Serious manifestations of ibuprofen toxicity including coma, apnea and/or metabolic acidosis occur in what percentage of adults and children?**

9% of adults and 5% of children.

○ **Which two NSAIDs will produce a false positive ferric chloride urine test (for salicylates)?**

Phenylbutazone and diflunisal.

○ **What is the half-life of ibuprofen? Naproxen? Indomethacin?**

The half-lives of ibuprofen, naproxen and indomethacin are 2-4 hours, 10-20 hours and 3-11 hours, respectively.

○ **What is the classic triad for opioid toxicity?**

Depressed mental status, miosis, and hypoventilation.

○ **Which opioid may induce wide complex dysrhythmias?**

Propoxyphene.

○ **Name three opioids more commonly associated with seizures.**

Meperidine, propoxyphene, tramadol.

○ **What is the duration of action of naloxone?**

Approximately 1 hr.

○ **How do opioids induce hypotension?**

Hypotension is mediated by histamine release. A combination of H1 and H2 antagonist is effective in improving hemodynamics effects of opioids in humans.

○ **Give the names of two opioids that have been associated with Serotonin Syndrome.**

Meperidine and dextromethorphan are both associated with serotonin syndrome.

○ **Which opioid in an overdose setting may result in an anticholinergic toxidrome?**

Diphenoxylate (Lomotil) is formulated with 0.025mg of Atropine.

○ **What is the potentially harmful neurotoxic metabolite of meperidine?**

Normeperidine.

○ **What is "Heroin Lung"?**

Noncardiogenic pulmonary edema, a complication of heroin overdose.

○ **What is the treatment of a narcotic overdose?**

Naloxone 0.4 to 2.0mg IV over 2-3min maximum 10mg *(.1mg/kg in a child)*. If patient responds favorably consider IV infusion at 2/3 the effective dose. Haddad (pediatric recommendation).

○ **What are the indications for use of naloxone?**

Respiratory depression (RR of 12 or less), coma or hypotension. Remember H1 and H2 blockers may also be effective in improving hypotension. Drowsiness alone is not an indication. In the setting of drowsiness, use of Narcan may result in withdrawal, and compromise of the airway, or aspiration pneumonia.

○ **Which drug is considered the prototype and standard for the opioid drugs?**

Morphine.

○ **What are the main pharmacological actions of morphine?**

Analgesia, respiratory depression, drowsiness and sedation, euphoria and tranquility, pupillary constriction, nausea and vomiting, and GI effects.

○ **What type of analgesia does morphine produce?**

It produces analgesia without loss of consciousness, it is more effective against continuous dull pain than sharp intermittent pain, and it acts at both the spinal level and at higher levels.

○ **What effect does morphine have on respiration?**

It produces respiratory depression primarily due to a decrease in sensitivity in the chemoreceptor centers to plasma $CO_2$.

○ **What effect does morphine have on the eye?**

It causes pupillary constriction.

○ **Does morphine effect the cardiovascular system?**

It has mild effects there such as orthostatic hypotension.

○ **How is morphine metabolized?**

It is mainly glucuronidated.

○ **What are the side effects of morphine use?**

Dependence, increased pressure in the biliary tract, dysphoria and excitement, histamine release.

○ **What type of withdrawal symptoms are seen with use of the opiates?**

It reflects an exaggerated rebound from the acute pharmacologic effects of the drug. The signs of withdrawal include rhinorrhea, lacrimation, yawning, chills, gooseflesh, hyperventilation, hyperthermia, mydriasis, muscular aches, vomiting, diarrhea, anxiety and hostility.

○ **Name two drugs that are opiate antagonists?**

Naltrexone and naloxone.

○ **What are the therapeutic uses of codeine?**

Mild to moderate pain and cough suppression.

○ **What effect does meperidine have on the eyes?**

Unlike most opiates it causes the pupils to dilate rather than constrict. This is related to its anticholinergic activity.

○ **What is diphenoxylate?**

A drug related to meperidine that is a potent anti-diarrheal agent.

○ **What is loperamide?**

It is also related to meperidine and is a potent anti-diarrheal agent.

○ **What is fentanyl?**

It is a synthetic opioid and a meperidine analog. Fentanyl and its derivatives including sufentanil are the most potent opioid agonists available.

○ **How is fentanyl used?**

It is a potent analgesic. It is also used to produce neuroleptanalgesia and is used in cardiovascular surgery.

○ **How is fentanyl administered?**

Either IV or transdermally or in lollipop form as preanesthetic medication for children.

○ **How does naloxone work?**

It is an opioid receptor antagonist. It binds all opiate receptors to displace bound opioid agonists.

○ **How does heroin differ from morphine?**

Heroin is hydrolyzed into morphine and therefore has many properties similar to morphine. It is however, more lipid soluble and can get across the blood brain barrier faster.

○ **How is naloxone used therapeutically?**

To reverse the respiratory depression and coma of opioid overdose.

○ **What are the therapeutic uses of naltrexone?**

It is useful for treating opioid dependence because it has a longer duration of action than naloxone.

○ **What are the adverse effects of naltrexone?**

Hepatotoxicity, nausea, sedation and headache.

○ **What happens if naloxone or naltrexone is given in the absence of an opiate agonist?**

Usually there is no physiologic effect in this situation.

○ **How do you treat an acute opioid overdose?**

Support respiration and use naloxone.

○ **What is the usual cause of death in patients with organophosphate poisoning?**

Respiratory failure secondary to central depression of respiratory drive as well as weakness of the muscles of respiration.

○ **Which group of pesticides forms generally reversible bonds with the cholinesterase enzyme?**

Carbamates.

○ **Hexachlorocyclohexane is the chemical name for which pesticide?**

Lindane.

○ **What are the two types of pyrethroid pesticides?**

Type I (do not contain a cyano group), Type II (contain a cyano group).

○ **What id the toxicity of Type II pyrethroids in humans?**

Paresthesia, nausea, vomiting, dizziness, seizures, and acute pulmonary edema.

○ **How are the paresthesias secondary to Type II pyrethroids treated?**

Vitamin E.

○ **Organophosphates, though less toxic to the environment, are _____ (more/less) toxic to humans acutely.**

More.

○ **Approximately what percentage of homes in the U.S. uses pesticides?**

90%.

○ **What are the routes of absorption of pesticides?**

Ingestion, inhalation, skin absorption.

○ **Which has a larger LD-50 in humans, malathion or parathion?**

Malathion (1,375 mg/kg) is "safer" than parathion (3 mg/kg).

○ **What is the mechanism by which organophosphate poisonings cause toxicity?**

Irreversible phosphorylation (inhibition) of acetylcholinesterase.

○ **What toxidrome does organophosphate and carbamate poisonings cause?**

Cholinergic.

○ **What is the difference in the mechanism of action between organophosphates and carbamates?**

Carbamates are reversible.

○ **The mnemonic 'DUMBELS' have been used to summarize the symptoms seen with excessive stimulation of which receptor subclass?**

Muscarinic.

○ **To what symptoms do the letters of the mnemonic 'DUMBELS' refer?**

D-diarrhea, U-urination, B-bronchospasm/bronchorrhea, E-emesis, L-lacrimation, S-salivation.

○ **Where are nicotinic cholinergic receptors found?**

Central Nervous System, autonomic ganglia, motor endplate.

○ **Organophosphate poisoned patients may experience loss of consciousness, delirium, respiratory depression, and seizures, by the stimulation of which receptors in the CNS?**

Nicotinic receptors in the CNS.

○    **Stimulation of which receptor in organophosphate poisoning results in muscle fasciculations?**

Nicotinic receptors at the motor endplate.

○    **In which group of patients may the typical cholinergic symptoms of acute organophosphate toxicity be absent?**

Children--often present only with neurobehavioral changes.

○    **What is the "delayed neurotoxic syndrome" of organophosphate poisoning?**

Paresthesias, and weakness in the distal extremities.

○    **When does this syndrome develop in relation to exposure?**

In 2-3 weeks.

○    **What type of electromyography pattern does it generate?**

Denervation.

○    **What is the "intermediate neurotoxic syndrome" of organophosphate poisoning?**

Weakness of the proximal limb muscles, muscles of respiration, and cranial nerve palsies.

○    **When with regards to exposure does this syndrome present?**

In 1-4 days.

○    **Can the weakness of the respiratory muscles be sufficiently severe to require mechanical ventilation?**

Yes.

○    **What pharmacokinetics mechanism may account for the intermediate neurotoxic syndrome?**

Delayed absorption or long half-life.

○    **Prolonged effect of succinylcholine as well as an exaggerated response to organophosphate poisoning may be seen in patients with a genetic deficiency of _____.**

Plasma cholinesterase (pseudocholinesterase).

○    **What percentage of the population is deficient in this enzyme?**

3%.

○    **Which of the two cholinesterases, plasma or RBC, is the preferred test in documenting exposure and monitoring resolution?**

RBC cholinesterase (true cholinesterase).

○    **How long does it take for the action of this enzyme to return after it has been poisoned by organophosphates?**

60-90 days or 1/2 to 1% per day, i.e., the rate of new RBC release from the bone marrow.

○ **Is there a clear relation in serum cholinesterase decrease and the severity of the symptoms of organophosphate poisoning?**

No.

○ **What is usually the cause of death in untreated organophosphate poisoning?**

Increased respiratory secretions resulting in respiratory failure.

○ **What is the first drug that should be given immediately in acute organophosphate poisoning?**

Atropine.

○ **How much of the drug must be given?**

Sufficient to dry the airways of secretion.

○ **What does pralidoxime and the other oximes do?**

They reversibly phosphorylate the acetylcholine receptors.

○ **Within what time-frame must it be given in an organophosphate poisoning.**

Within 24-48 hours.

○ **What are the possible side effects if given too rapidly.**

It should be given 1-2 g (20-50 mcg/kg in children) intravenously 30 min. It may cause tachycardia, laryngeal spasm, and muscle rigidity.

○ **What is the time course of carbamate poisoning?**

Onset 15 min - 20 min. Resolution within 24 hours.

○ **What is the effect of pralidoxime (2-PAM) in carbamate poisoned patients?**

It may enhance the acetylcholinesterase inactivation.

○ **What is the most commonly used organochlorine pesticide in the U.S.?**

Lindane.

○ **What enzyme does lindane inhibit, causing seizures?**

Gamma Amino Butyric Acid (GABA).

○ **What oral treatment may increase the excretion of organochlorines?**

Cholestyramine.

○   **Synthetic pyrethroids, such as permethrin, are synthetic versions of pyrethrum, which is an oleoresin extract of _____.**

*Chrysanthemum cinerariaefolium.*

○   **What are the symptoms of pyrethrin poisoning?**

Tremor, incoordination, salivation, diarrhea, and rarely death.

○   **Paraquat is especially toxic to _____.**

Lungs.

○   **What routine treatment given in ambulances and in emergency departments is contraindicated in paraquat poisoning?**

Oxygen.

○   **Why?**

Generation of hydrogen peroxides and free radicals are increased.

○   **What effect does paraquat have on skin, and gastrointestinal tract?**

Caustic.

○   **What is the difference between diquat and paraquat?**

Less toxicity with diquat, not as concentrated in the lung.

○   **What is the mechanism of toxicity from *Dieffenbachia* species?**

*Dieffenbachia* species contain calcium oxalate crystals and proteolytic enzymes that are packaged in raphides and bundled into idioblasts. When pressure is placed on the idioblasts, the crystals project outward and inject the enzymes under the skin or mucosa. The enzymes increase histamine and bradykinin release leading to local pain and swelling. Most exposures occur in small children who bite the leaves.

○   **What is the toxicity of poinsettia (*Euphorbia pulcherrima*)?**

Poinsettia contains diterpene esters which may cause some local irritation or nausea and vomiting.

○   **Are *Philodendron* species toxic?**

*Philodendron* species can rarely cause local or gastrointestinal irritation.

○   **What is the laboratory abnormality associated with pokeweed (*Phytolacca americana*) toxicity?**

Leukocytosis. *Phytolacca americana* contains phytolaccine, a gastrointestinal irritant, and pokeweed mitogen, which causes lymphoid mitosis leading to leukocytosis on days 2-10. Toxicity is often avoided by double boiling (parboiling) the plant prior to ingestion.

○   **What is the antigenic substance in the *Toxicodendron* species (poison ivy, poison oak and poison sumac)?**

Urushiol.

O   **What is the toxicity of *Datura stramonium* (Jimson Weed)?**

Jimson Weed contains belladonna alkaloids, including atropine, scopolamine and hyoscyamine, that cause anticholinergic toxicity.

O   **How much atropine is present in 100 seeds of *Datura stramonium*?**

100 *Datura stramonium* seeds contain the equivalent of 6mg of atropine.

O   **What is the pattern of liver necrosis seen with Ackee fruit (*Blighia sapida*) toxicity?**

Centrilobular necrosis.

O   **What is the antidote for Oleander toxicity?**

Oleander (*Nerium oleander*) contains cardiac glycosides and produce a digitalis-like toxicity. Digoxin-specific antibody fragments can be used to reverse toxicity, but particularly high doses may be necessary because of incomplete cross-reactivity.

O   **Are Digoxin levels accurate in plant-based cardiac glycoside toxicity (e.g. ingestion of lily of the valley)?**

Digoxin levels may be elevated in a patient with cardiac glycoside toxicity from ingestion of lily of the valley. However, digoxin levels may be lower than expected for the patient's toxicity because of incomplete cross-reactivity of naturally occurring glycosides and digoxin.

O   **What is the toxic substance in water hemlock (*Cicuta maculata*)?**

Cicutoxin.

O   **What is the toxicity of *Cicuta maculata* (water hemlock)?**

Water hemlock causes nausea, vomiting, abdominal cramping and status epilepticus. The seizures may be refractory to standard therapy and is the probable cause of death in most cases.

O   **Describe a death by poison hemlock (*Conium maculatum*).**

*Conium maculatum* contains coniine, a piperidine alkaloid similar to nicotine, that causes gastrointestinal upset, tachycardia, tremors, mydriasis, and seizures followed by bradycardia, and ascending muscle paralysis. Death is generally from paralysis.

O   **What is the toxin contained in the *Prunus* species?**

Amygdalin.

O   **What is the toxicity of Amygdalin?**

Amygdalin is found in the leaves or seeds of the *Prunus* species (e.g. apple seeds, apricot, cassava, cherry laurel, hydrangea, peach, plum and western chokecherry). Amygdalin is metabolized by the enzyme emulsin to form hydrocyanic acid. Toxicity is identical to cyanide toxicity.

O   **What is the mechanism of action of Ricin?**

Ricin inhibits the 60S ribosomal subunit preventing binding of elongation factor 2 and inhibiting protein synthesis.

○ **What is the toxic chemical found in 'deadly nightshade'?**

Atropine and anticholinergic alkaloids.

○ **What is *Melaleuca alternifolia*?**

*Melaleuca alternifolia* is Tea Tree Oil and can cause sedation and ataxia.

○ **What is the toxicity from Dogbane?**

Digoxin-like cardiac glycoside toxicity.

○ **What is catnip?**

Catnip contains *Nepeta cataria* which is a mild hallucinogen.

○ **What are the indications for hemodialysis in salicylate toxicity?**

Renal failure.
Noncardiogenic pulmonary edema.
Severe acid-base or electrolyte imbalance, despite appropriate and aggressive therapy.
Coagulopathy secondary to hepatic failure.
Salicylate level > 100 mg/dL (in acute overdose).
Congestive heart failure (relative).
Progressive deterioration in vital signs.

○ **Oil of wintergreen contains what toxic substance?**

Oil of wintergreen contains 1,4 g/cc of salicylates.

○ **Which type of acid base disturbance initially occurs with a salicylate overdose?**

Respiratory alkalosis. Approximately 12 hours later, an anion gap metabolic acidosis or mixed acid base picture may occur.

○ **Is hyperglycemia or is hypoglycemia expected with a salicylate overdose?**

Expect either hyperglycemia or hypoglycemia.

○ **A patient presents with an acute salicylate ingestion. What symptoms are expected with a mild, a moderate, and a severe overdose?**

1. Mild: Lethargy, vomiting, hyperventilation, and hyperthermia.
2. Moderate: Severe hyperventilation and compensated metabolic acidosis.
3. Severe: Coma, seizures, and uncompensated metabolic acidosis.

○ **What is the treatment for a salicylate overdose?**

Decontaminate, lavage and charcoal, replace fluids, supplement with potassium, alkalize the urine with bicarbonate, cool for hyperthermia, administer glucose for hypoglycemia, place on oxygen and PEEP for pulmonary edema, prescribe multiple dose activated charcoal, and initiate dialysis.

○ **What are the acid-base disturbances commonly present in salicylate overdose?**

Respiratory alkalosis and metabolic acidosis.

○ **How do salicylates cause a respiratory alkalosis?**

Stimulation of the respiratory center of the brain.

○ **How does the acid-base disturbance after salicylate overdose in pediatric patients differ from that in adults?**

In children the respiratory alkalosis is often transient and the metabolic acidosis more prominent.

○ **What is the first acid-base change after salicylate overdose?**

The respiratory alkalosis.

○ **What are the main metabolic effects of salicylate toxicity?**

Uncoupling of oxidative phosphorylation increased lactate production.

○ **What effect may salicylate toxicity have on the lungs?**

Non-cardiogenic pulmonary edema.

○ **What liver disease in children has been associated with salicylate use?**

Reye's syndrome.

○ **What risk factors have been associated with the development of pulmonary edema after salicylate overdose?**

Chronic overdose, neurologic symptoms, and smoking.

○ **What neurologic effects may occur with salicylate toxicity?**

Tinnitus and hearing loss, vertigo, hyperventilation, agitation, convulsions.

○ **What is the $pK_a$ of salicylate?**

3.5.

○ **What GI effects may be seen in salicylate toxicity?**

Nausea, vomiting, gastritis, pylorospasm.

○ **What is the therapeutic range for salicylate?**

15 to 30 mg/dL.

○ **What is the normal protein binding of salicylate and how does it change after overdose?**

The normal protein binding of 90% falls to 75% with high serum levels.

○ **What percentage of salicylate is excreted unchanged in the urine?**

2.5%.

○ **What changes occur in the elimination of salicylate after overdose?**

Half-life is prolonged due to saturation of elimination pathways and change from first order to zero order kinetics.

○ **Is the Done nomogram useful in predicting toxicity in salicylate overdoses?**

Rarely- the nomogram may be used only if very strict criteria are met including single overdose, non-enteric coated formulation, and serum pH 7.4 or higher.

○ **Why does a low blood pH worsen salicylate toxicity?**

Low pH enhances salicylate concentration in body tissues such as the CNS.

○ **Why does alkalinization of the urine enhance salicylate excretion?**

Alkalinization of the urine causes salicylate to become ionized in the urine, preventing re-absorption in the non-ionized state. This is referred to as "ion trapping".

○ **What patients are at risk for chronic salicylate toxicity?**

The elderly and young children.

○ **How do the symptoms of chronic salicylate toxicity differ from those in acute toxicity?**

Symptoms are similar, except that chronic toxicity most often manifests more pronounced neurologic symptoms and is more likely to cause pulmonary edema.

○ **What qualitative bedside test may be used to detect salicylate?**

Addition of ferric chloride to urine will result in a dark purple color if salicylate is present.

○ **What abnormality may be seen on urinalysis after salicylate overdose?**

Ketonuria and proteinuria.

○ **Why is acetazolamide not indicated for alkalinizing the urine after salicylate overdose?**

Acetazolamide will increase the acidity of the blood and enhance distribution of salicylate to the body tissues.

○ **What is the target urine pH level of the urine when alkalinizing to enhance salicylate elimination?**

7.5 to 8.

○ **What electrolyte abnormality may make urinary alkalinization more difficult?**

Hypokalemia.

○ **What is the treatment for severe salicylate toxicity?**

Hemodialysis.

○ **What serum concentrate of salicylate is an indication for hemodialysis?**

100 mg/dL.

○ **What dose of aspirin is equivalent in salicylate to one cc of methyl salicylate?**

1.4 gm.

○ **What is the active ingredient of oil of wintergreen?**

Methyl salicylate.

○ **What is the half-life of a therapeutic dose of salicylate?**

2 to 4 hours.

○ **Why may endotracheal intubation acutely worsen salicylate toxicity?**

During intubation, a patient who has been breathing rapidly to maintain a normal or near-normal pH may become acidotic due to decreased ventilation. Acidosis will enhance tissue distribution of salicylate.

○ **Salicylate is structurally similar to what vitamin?**

Vitamin K.

○ **What are the effects of salicylate toxicity on blood clotting?**

Hypoprothrombinemia and decreased platelet function.

○ **What effect does theophylline have on cyclic AMP?**

Increases it.

○ **What are the differences between theophylline and aminophylline?**

Aminophylline is the ethylenediamine salt of theophylline. Aminophylline may be given IV, theophylline by mouth only.

○ **To what class of drugs does theophylline belong?**

Methylxanthines.

○ **In what forms is theophylline used?**

Commonly as a sustained-release formulation, also as immediate release theophylline and aminophylline.

○ **What are the likely mechanisms of action of theophylline?**

Phosphodiesterase inhibition, adenosine antagonism, catecholamine release.

○ **What is the $V_d$ of theophylline?**

0.5 L/kg.

○ **What are the metabolic effects of acute theophylline toxicity?**

Hypokalemia, hypophosphatemia, hypomagnesemia, lactic acidosis, hyperglycemia.

○ **Above what serum theophylline level is serious acute toxicity likely to occur?**

90 to 100 ug/L.

○ **Above what serum theophylline level is serious toxicity likely to occur in a chronic overdose?**

40 ug/mL.

○ **What are the cardiovascular effects of acute theophylline toxicity?**

Sinus tachycardia, supraventricular tachycardia, atrial fibrillation, multifocal atrial tachycardia, hypotension, widened pulse pressure, ventricular arrhythmias.

○ **What are the CNS effects of acute theophylline toxicity?**

Anxiety, hyperventilation, tremor, seizure, status epilepticus.

○ **What is the cause of hypotension in theophylline overdose?**

Beta-adrenergic mediated vasodilation.

○ **What is the treatment for theophylline induced hypotension?**

IV fluids, Alpha-adrenergic agonists, Beta-adrenergic blockers.

○ **What methods of enhanced elimination are proven to lower serum levels of the drug?**

Charcoal hemoperfusion, hemodialysis, and multi-dose activated charcoal.

○ **What is the preferred method of enhanced elimination in severe theophylline toxicity?**

Charcoal hemoperfusion.

○ **What is the clearance of theophylline by charcoal hemoperfusion?**

225 mL/min.

○ **What is the mechanism of theophylline-induced hypokalemia?**

Shift of potassium into cells via beta-adrenergic stimulation.

○ **What percentage of theophylline is bound to plasma proteins?**

50%.

○ **Name the three common methylxanthines.**

Theophylline, caffeine, theobromine.

○ **Theophylline is an active metabolite of what drug?**

Caffeine - particularly in neonates.

○ **Name four elimination products of theophylline.**

3-methylxanthine, 1,3-dimethyluric acid, 1-methylxanthine (which is further metabolized to 1-methyluric acid).

○ **What is the active metabolite of theophylline?**

1,3-dimethyluric acid.

○ **Why may orogastric lavage be ineffective in removing pills after a theophylline overdose?**

The pills are usually too large to fit into even large bore orogastric tubes.

○ **What toxic effect of theophylline overdose may make therapy with activated charcoal difficult?**

Severe nausea and vomiting.

○ **How often should activated charcoal be administered to a patient with severe theophylline toxicity?**

Every hour.

○ **What is two possible adverse effect of charcoal administration in a sustained-release theophylline overdose?**

Vomiting, bezoar formation.

○ **What is one possible problem with whole-bowel irrigation with PEG solution in a patient with sustained-release theophylline overdose?**

Decreased effectiveness of activated charcoal.

○ **Should phenytoin be administered to a patient with theophylline-induced seizures?**

No.

○ **How often should theophylline levels be checked after overdose?**

Every one to two hours.

○ **What level of theophylline is an indication for charcoal hemoperfusion?**

90 ug/mL.

○ **Name some indications for charcoal hemoperfusion in theophylline toxicity?**

Seizures, hypotension unresponsive to IV fluids, ventricular dysrhythmias, vomiting despite antiemetic therapy.

○ **In what other instances may charcoal hemoperfusion be indicated?**

Rapidly rising theophylline level, significant underlying medical issues.

○   **What abnormality may be seen on the CBC in theophylline overdose?**

Increased white blood cell count.

○   **Which age groups of patients are at higher risk of toxicity in theophylline overdose?**

Neonates and the elderly.

○   **What two mechanisms make activated charcoal effective in theophylline overdose?**

It binds the unabsorbed theophylline in the gut and decreases serum levels by "gastrointestinal dialysis".

○   **What is the initial dose of fomepizole in ethylene glycol toxicity?**

15 mg/kg.

○   **What is the toxic metabolite of methanol?**

Methanol is metabolized by alcohol dehydrogenase to formaldehyde which is metabolized by aldehyde dehydrogenase to formic acid. Formic acid causes the severe metabolic acidosis and blindness.

○   **Which is the most intoxicating: methanol, ethylene glycol or isopropanol?**

CNS intoxication from alcohols is directly related to their number of carbon atoms.
Isopropanol > ethylene glycol, ethanol > methanol.

○   **What are the indications for ethanol of fomepizole therapy in acute ethylene glycol ingestion?**

Ethylene glycol > 20mg/dL, osmol gap > 5 mosm/L and metabolic acidosis.

○   **Which toxic alcohol ingestion is not effectively treated with 4-MP?**

Isopropyl.

○   **What are the indications for hemodialysis in acute ethylene glycol ingestion?**

Ethylene glycol > 20 mg/dL, osmol gap > 10 mosm/L, metabolic acidosis and renal failure.

○   **Which commercial products contain methanol?**

Windshield washing fluid, deicing solutions, carburetor cleaners, paint removers/thinners, model airplane fuels, antifreeze and gasohol.

○   **How is methanol excreted?**

10% is excreted unchanged in the lungs. 3% is excreted unchanged in the kidneys and most is metabolized in the liver to $CO_2$ and $H_2O$.

○   **Which commercial products contain ethylene glycol?**

Ethylene glycol is most commonly associated with antifreeze, but is also found in fire extinguishers, inks, pesticides, adhesives and in air conditioning and solar heating systems.

○ **How is ethylene glycol excreted?**

Ethylene glycol is metabolized in the liver and 20% is excreted unchanged in the urine. This renal excretion accounts for all of the excretion of the drug in patients who are receiving ethanol or fomepizole.

○ **What is the first metabolite of ethylene glycol?**

Ethylene glycol is metabolized by alcohol dehydrogenase to glycoaldehyde. Glycoaldehyde is metabolized to glycolic acid, then glyoxylic acid and then oxalic acid.

○ **Which toxic alcohol is metabolized to lactic acid and maybe associated with both an osmolal gap and a severe anion gap metabolic acidosis?**

Propylene glycol.

○ **What is "sudden sniffing death"?**

Inhalation of hydrocarbons for their euphoric effects, particularly halogenated hydrocarbons like trichloroethane, may sensitize the myocardium to the effects of catecholamines. Intense activity after "sniffing" or "huffing" may lead to ventricular fibrillation and sudden death.

○ **What quality of hydrocarbon compounds describes the tendency of a liquid to become a gas?**

Volatility.

○ **What quality of hydrocarbon compounds describes the tendency of a liquid to resist flow?**

Viscosity.

○ **Hydrocarbon ingestions account for what percent of poison center calls in the U.S.?**

About 5%.

○ **What is the primary target organ in serious petroleum distillate ingestions?**

The lungs.

○ **Following ingestion of petroleum products, how do they enter the lungs?**

By aspiration, not via systemic spread.

○ **What do aspirated hydrocarbons do in the lung?**

They interfere with surfactant activity.

○ **What type of pneumonia results from the aspiration of the higher density hydrocarbons?**

Lipoid pneumonia.

○ **What is the most worrisome cardiac effect following inhalation of halogenated hydrocarbons?**

Myocardial sensitization and lethal arrhythmias.

○ **T/F: The findings on chest x-ray correlate well with symptoms following hydrocarbon aspiration.**

False.

○ **What is turpentine made from?**

Pine oil.

○ **What is the major toxicity of petroleum distillates?**

Pneumonitis.

○ **What characteristics (surface tension, viscosity, and volatility) of petroleum distillates increase the risk of aspiration?**

Low surface tension, low viscosity, and high volatility.

○ **Which is the most important of these?**

Viscosity.

○ **Do petroleum distillates arrive at the lung, where they are toxic, through gastrointestinal absorption (and transport via the blood stream) or through aspiration.**

Aspiration.

○ **Do substances with viscosity >100 Saybolt Seconds Universal (SSU) have a high or low aspiration potential?**

Low.

○ **What do petroleum distillates do to the lung when aspirated?**

Inhibit surfactant and also directly damage.

○ **Does the inhalation of petroleum distillates do the same?**

No.

○ **What is the cardiac toxicity of hydrocarbons that are ingested?**

Sensitization to catecholamines, and resultant malignant arrhythmias.

○ **Are there always chest radiograph abnormalities in significant hydrocarbon aspirations within the first few hours after ingestion?**

No.

○ **If a patient after having ingested gasoline remains asymptomatic for 6 hours after ingestion, is it likely that the pulmonary toxicity will develop?**

No.

○ **Is gastric decontamination (lavage, charcoal) recommended for petroleum distillates?**

No.

○ **Why?**

Absorption is minimal, systemic toxicity is minimal, and decontamination increases the risk of aspiration.

○ **Because terpenes (such as pine oil, or turpentine) are more viscous, they are less of an aspiration risk, but they have more toxic than other hydrocarbons to which two organ systems?**

CNS, GI.

○ **All chlorinated short chain aliphatic hydrocarbons affect which two organ systems?**

CNS, skin.

○ **What is "degreaser's flush"?**

Skin flushing seen when workers exposed to trichloroethylene drink ethanol.

○ **What is the biochemical basis for this reaction?**

Competitive inhibition of aldehyde dehydrogenase.

○ **What is the usual cause of death in acute poisoning from chlorinated hydrocarbons?**

Solvent induced narcosis.

○ **Why is the liver toxicity of chlorinated hydrocarbons delayed by at least hours if not days?**

Toxicity is from bioreactive metabolites such as free radicals or epoxides.

○ **A teenager presenting with severe generalized weakness, with the smell of paint/glue on him, has been abusing _____.**

Toluene.

○ **How does this cause the severe weakness or paralysis?**

Toluene causes Type I (distal) Renal Tubular Acidosis and severe acute hypokalemia.

○ **What is the main serious toxicity of camphor?**

Seizures.

○ **Can 1 g (10 mL of Campho-Phenique) cause death in a child?**

Yes.

○ **This 10-year-old boy was playing with his mother's epi-penTM when it discharged into his finger. His thumb is erythematous and painful at the base, but pale and numb at the tip. He has no capillary refill in the tip of the finger. Is there a therapy for this?**

Phentolamine given subcutaneously may relieve the alpha vasoconstriction. Phentolamine was injected subcutaneously in this child's finger and capillary refill was regained in a few minutes.

○ **What is the dose in an epi-penTM?**

Epi-penTM contains 0.3 cc of 1:1000 epinephrine, or 0.3mg of epinephrine.

○ **You see this snake in North America. Is it poisonous?**

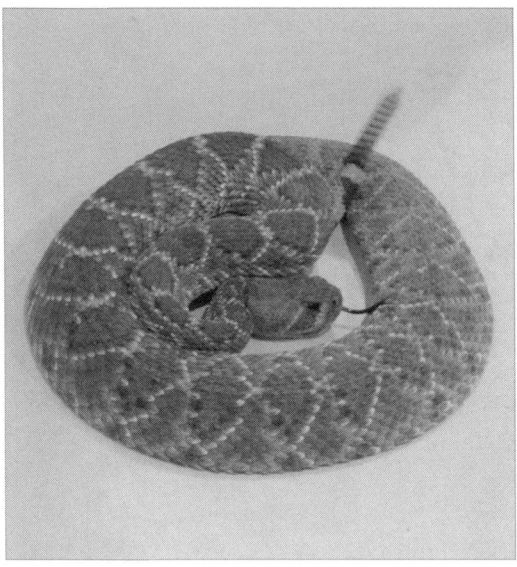

Yes. This snake can be identified as a pit viper by several characteristics: a pit located just below the halfway point between its eye and nostril, elliptical-shaped pupils, triangular head, and its rattle.

○ **Is this snake's bite always poisonous?**

Rattlesnakes have about a 20% rate of 'dry bites', or bites that do not inject venom. Dry bites are more likely in defensive bites, rather than when the snake is hunting.

○ **What is the possible toxicity related to a bite from this snake?**

Local toxicity will include swelling and pain. Systemic symptoms include nausea, vomiting, lightheadedness, metallic taste in mouth as well as thrombocytopenia, coagulopathy, renal failure, and hemolysis.

○ **Would the Crotalidae Polyvalent Anti-venin (Wyeth) treat this bite?**

Yes, the Crotalidae Polyvalent Anti-venin is active against rattlesnakes (crotalus and sistrurus), agkistrodon species (copperheads, water moccasins) and some South American and Asian snakes. This snake is a western diamondback.

○ **How is the Crotalidae Polyvalent Anti-venin produced?**

The polyvalent anti-venin is produced with the venom of the western diamondback, eastern diamondback, tropical rattlesnake and the fer-de-lance. These venoms are injected into horses. The horse's serum is then used to isolate the IgG. Unfortunately, may patients have allergic reactions to this anti-venin and most patients who have several vials will develop serum sickness.

○ **What are the toxicologic causes of basal ganglia infarct in children?**

Carbon monoxide and methanol.

O **This patient has a carboxyhemoglobin level of 40% and is unconscious. What therapy is indicated?**

The patient should be placed on 100% oxygen as soon as possible. If the patient is at a center that has rapid access to a hyperbaric chamber, hyperbaric oxygen therapy may be helpful, particularly if the patient lost consciousness.

# METABOLIC, ENDOCRINE AND NUTRITION

○ **What are the causes of factitious hyponatremia?**

Hyperglycemia, hyperlipidemia, or hyperproteinemia.

○ **How does hyperglycemia lead to hyponatremia?**

Because glucose stays in the extracellular fluid, hyperglycemia draws water out of the cell into the extracellular fluid. Each 100 mg/dL increase in plasma glucose decreases the serum sodium by 1.6 to 1.8 mEq/L.

○ **What is the most common cause of hypovolemic hyponatremia in children?**

Viral gastroenteritis. Vomiting and/or diarrhea occurs with this condition.

○ **What is the most common cause of euvolemic hyponatremia in children?**

Syndrome of inappropriate secretion of antidiuretic hormone (SIADH). Causes include CNS disorders, medications, tumors, and pulmonary disorders.

○ **What are the signs and symptoms of hyponatremia?**

Weakness, nausea, anorexia, vomiting, confusion, lethargy, seizures, and coma.

○ **What are the most common causes of hypotonic fluid loss leading to hypernatremia?**

Diarrhea, vomiting, hyperpyrexia, and excessive sweating.

○ **What are the signs and symptoms of hypernatremia?**

Confusion, muscle irritability, seizures, respiratory paralysis, and coma.

○ **What are the ECG findings of a patient with hypokalemia?**

Flattened T-waves, depressed ST segments, prominent P- and U-waves, and prolonged QT and PR intervals.

○ **What are the ECG findings for a patient with hyperkalemia?**

Peaked T-waves, prolonged QT and PR intervals, diminished P-waves, depressed T-waves, QRS widening, levels exceeding 10 mEq/L, and a classic sine wave.

○ **What is the first ECG finding for a patient with hyperkalemia?**

The development of tall peaked T-waves at levels of 5.6–6.0 mEq/L, which is best seen in the precordial leads.

○ **What is the quickest way to stabilize the myocardium in a patient with hyperkalemia?**

Administration of calcium gluconate (10%) 10-20 mL, IV with an onset of action of 1-3 minutes.

○ **What are some causes of hyperkalemia?**

Acidosis, tissue necrosis, hemolysis, blood transfusions, GI bleed, renal failure, Addison's disease, primary hypoaldosteronism, excess po K+ intake, RTA IV, and medication (such as succinylcholine, β-blockers, captopril, spironolactone, triamterene, amiloride, and high dose penicillin).

○ **What are the causes of hypocalcemia?**

Shock, sepsis, multiple blood transfusions, hypoparathyroidism, vitamin D deficiency, pancreatitis, hypomagnesemia, alkalosis, phosphate overload, chronic renal failure, hypoalbuminemia, and medication, such as Dilantin, phenobarbital, heparin, theophylline, cimetidine, and gentamicin.

○ **What is the most common cause of hyperkalemia?**

Lab error. Chronic renal failure is the most common cause of "true hyperkalemia."

○ **What are the most common causes of hypercalcemia?**

In descending order, malignancy, primary hyperparathyroidism, and thiazide diuretics.

○ **What are the signs and symptoms of hypercalcemia?**

The most common gastrointestinal symptoms are anorexia and constipation. A classic mnemonic can be used to remember them:

Stones:          renal calculi.
Bones:           osteolysis.
Abdominal groans: peptic ulcer disease and pancreatitis.
Psychic overtones: psychiatric disorders.

○ **What is the initial treatment for hypercalcemia?**

Patients with hypercalcemia are dehydrated because high calcium levels interfere with ADH and the ability of the kidney to concentrate urine. Therefore, the initial treatment is restoration of the extracellular fluid with 2 times maintenance level of normal saline within 24 hours. After the patient is rehydrated, administer Furosemide in doses of 1 to 3 mg/kg.

○ **What is the most common cause of hyperphosphatemia?**

Acute and chronic renal failure.

○ **What are the two primary causes of primary adrenal insufficiency?**

Tuberculosis and autoimmune destruction account for 90% of the cases.

○ **What are the signs and symptoms of primary adrenal insufficiency?**

Fatigue, weakness, weight loss, anorexia, hyperpigmentation, nausea, vomiting, abdominal pain, diarrhea, and orthostatic hypotension.

○ **What characteristic lab findings are associated with primary adrenal insufficiency?**

Hyperkalemia, hyponatremia, hypoglycemia, azotemia (if volume depletion is present), and a mild metabolic acidosis.

○ **How should acute adrenal insufficiency be treated?**

Administration of hydrocortisone (2 mg/kg) and crystalloid fluids containing dextrose.

○ **What are the main causes of death during an adrenal crisis?**

Circulatory collapse and hyperkalemia-induced arrhythmias.

○ **What are the causes of acute adrenal crisis?**

It occurs secondary to a major stress, such as surgery, severe injury, or any other illness in a patient with primary or secondary adrenal insufficiency.

○ **What is thyrotoxicosis, and what are the causes?**

A hypermetabolic state that occurs secondary to excess circulating thyroid hormone caused by thyroid hormone overdose, thyroid hyperfunction, or thyroid inflammation.

○ **What is the most common cause of hypoglycemia seen in the ED.**

An insulin reaction in a diabetic patient.

○ **What is the role of phosphate replacement during the treatment of DKA?**

Phosphate is only required if serum phosphate is <1.0 mg/L.

○ **What is the most important "initial" step for the treatment of DKA?**

Fluid administration with 20 cc/kg normal saline.

○ **In the first two years of life, what is the most common cause of drug-induced hypoglycemia?**

Salicylates. Between 2 and 8, alcohol is the most likely cause, and between 11 and 30, insulin and sulfonylureas are the culprits.

○ **What is the most common type of hypoglycemia in a child?**

Ketotic hypoglycemia. Attacks usually occur when the child is stressed by caloric deprivation. This condition usually develops in boys between 18 months and 5 years of age. Attacks may be episodic and are more frequent in the morning or during periods of illness.

○ **What are the neurologic signs and symptoms of hypoglycemia?**

Hypoglycemia may produce mental and neurologic dysfunction. Neurologic manifestations can include paresthesias, cranial nerve palsies, transient hemiplegia, diplopia, decerebrate posturing, and clonus.

○ **What are the complications of bicarbonate therapy in DKA?**

Paradoxical CSF acidosis, cardiac arrhythmias, decreased oxygen delivery to tissue, and fluid and sodium overload and possible cerebral edema.

❍ **What lab findings are expected with diabetic ketoacidosis?**

Elevated ß-hydroxybutyrate, acetoacetate, acetone, and glucose. Ketonuria and glucosuria are present. Serum bicarbonate levels, $pCO_2$, and pH are decreased. Potassium may be initially elevated but falls when the acidosis is corrected.

❍ **Outline the basic treatment for DKA.**

Administer fluids. Start with normal saline (20 cc/kg bolus), followed by potassium (100-200 mEq in the first 12-24 hours). Prescribe insulin, 0.1 units/kg bolus, then 0.1 units/kg/hr infusion. (Ed. Note: Many physicians no longer give bolus.) Add glucose to the IV fluid when the glucose levels fall below 250 mg/dL and give the patient potassium phosphate as supplement.

❍ **What is the most common cause of secondary adrenal insufficiency and adrenal crisis?**

Iatrogenic adrenal suppression from prolonged steroid use. Rapid withdrawal of steroids may lead to collapse and death.

❍ **An increase of $pCO_2$ of 10 mm Hg leads to an expected decrease in pH of about:**

0.08.

❍ **A decrease of $pCO_2$ of 10 mm Hg leads to an expected increase in pH of about:**

0.13.

❍ **What expected increase in pH is associated with a rise in $HCO_3$ of 5.0 mEq/L?**

0.08.

❍ **What expected decrease in pH is associated with a decrease in $HCO_3$ of 5.0 mEq/L?**

0.10.

❍ **How is the anion gap calculated from electrolyte values?**

Anion gap = $Na-Cl-CO_2$. The normal gap is $12^{+/-} 4$ mEq/L.

❍ **What is the most common endocrine disorder of childhood and adolescence?**

Diabetes mellitus (DM).

❍ **What are the two primary causes of metabolic alkalosis?**

Loss of hydrogen and chloride from the stomach and overzealous diuresis with loss of hydrogen, potassium, and chloride.

❍ **What are the peak age groups in children who develop IDDM?**

Between the ages of 5 and 7 and at puberty.

❍ **What is the equation for determining serum osmolarity?**

Osmserum = [serum Na+(mEq/L) + K+(mEq/L)] x 2 + (glucose(mg/dL) / (18) + (BUN(mg/dL) / (3).

○    **What condition should be suspected in a child who presents with lethargy, weight loss, and new onset enuresis in a previously toilet trained child?**

New onset DM.

○    **How does a child with DKA present?**

The child will present with vomiting, polyuria, dehydration, Kussmaul breathing and abdominal pain.

○    **What are the dangers of administering $HCO_3^-$ to a child with DKA?**

Alkalosis shifts the oxygen distribution curve to the left ultimately diminishing the release of oxygen to peripheral tissue. Also, use of $HCO_3^-$ can result in a paradoxical cerebral acidosis and is associated with cerebral edema.

○    **What is the Primary life threatening complication in the aggressive treatment of DKA?**

Cerebral edema. It occurs in < 1% of pediatric patients in DKA. It carries a 40% - 90% mortality and is responsible for 50% - 60% of deaths due to DKA.

○    **What signs and symptoms should a physician look for when considering cerebral edema in a patient being treated for DKA?**

Change in mental status, "delirious outbursts", bradycardia, vomiting, decreased reflexes, and changes in pupillary response.

○    **What percent of pediatric patients have DKA at their first hospital presentation?**

DKA is present at 25% - 40% of initial presentations of newly diagnosed juvenile onset diabetics.

○    **What is the most serious immediate life threatening risk to a child with DKA?**

Dehydration. While patients may have hyperglycemia and metabolic acidosis, dehydration is the most serious life threatening condition.

○    **When a child in DKA presents to the emergency department, The K+ will be increased, decreased, or normal?**

Total body K+ is depleted though serum levels may be normal. Transcellular shifts during acidosis move K+ extracellular in exchange for H+ ions. The osmotic diuresis due to the hyperglycemia results in overall K+ loss. In addition, the dehydration stimulates aldosterone secretion which further contributes to K+ excretion.

○    **What are the risk factors for development of cerebral edema in a patient in DKA?**

High $CO_2^-$ and BUN at presentation, and $HCO_3^-$ use.

○    **How do you calculate the water deficit in a patient with DKA?**

The fluid deficit is estimated to be approximately 10% of the patient's weight in kilograms.

○    **How do you determine if a child in DKA requires $HCO_3^-$?**

It should not be used unless the pH is < 6.8. Acidosis will be corrected with fluids and insulin.

○ **When should glucose be added to the IVF in the treatment of DKA?**

When the blood glucose level reaches 250 mg/dL the IVF should be changed to D5.45%NS.

○ **How often should you monitor the serum K+ in a child with DKA?**

The K+ should be checked every 2 - 4 hours until acidosis is corrected.

○ **Why do DKA patients experience changes in vision following the initiation of therapy?**

Rehydration in conjunction with the correction of hyperglycemia causes fluid shifts in the eyes with reversible lens distortion.

○ **What are the signs and symptoms of hypoglycemia?**

They are nonspecific but may include seizures, tremulousness, confusion, palpitations, sweating, and irritability.

○ **How is a child with hypoglycemia treated?**

Administer 2.5 ml/kg of 10% dextrose. If convulsions are present increase to 4ml/kg of 10% dextrose. Maintain the blood glucose level using 8 mg/kg/min of a 10% dextrose solution.

○ **What is the most common cause for hypothyroidism in the neonate?**

Thyroid dysgenesis.

○ **What is the most common thyroid anomaly in childhood?**

The thyroglossal duct cyst which is remnant of the thyroglossal duct.

○ **Are infants born with complete thyroid agenesis symptomatic at birth?**

No. Transplacental T4 provides adequate thyroid hormone however the TSH level will still be elevated enough for detection of the abnormality.

○ **A mass at the base of the tongue in a newborn with adequate T4 levels is suggestive of what disorder?**

A sublingual thyroid or a thyroglossal duct cyst.

○ **What is the possible cause for a transient congenital hypothyroidism?**

Maternal antibodies that inhibit TSH binding.

○ **What are the signs of neonatal hypothyroidism?**

Poor appetite, sluggishness, macroglossia, somnolence, large abdomen, hypothermia, molted skin, constipation, edema and bradycardia.

○ **What is the treatment for neonatal hypothyroidism?**

Sodium-L-Thyroxine (10 - 15 mcgs/kg in neonates).

○   **What is the most common cause of a acquired hypothyroidism?**

Lymphocytic thyroiditis.

○   **What is the most common clinical manifestation of lymphocytic thyroiditis?**

The appearance of a goiter.

○   **What is the differential diagnosis of a congenital goiter?**

Antithyroid drugs or iodine containing medications used during pregnancy, hyperthyroid infants, iodine deficient infants and rarely congenital teratoma.

○   **Is Grave's disease more common in boys or girls?**

Girls are affected five times as much as boys.

○   **What are the classical signs and symptoms of Grave's disease?**

Emotional lability, autonomic hyperactivity, exophthalmos, tremor, weight loss or increased appetite with no weight gain, diarrhea, and a goiter in nearly all affected individuals.

○   **How is Grave's disease confirmed by laboratory testing?**

One would find increased bound and free T3 and T4 with decreased TSH.

○   **What treatment options exist for children with Grave's disease? What treatment is recommended?**

Children can be managed medically with propylthiouracil(PTU) or methimazole, surgically with a subtotal thyroidectomy or with radioiodine therapy. Medical management is the treatment of choice.

○   **What are the differences between PTU and methimazole?**

Methimazole is ten times more potent on a weight basis allowing it to be a once a day medication. PTU is predominately protein bound making it a better choice in pregnant and nursing mothers as its ability to cross the placental membrane is limited.

○   **What are the respective doses of PTU and methimazole?**

PTU is given at 5 - 10 mg/kg/d dived T.I.D. while methimazole is .5 - 1.0 mg/kg/d given either QD. or B.I.D.

○   **What is the most common physical finding in Grave's disease?**

Goiter.

○   **What medication is available to treat the autonomic hyperactivity associated with Grave's disease?**

Propranolol, a beta blocker dosed at .5 - 2.0 mg/kg/d divided T.I.D.

○   **What is the most common cause for congenital hyperthyroidism?**

Transplacental passage of thyroid receptor antibodies from a mother with Grave's disease.

○ **What are the three largest concerns with surgical management of Grave's disease?**

Hyper or hypothyroidism depending on the amount of tissue removed, hypoparathyroidism, and vocal cord paralysis.

○ **What is the most common disorder of thyroid gland function in children presenting to the ED?**

Thyrotoxicosis.

○ **What commonly occurs in the newborn whose mother suffered from hyperparathyroidism during pregnancy?**

Hypocalcemia resulting from suppression of the fetal parathyroids due to the elevated serum calcium in the maternal circulation.

○ **What is the most common disorder causing thyrotoxicosis in children?**

Grave's disease.

○ **What percent of children with hyperthyroidism experience a thyroid storm?**

Approximately 1%.

○ **What are the symptoms of child suffering from a thyroid storm?**

Tachycardia, systolic hypertension, tremulousness, delirium and hyperthermia.

○ **How do you manage acute thyrotoxicosis?**

Propranolol at 10 mg/kg IV over 10 - 15 minutes for hypertension and increased metabolic rate. Lugol's iodide, 5 drops PO every eight hrs or Na+ iodide 125 - 250 mg/d IV over 24 hrs will stop thyroxine production.

○ **What measures can be taken to further reduce peripheral conversion of T4 to T3?**

Oral dexamethasone at .2 mg/kg or oral hydrocortisone 5 mg/kg.

○ **What is the differential diagnosis of acute primary adrenal insufficiency?**

Congenital adrenal hypoplasia, autoimmunity, TB, infection, trauma, and adrenal hemorrhage.

○ **What are the clinical manifestations of adrenocortical insufficiency?**

Low blood pressure, muscular weakness, weight loss, anorexia and salt craving.

○ **What emergency should be suspected in patients who present with cyanosis, cold skin, thready pulse, hypotension and tachypnea?**

Addison's crisis.

○ **What conditions have been implicated in precipitating adrenal crisis?**

Infection, trauma, fatigue, and various medications.

## METABOLIC, ENDOCRINE AND NUTRITION

○ **Which symptom is most commonly seen in children with Addison's disease?**

Hypoglycemia.

○ **What is the Waterhouse-Friderichsen Syndrome?**

Primary adrenal insufficiency due to adrenal hemorrhage. It is often secondary to meningococcemia induced shock.

○ **What are the causes of secondary adrenal insufficiency?**

Diminished ACTH levels secondary to long term glucocorticoid treatment.

○ **At what decreased Na+ concentration do children generally become symptomatic?**

When the serum Na+ is less than 120 mEq/L.

○ **What syndrome is likely to be present in a 7-year-old child who presents with nausea, vomiting, and a single seizure with laboratory results consistent with hyponatremia and increased urine osmolarity?**

The syndrome of inappropriate antidiuretic hormone (SIADH).

○ **What is SIADH?**

It is a the syndrome of inappropriate ADH(antidiuretic hormone) secretion. It occurs when the plasma vasopressin levels are abnormally elevated for the corresponding plasma osmolarity.

○ **What is the most common cause of SIADH in children?**

Infection. 50% of children with bacterial meningitis have concomitant SIADH.

○ **How is SIADH treated?**

Most important is treating the underlying condition. Fluid restriction and demeclocycline have been proven to increase serum Na+. In emergent situations, furosemide, in conjunction with 300 ml/M2 of 1.5% NaCl may be used.

○ **What is the emergent treatment for a hyponatremic child suffering from SIADH?**

3 ml/kg of 3% saline q10-20 minutes until the symptoms resolve. A single dose of 1 mg/kg of furosemide may be used. 5 - 10 mg/kg of phenytoin IV can be used to inhibit ADH secretion as well as help to prophylax against possible seizures. Treating the underlying condition however is still the most important consideration.

○ **What is the danger of correcting the Na+ too vigorously?**

Central pontine myelinolysis.

○ **How is the diagnosis of diabetes insipidus made in a child?**

By finding hypernatremia, increased serum osmolarity and decreased urine osmolarity.

O **What is the danger of vigorously hydrating a patient who has hypernatremia due to diabetes insipidus?**

Cerebral edema, seizures and death.

O **What additional adjuncts can be used in addition to volume replacement in a patient with diabetes insipidus?**

Intranasal administration of DDAVP at 0.4 g/kg.

O **Is Cushing's disease different from Cushing's syndrome?**

Cushing's disease results from pituitary adenomas while Cushing's syndrome is elevated cortisol levels from various causes including; paraneoplastic syndromes, primary adrenal tumors, and exogenous use of cortisol.

O **What is the most common cause of excess cortisol production in infants?**

A functioning adrenocortical tumor.

O **What is the most common cause of childhood hyperparathyroidism?**

A single parathyroid adenoma.

O **What are the clinical manifestations of hyperparathyroidism regardless of cause?**

Anorexia, nausea, vomiting, constipation, polydipsia, polyuria, fever, weight loss, kidney stones and muscular weakness.

O **What is the most common cause for secondary hyperparathyroidism in children?**

Chronic renal disease. The formation of the active form of vitamin D takes place in the kidney. With diseased kidneys the active form of vitamin D is not made resulting in decreased intestinal absorption of calcium.

O **What is the treatment of choice for symptomatic hypercalcemia (>15 mg/dL)?**

Isotonic saline is the first treatment.

O **In a child with resolving DKA, when do you cease insulin infusion?**

When ketones have been cleared, metabolic acidosis has resolved, blood glucose has normalized and the patient can eat and drink.

O **A child is brought in obtunded and with acute hypoglycemia, what should be the first treatment modality?**

IV glucose infusion (2-3 mg/kg of $D_{10}W$ or 1ml/kg of $D_{25}W$).

O **What causes pseudohyponatremia?**

High glucose, triglycerides, or protein.

○ **What are the daily sodium requirements of premature and full term newborns?**

3-4 mEq/kg/d for premature and 1-2 mEq/kg/d for full term.

○ **In which conditions are electrolytes considered high yield?**

Age <6 months, vomiting, tachycardia, dry mucous membrane, and capillary refill >2 seconds. The presence any of these criteria is 100% sensitive for significant abnormalities.

○ **What is the formula for obtaining the true calcium level with hypoalbuminemia?**

Subtract 0.8 mg/dL from total serum calcium for each 1 g/dL decrease in serum albumin below normal.

○ **What are the clinical findings in patient with hypocalcemia?**

Chvostek sign (tapping on facial nerve causes twitch), Trousseau sign (carpal spasm after inflating BP cuff for 3 minutes), hyperactive reflexes, low BP, or CHF.

○ **What is the relationship between acidosis and hyperkalemia?**

A decrease in the pH of 0.1 will increase K+ 0.3-1.3 mEq/L due to the H+/K+ exchange pump.

# SUDDEN INFANT DEATH SYNDROME AND APPARENT LIFE-THREATENING EVENT

○ **Sudden Infant Death Syndrome (SIDS) is the most common cause of death for infants in the first year of life. It occurs at a rate of 2/1000, or 10,000/year. What are 6 risk factors associated with SIDS?**

1) Prematurity with low birth weight.
2) Previous episode of apnea or apparent life-threatening event (ALTE).
3) Mother is a substance abuser.
4) Family history of SIDS.
5) Male gender.
6) Low socioeconomic status.

○ **What are three modifiable risk factors for sudden infant death syndrome (SIDS).**

Prone sleeping position, maternal smoking, lack of breastfeeding.

○ **SIDS has a bimodal distribution. At what ages do the peaks occur?**

2.5 and 4 months.

○ **Define failure to thrive (FTT).**

FTT is defined as infants who are below the third percentile in height or weight or whose weight is less than 80% of the ideal weight for their age. Almost all patients with FTT are under 5 years old, while the majority of children are 6–12 months old.

○ **What is the most common cause of FTT?**

Poor intake is responsible for 70% of FTT cases. One third of these cases are educational problems, ranging from inaccurate knowledge of what to feed a child to over-diluting formula to "make it stretch further."

○ **What is the prognosis for patients with FTT?**

Only 1/3 of patients with FTT due to environmental factors have a normal life. The remainder grow up small for their size, and the majority also have developmental, psychological, and educational deficiencies.

○ **What is the definition of apnea in an infant?**

Apnea is either cessation of breathing for more than 20 seconds, or a shorter period associated with cyanosis or bradycardia.

○ **What is the definition of ALTE?**

An Apparent Life Threatening Event is apnea associated with color change (cyanosis or redness), a loss of muscle tone, and choking or gagging.

○ **Compared to an otherwise healthy infant, how much more likely is a child with a history of ALTE to go on to have SIDS?**

About 3-5 times more likely.

○ **What percentage of infants who have SIDS had a prior ALTE?**

About 5%.

○ **What is the disposition for a patient diagnosed with an ALTE?**

Admit to a monitored bed.

# NEUROLOGY

○ **What are causes that predispose a child to stroke?**

Prematurity, Sickle Cell anemia, cyanotic congenital heart disease, coagulation disorders, trauma and arterial venous malformation.

○ **What data exist about the use of TPA for the treatment of stroke in neonates, infants and children?**

There is little data regarding the use of TPA for the treatment of strokes in patients less than 18 years of age. However, thrombolytic drugs may have some role in very select and unusual pediatric clinical entities.

○ **What are signs of increased intracranial pressure?**

Altered mental status (combativeness, irritability, somnolence), abnormal pupils (pupillary dilatation, lack of response to light, unequal size), and abnormal motor posturing.

○ **What are indications for intubation of a comatose child?**

Depressed mental status can be associated with hypoventilation (and the development of hypoxia and hypercarbia), loss of protective air reflexes and increased intracranial pressure. Intubation is indicated for oxygenation, control of intracranial hypertension (through mild hyperventilation) and protection of the airway.

○ **What is Cushing's triad?**

Cushing's triad is the combination of bradycardia, hypertension and irregular ineffective respiration. It is a late sign of increased intracranial pressure and impending herniation.

○ **What three bacterial illnesses present with peripheral neurologic findings?**

Botulism, tetanus, and diphtheria.

○ **A child complains of blurry vision. On exam she has an abnormal pupil reflex and a white reflex on funduscopic examination. What is the treatment?**

Surgical removal of the eye. This is a retinoblastoma that can grow to other sites in the brain or body. This is an inheritable condition, and she should be counseled on the dangers when she is ready for children.

○ **What area of the brain is dysfunctional when a patient has Cheyne-Stokes respirations?**

The cortex. The nervous system is relying on diencephalic control.

○ **A 15-year-old presents with a history of being knocked unconscious for 10 seconds while playing touch football one week ago. Since then, he has had intermittent vertigo, nausea, vomiting, blurred vision, a headache, and malaise. His neuro exam and CT are normal. What is the diagnosis?**

Post concussive syndrome. Most individuals recover fully over a 2 to 6 week time span. However, a few of these cases have persistent deficits.

○ **A 16-year-old presents with progressively severe intermittent vertigo for 6 months and progressive unilateral hearing loss for 3 months. What is the diagnosis?**

Cerebellopontine angle tumor. Confirm diagnosis with a MRI scan.

○ **Differentiate between decerebrate and decorticate posturing.**

Decerebrate posturing is when the elbows and legs are extended which is indicative of a midbrain lesion.

Decorticate posturing is when the elbows are flexed and the legs are extended. This suggests a lesion in the thalamic region. Remember: DeCORticate = hands by the heart (cor).

○ **Differentiate between partial seizures and generalized seizures.**

Partial seizures arise from a single focus and may spread out, whereas generalized seizures involve the whole cerebral cortex. Absence and grand mal seizures are examples of generalized seizures.

○ **Recurrent seizures in patients with a history of febrile seizures generally occur in what time frame?**

About 85% occur within the first 2 years. The younger the child, the more likely recurrence will happen. If a patient has a febrile seizure in the first year of life the recurrence rate is 50%. If it occurs in the second year, the recurrence is only 25%.

○ **What will happen if you shine a light in the eyes of a patient who is in a diabetic coma?**

The pupils will constrict.

○ **Which is more common, a subdural hemorrhage or an epidural hemorrhage?**

A subdural. Subdurals can result from the tearing of the bridging veins. Bleeding occurs less rapidly because the veins, not arteries, are damaged.

○ **A 16-year-old woman complains of a throbbing, dull, unilateral headache that lasts for hours then goes away with sleep. She also has been nauseous and has vomited twice. She reports small areas of visual loss plus strange zigzag lines in her vision. What is the diagnosis?**

A classic migraine headache.

○ **What factors may precipitate migraine headaches?**

Bright lights, cheese, hot-dogs and other foods containing tyramine or nitrates, menstruation, monosodium glutamate, and stress.

○ **Describe the key signs and symptoms of a classic, a common, an ophthalmoplegic, and a hemiplegic migraine headache.**

1. Common: This headache is indeed the most common. It is a slow evolving headache that lasts for hours to days. A positive family history as well as two of the following are prevalent: Nausea or vomiting, throbbing quality, photophobia, unilateral pain, and increase with menses. Distinguishing feature from "Classic" migraine is the lack of visual symptoms.

2. Classic: Prodrome lasts up to 60 minutes. Most common symptom is visual disturbance, such as homonymous hemianopsia, scintillating scotoma, fortification spectra, and photophobia. Lip, face, and hand tingling, as well as aphasia and extremity weakness may occur. Nausea and vomiting may also result.

3. <u>Ophthalmoplegic</u>: Most frequently manifests in young adults. Patient has an outwardly deviated, dilated eye, with ptosis. The third, sixth, and fourth nerves are typically involved.

4. <u>Hemiplegic</u>: Unilateral motor and sensory symptoms, mild hemiparesis to hemiplegia are exhibited with this type of headache.

❍ **What elements in a patients history suggest an intracranial tumor?**

(1) Wake patients from their sleep (2) worse in the morning, (3) increase in severity with postural changes or Valsalva maneuvers, (4) are associated with nausea and vomiting (5) associated with focal defects or mental status changes, and (6) occur with a new onset of seizures.

❍ **A 17-year-old woman with a history of flu like symptoms (URI) one week ago now presents with vertigo, nausea, and vomiting. No auditory impairment or focal deficits are noted. What is the most likely cause of her problem?**

Labyrinthitis or vestibular neuronitis.

❍ **A 16-year-old female complains of weakness and tingling in her right arm and leg for 2 days. She reports an episode of right eye pain and blurred vision that resolved over one month, but the onset of that pain started 2 years ago. She also recalls a two week episode of intermittent blurred vision the previous year. What is the diagnosis?**

Presumptive multiple sclerosis. Confirm with MRI and CSF (look for oligoclonal bands).

❍ **What neoplastic process is most commonly associated with myasthenia gravis?**

Thymoma.

❍ **Which is the most common medication associated with Neuroleptic Malignant Syndrome?**

Haloperidol. Other drugs, especially antipsychotic medications, are also causative.

❍ **What is the hallmark motor finding in Neuroleptic Malignant Syndrome?**

"Lead pipe" rigidity.

❍ **What is the most common cause of syncope in children?**

Vasovagal or simple fainting (50%).

❍ **What is the significance of bilateral nystagmus with cold caloric testing?**

It signifies that an intact cortex, midbrain, and brainstem are present.

❍ **How are upper motor neuron (UMN) lesions of CN VII (facial nerve) distinguished from peripheral lesions?**

1. <u>UMN</u>: A unilateral weakness of the lower half of the face.
2. <u>Peripheral</u>: Involves the entire half of the face.

❍ **What symptoms form the classic tetrad seen in kernicterus?**

Choreoathetosis, supernuclear ophthalmoplegia, sensorineural hearing loss, and enamel hypoplasia.

○ **What is the most common cause of intermittent ataxia in children?**

Migraine headaches involving the basilar artery

○ **What are the most common cause of acute ataxia (onset < 24 hours)?**

Drug toxicity and infection.

○ **What are the three most common predisposing factors in the formation of a brain abscess?**

Cyanotic heart disease, otitis and sinusitis.

○ **What is the most common cranial neuropathy seen in Lyme disease?**

Unilateral or bilateral facial palsy. Less frequently, The VIII nerve can also be affected.

○ **What are growing skull fractures?**

These are seen as a complication of skull fracture in children under three years of age. They are caused by the presence of leptomeningeal cyst that is formed by an unrecognized dural laceration. It prevents the two sides of the bone from aligning together during recovery.

○ **When should steroids be used in the treatment of increased intracranial pressure (ICP)?**

Steroids are beneficial in the treatment of vasogenic edema, so should be used to treat increased ICP associated with tumors.

○ **What is the main difference in the history obtained between seizures and breath-holding spells?**

Breath-holding spells are always provoked. Cyanotic breath-holding spells are provoked by crying precipitated by fright, anger, pain, or frustration. Pallid breath-holding spells are provoked by pain, especially a minor bump to the head.

○ **Ophthalmoplegic migraine affects which cranial nerve?**

Cranial nerve III.

○ **Which toxic neuropathy can be clinically misdiagnosed in infants as Guillain-Barré syndrome?**

Botulism. Unlike in older patients that ingest the toxin, infants are usually colonized by the bacteria. A risk factor seems to be feeding the infant honey.

○ **What components of the history are the most important in evaluating a child with neurological problems?**

Developmental, perinatal, birth and family.

○ **What is the significance of a mildly depressed and pulsatile fontanelle in an infant?**

Nothing. This is normal.

○ **What is Gower's sign?**

A specific way to rise to standing from the supine position that is seen in certain forms of muscular dystrophy. The child first rolls over onto hands and knees. Then the child stands up by "walking" his/her hands up the leg.

○ **An adolescent presents to the ED with complaints of left lower leg weakness. CSF analysis shows elevated protein but normal WBC count. What idiopathic disease might be at work here?**

Guillain-Barré syndrome.

○ **What is the most useful test to diagnose multiple sclerosis in children?**

MRI showing multiple white matter plaques in the periventricular regions.

○ **In a child in a coma you elicit positive doll's eyes reflex. Does this mean the eyes move with the head, or away from the head?**

Away from the movement of the head. This sign determines viability of the brainstem. A positive sign means the brainstem is working properly.

○ **Which way do the eyes move in normal caloric testing?**

Remember the mnemonic COWS- Cold Opposite, Warm Same. Absence of the nystagmus occurs with eighth nerve damage.

○ **What is the most common cause of acute onset, painless monocular blindness in patients between 15-18?**

Optic neuritis. 60% of these patients eventually develop multiple sclerosis.

○ **How do older children with stroke present?**

Acute hemiplegia.

○ **What are the most common causes of childhood stroke?**

Congenital heart disease and sickle cell disease.

○ **T/F Ischemic strokes are more common in children than hemorrhagic strokes?**

False: Ischemic strokes and hemorrhagic strokes occur with equal frequency.

○ **What is the most common vascular etiology of childhood stroke?**

Moyamoya. This is a vascular condition that leads to occlusion of intracranial arteries.

○ **What is the most common cause of a hemorrhagic stroke in children?**

Arterial vascular malformation.

○ **What is the incidence of stroke reoccurrence in sickle cell patients not receiving adequate therapy?**

50%

❍   **What therapeutic measure decrease the reoccurrence of stroke in a patient with sickle cell disease?**

Chronic periodic blood transfusions and possible hydroxyurea.

❍   **A Babinski sign is indicative of an abnormality of what tract?**

Corticospinal. It is indicative of an upper motor neuron lesion.

❍   **What is the incidence of a child with a history of febrile seizures developing a convulsive disorder compared with a child who has never had a febrile seizure?**

It is the same.

❍   **What is the drug of choice for febrile seizures?**

No treatment is usually given, aside from reducing the fever.

❍   **A child is brought in with a new onset "tic". What is your treatment?**

None at this time. Simple clonic motor tics usually resolve spontaneously in less than a year.

❍   **What can you give to ameliorate the dystonic reactions sometimes seen in a patient taking haloperidol?**

Benztropine (Cogentin), trihexyphenidyl (Artane), and diphenhydramine (Benadryl).

❍   **What metabolic abnormalities can cause neonatal seizures?**

Hypoxemia, hypoglycemia, hypocalcemia, hypomagnesemia and hyponatremia.

❍   **What is the definition of ataxia?**

Ataxia is an impairment in the coordination of movement without the loss of muscle strength.

❍   **What is the most common posterior fossa tumor ?**

Astrocytoma.

❍   **Can ataxia be a manifestation of Guillain-Barré syndrome?**

Yes- if there is a significant sensory neuropathy present, there may be an impairment of afferent sensory input to the cerebellum, causing a "sensory ataxia", in addition to the muscle weakness and areflexia seen in these patients.

❍   **What clinical features define a simple febrile seizure?**

1. Brief duration, usually less than 15 minutes.
2. Generalized seizure.
3. Occur within the first 24 hours of a febrile illness.
4. Occur in children between 6 mo - 5 years of age.
5. Normal neurologic development.
6. Normal neurologic examination after the seizure.

○ **Will a child with simple febrile seizures have a normal electroencephalogram (EEG)?**

Yes.

○ **What clinical features characterize children with benign paroxysmal vertigo?**

1) Age less than 4 years; 2) sudden onset of vertigo; 3) autonomic symptoms, such as nausea, vomiting and sweating; 4) nystagmus.

○ **What symptoms and signs distinguish transverse myelitis from Guillain-Barré syndrome?**

Both transverse myelitis and acute polyneuritis share the acute onset of lower extremity weakness and paresthesias as presenting symptoms and signs. Patients with transverse myelitis will initially complain of back pain (in the absence of trauma) and urinary retention. Patients with acute polyneuritis will have bowel and bladder dysfunction later in the course. On physical examination of patients with transverse myelitis, a distinct "sensory level" will also be elicited; impairment of touch, pain and temperature sensation will be seen, but proprioception will remain intact.

○ **What is the pathophysiology of Guillain-Barré syndrome?**

The pathologic hallmark of acute polyneuritis is demyelination of motor and sensory nerves, thought to be due to an autoimmune process, causing the classic ascending paralysis, areflexia and paresthesias seen in these patients.

○ **What is the pathophysiology of myasthenia gravis?**

Antibodies against the acetylcholine receptor of the post-synaptic neuromuscular junction-this results in failure of neuromuscular transmission, with consequent fluctuating muscle weakness.

○ **What are the presenting signs and symptoms of juvenile myasthenia gravis?**

The juvenile form of myasthenia gravis accounts for 25% of all cases and is the predominant form seen in the pediatric population, usually in school-age children. Most patients will have ptosis, oculomotor palsies and truncal or limb weakness that becomes progressively worse with continued muscle activity.

○ **What is the "Tensilon test"?**

The Tensilon test secures the diagnosis of myasthenia gravis. Edrophonium (Tensilon), which is an anticholinesterase drug, is given slowly by the intravenous route. Patients with myasthenia gravis will have a brief, but dramatic, resolution of their muscle weakness.

○ **A 4-year-old presents with the acute onset of unsteadiness of gait. He has otherwise been well, except for a recent upper respiratory infection. Examination reveals ataxia, tremor and bilateral dysmetria. What is the most likely diagnosis?**

Acute cerebellar ataxia, which is characterized by the acute onset of ataxia in an otherwise healthy child, usually between the ages of 1 and 4 years. Antecedent viral infections precede the onset of symptoms in over half of patients. Resolution of symptoms usually occurs within 2 weeks of the onset of symptoms.

○ **What must be excluded in the above patient before the diagnosis of acute cerebellar ataxia?**

A posterior fossa mass or tumor.

○ **Is Lyme disease a common cause of seventh nerve palsy?**

Yes-there is a subset of patients with Lyme disease who present solely with an isolated seventh nerve palsy.

○ **What is the likelihood that a patient with Bell's Palsy will completely recover?**

Complete recovery is seen in up to 80% of patients, usually within three weeks of the onset of symptoms.

○ **What is the definition of " non-communicating" hydrocephalus?**

If the obstruction to the flow of cerebrospinal fluid occurs within the ventricular system, then non-communicating hydrocephalus results.

○ **What is the definition of "communicating" hydrocephalus?**

If the obstruction to the flow of cerebrospinal fluid occurs outside the ventricular system at the level of any of the exit foramina or if there is an excessive production of cerebrospinal fluid, then communicating hydrocephalus results.

○ **What is the most common cause of neonatal seizures?**

Hypoxic-ischemic encephalopathy, which accounts for nearly 60% of cases.

○ **What agents are useful to decrease the production of cerebrospinal fluid (CSF) in patients with hydrocephalus?**

Acetazolamide, furosemide and glycerol have all been used to decrease CSF production.

○ **What is "benign intracranial hypertension" (pseudotumor cerebri)?**

A syndrome in which patients have symptoms and signs (headache, papilledema) of increased intracranial pressure; however, physical examination shows no focal neurologic deficits or encephalopathy and there is no evidence of an intracranial mass or obstruction to the flow of CSF. CSF analysis will be normal except for increased opening pressure.

○ **What drugs are thought to be associated with the development of benign intracranial hypertension (pseudotumor cerebri)?**

Antibiotics, such as tetracycline, minocycline, penicillin, gentamicin; oral contraceptives; steroids; NSAIDS such as indomethacin; thyroid; lithium carbonate.

○ **What is the most common complication from a linear skull fracture?**

A subgaleal hematoma is the most common complication. These hematomas can become very large, especially if they liquefy and dissect through the subgaleal space.

○ **A 10-year-old presents with a large scalp laceration with an underlying depressed skull fracture that needs to be elevated in the OR; however, this will not occur for several hours. The child is otherwise stable. Should the overlying laceration be repaired before the child goes to the OR?**

Yes: rarely is the site of the laceration the site of incision to repair the depressed skull fracture. Meticulous wound care and closure will prevent hemorrhage and prolonged exposure of the fracture site to skin organisms, especially if there is a delay in definitive operative treatment. Antibiotic treatment to cover skin flora is also recommended.

○ **A child with a significant closed head injury develops generalized seizures. Which (intravenous) anticonvulsant should be administered?**

Phenytoin, as it will not cloud the sensorium or cause sedation, so that subsequent neurologic examinations can be done easily.

O   **A 5-month-old child presents with coma. There is no history of reported trauma or viral prodrome. On examination the child is afebrile, comatose, with decerebrate posturing and fixed, dilated pupils and a bulging fontanel. What other physical examination finding would help to confirm the diagnosis?**

Funduscopic examination-if retinal hemorrhages are present, then this is most likely a case of a shaking-impact injury. A CT scan may show subdural or intracranial hemorrhage.

O   **A child presents with severe somnolence and a two week history of gradually worsening headache. On examination he is somnolent and responsive only to pain. He also has bilateral sixth nerve palsies. What is the cause of his symptoms?**

A diffuse increase in intracranial pressure, probably the result of an intracranial mass.

O   **What type of breathing pattern is seen in patients with "Cheyne-Stokes" respirations?**

Patients with Cheyne-Stokes respirations will have periods of hyperpnea followed by shorter periods of apnea.

O   **Where is the dysfunction in the CNS in patients who have Cheyne-Stokes respirations?**

Patients with Cheyne-Stokes respirations have bilateral cerebral hemisphere dysfunction with normal brainstem function.

O   **In patients with true vertigo, at what levels of the CNS may the defect occur?**

Patients who have true vertigo have a vestibular defect that may be peripheral (involving the labyrinth in the inner ear or the vestibular nerve) or central (involving the vestibular nuclei and its central pathways).

O   **Can otitis media be a cause of vertigo in children?**

Yes.

O   **What is the most common cause of labyrinthitis in children?**

Viral disese like influenza, measles and mumps.

O   **Which symptoms help to distinguish vestibular neuronitis from labyrinthitis in children?**

Children with labyrinthitis will have hearing loss, while those with vestibular neuronitis will not.

O   **What clinical features characterize children with cyclic vomiting?**

Cyclic vomiting is a migraine variant that maybe present in young children. These patients will have cyclic, or even monthly, episodes of vomiting with abdominal pain that are alleviated by periods of deep sleep. Later in life, these children often develop migraine headaches.

O   **What clinical features characterize children with acute confusional states?**

Acute confusional states are migraine variants that have unusual presentations, such as the onset of headache that is followed by a period of vomiting, lethargy and confusion, disorientation and unresponsiveness. These episodes of "acute confusion" may last for several hours, after which the patient may have no memory of the event. There will be a family history of migraine headache.

O   **How does one make the diagnosis of acute confusional state?**

History of headache followed by a period of confusion or unresponsiveness that is not due to any organic cause and a family history or migraine headaches.

O   **A healthy 5-month-old infant presents with episodes of sudden flexion of the neck and upper extremities, occurring upon awakening. The child has been developing normally, the pregnancy and delivery were uneventful. The child has a normal neurologic exam, as well as a CT of the head which shows no abnormalities?**

This patient has infantile spasms, which often has an excellent prognosis for normal neuro-development.

O   **What drug(s) is(are) preferred for the management of infantile spasms?**

Adrenocorticotrophic hormone (ACTH) or prednisone-the dosage and length of therapy are controversial.

O   **What is the most common movement disorder in childhood?**

Transient tic disorder, which presents most often in boys. The movements consist of eye-blinking, throat clearing or other repetitive facial movements. These "tics" usually regress after one year and do not require drug treatment.

O   **A 6-month-old infant presents with a progressively enlarging, pulsating mass on his skull. He had fallen off the changing table and hit his head on the floor one month earlier, but did not seek medical care at the time. What is the most likely diagnosis?**

A leptomeningeal cyst, which is an unusual complication of linear skull fractures. The cyst is caused by interposition of the leptomeninges and occasionally, traumatized brain, through the interrupted dura and edges of the fracture. The mass will then expand because of communication with the CSF space and the cyst.

O   **A 6-year-old child falls 5 feet, hitting his head on concrete and then has a generalized seizure lasting less than 1 minute. His neurological exam is completely normal. What is the most likely diagnosis?**

Post-traumatic seizure.

O   **His parents want to know the likelihood of another seizure. What do you tell them?**

Approximately 25% of children with post-traumatic seizure will have additional seizures beyond one week after the injury.

O   **A 3-year-old child presents with coma. He had intractable, non-bilious vomiting for 24 hours prior to the onset of coma. There is no history of trauma. SGOT and SGPT are elevated but the serum bilirubin is normal. What is the most likely diagnosis?**

Reye's syndrome.

O   **What is Horner's syndrome?**

Miosis, ptosis, and anhydrosis (lack of sweat).

O   **What is the definition of status epilepticus?**

Continuous generalized convulsive seizures for at least 5 minutes, intermittent seizures for at least 15 minutes, or continuous EEG seizures for at least 15 minutes.

○   A 16-year-old obese girl with a history of irregular menses presents with a severe headache and blurry vision. Your physical exam is unremarkable except for papilledema. Her head CT is negative. An LP is done and opening pressure is 380 mm H$_2$O. What is the diagnosis and treatment?

Pseudotumor cerebri. Draining some fluid is therapeutic. Also, start her on a course of steroids.

○   What is the agent of choice for treating status epilepticus?

Stopping the seizure is the primary goal, because the longer the seizure continues, the harder it is to stop. Lorazepam (Ativan) is preferred over diazepam (Valium) because of its longer duration of action.

○   What is the most common arrhythmia causing syncope in patients with a structurally normal heart?

Supraventricular tachycardia (SVT).

○   Which MRI findings are suggestive of herpes simplex encephalitis?

Edema or hemorrhage in the temporal lobes.

○   What are the features required to diagnose Guillain-Barré Syndrome?

Progressive motor weakness and areflexia.

○   What is the hallmark in cerebrospinal fluid which indicate that the patient might have Guillain-Barré Syndrome?

Albumino-cytologic dissociation, which is found as early as the third day into the illness, but may occur as late as the second or third week.

○   Aside from measures intended to stop seizures, what is the major therapeutic priority in the management of status epilepticus?

Maintenance of oxygenation, adequate ventilation, and the prevention of hypoxia.

○   In what disease is cerebrospinal fluid albuminocytologic dissociation seen and what does it mean?

Guillain-Barré Disease. An increase in cerebrospinal fluid protein without a corresponding increase in cerebrospinal fluid white cells is referred to as albuminocytologic dissociation.

# RHEUMATOLOGY, IMMUNOLOGY AND ALLERGY

○ **Which drug is the most common pharmaceutical cause of true allergic reactions?**

Penicillin.

○ **Anaphylaxis-related deaths are primarily caused by penicillin. What is the second most common cause?**

Insect stings.

○ **Most children with mucocutaneous lymph node syndrome (MLNS) are below what age?**

MLNS, or Kawasaki disease, is predominantly found in children under 9 years of age.

○ **What percentage of patients with MLNS also develop acute carditis?**

Fifty percent will develop carditis, usually myocarditis with mild to moderate congestive heart failure. Pericarditis, conduction abnormalities, and valvular disturbances may occur but are less common.

○ **A patient presents with fever, acute polyarthritis, or migratory arthritis a few weeks after a bout of Streptococcal pharyngitis. What disease should be suspected?**

Acute rheumatic fever.

○ **What treatment should be started after the diagnosis of acute rheumatic fever has been made?**

Penicillin or erythromycin should be given even if cultures for Group A *Streptococcus* are negative. High-dose aspirin therapy is used at an initial dose of 75-100 mg/kg/day. Carditis or congestive heart failure is treated with prednisone, 1-2 mg/kg/day.

○ **Myocardial infarction can occur with which two rheumatic diseases?**

Kawasaki disease and polyarteritis nodosa (PAN).

○ **What is the most common cause of anaphylactoid reactions?**

Intravenous iodinized radiographic contrast media.

○ **What is required to make a diagnosis of mucocutaneous lymph node syndrome, or Kawasaki disease, in a young patient with a prolonged fever?**

The diagnosis requires four of these five common clinical findings:

1. Conjunctival inflammation.
2. Rash.
3. Adenopathy.
4. Strawberry tongue and injection of the lips and pharynx.
5. Erythema and edema of extremities.

Desquamation of the fingers and the toes may be striking, but it is a late finding and is not one of the key clinical features of the disease.

O    **What is the treatment of choice for the patient in anaphylactic shock?**

Epinephrine, 0.3-0.5 mg intravenously.

O    **How long should a patient with a generalized anaphylactic reaction be observed?**

24 hours because recurrence of hemodynamic collapse and airway compromise is common.

O    **What cardiac complication commonly occurs with SLE as well as with juvenile rheumatoid arthritis and rheumatoid arthritis?**

Pericarditis.

O    **What are the articular symptoms of late, Stage III, Lyme disease?**

Chronic arthritis, especially in the knee, periostitis, and tendonitis.

O    **What are the articular symptoms of late, Stage III, Lyme disease?**

Chronic arthritis, especially in the knee, periostitis, and tendonitis.

O    **A 10-year-old child presents limping and complaining of several weeks of groin, hip, and knee pain that worsens with activity. What diseases should be considered?**

Transient tenosynovitis of the hip, slipped capital femoral epiphysis, Legg-Calvé-Perthes, suppurative arthritis, rheumatic fever, juvenile rheumatoid arthritis, and tuberculosis of the hip.

O    **What disease is suspected in an adolescent with a tender, purpuric dependent rash, colicky abdominal pain, migratory polyarthritis, and microscopic hematuria?**

Henoch-Schönlein purpura, a leukoblastic vasculitis. Intestinal or pulmonary hemorrhage may occur, and 7–9% percent of the cases will develop chronic renal sequelae. Salicylates are effective for the arthritis. Other treatment is directed at the symptoms. Steroids are not particularly effective.

O    **A child has painful swollen joints along with a spiking high fever, shaking chills, signs of pericarditis, and a pale erythematous coalescing rash on the trunk, palms, and soles. Hepatosplenomegaly is found. What is the diagnosis?**

Systemic juvenile rheumatoid arthritis.

O    **What treatment besides aspirin is effective in preventing the complications of Kawasaki disease?**

Intravenous immunoglobulins can reduce the incidence of coronary artery aneurysms to less than 5%.

O    **What disease classically produces erythematous plaques with dusky centers and red borders resembling a bulls-eye target?**

Erythema multiforme. This disease can also produce non-pruritic urticarial lesions, petechiae, vesicles, and bullae.

❍ **Which joint is typically involved in the <u>most</u> <u>common</u> form of juvenile rheumatoid arthritis?**

Knee

❍ **What autoimmune disease produces lesions that are sometimes urticarial in appearance yet are not pruritic?**

Erythema multiforme.

❍ **Which drugs are <u>most</u> <u>commonly</u> implicated in toxic epidermal necrolysis?**

Sulfonamides and sulfones, phenylbutazone and related drugs, barbiturates, other antiepileptic drugs, and antibiotics.

❍ **What is the appropriate management for TEN?**

Admit for management similar to that required for extensive second-degree burns.

❍ **What can cause erythema multiforme?**

EM can be triggered by viral or bacterial infections, by drugs of nearly all classes, and by malignancy.

❍ **What is the <u>most</u> <u>common</u> cause of allergic contact dermatitis?**

*Toxicodendron* species, such as poison oak, poison ivy, and poison sumac are responsible for more cases of contact dermatitis than all the other allergens combined.

❍ **Why does scratching spread poison oak and poison ivy?**

The antigenic resin contaminates the hands and fingernails and is thereby spread by rubbing or scratching. A single contaminated finger can produce more than 500 reactive groups of lesions.

❍ **How is the antigen of poison oak or poison ivy inactivated?**

Careful washing with soap and water destroys the antigen. Special attention must be paid to the fingernails, otherwise the antigenic resin can be carried for weeks.

❍ **What underlying illnesses should be considered in a patient with nontraumatic uveitis?**

Collagen vascular diseases, sarcoid, ankylosing spondylitis, Reiter's syndrome, tuberculosis, syphilis, toxoplasmosis, juvenile rheumatoid arthritis, and Lyme disease.

❍ **What is the difference between episcleritis and scleritis?**

Both are associated with collagen vascular disorders; episcleritis is a benign superficial inflammation of the tissues between the sclera and the conjunctive. Scleritis is a more severe and more painful inflammation of the deep sclera which can result in visual loss.

❍ **What is the probable diagnosis of a patient with myalgias, arthralgias, headache, and an annular erythematous lesion accompanied by central clearing?**

Stage I Lyme disease with the classic lesion of Erythema Chronicum Migrans (ECM).

❍   **What rheumatologic ailments can produce acute airway obstruction?**

Relapsing polychondritis and rheumatoid arthritis.

❍   **How is septic bursitis contracted?**

A puncture wound or an overlying cellulitis are the typical sources for septic bursitis.

❍   **What type of infections are newborns most susceptible to and why?**

Gram negative organisms. Since there is no passive transfer of IgM, which are heat stable opsonins, the opsonization process is impaired.

❍   **So then, why aren't infants more susceptible to gram positive organisms?**

Passively transferred IgG serves as effective opsonins.

❍   **What four infectious agents are most commonly associated with asplenic individuals?**

*S. pneumoniae, Neisseria* sp., *H. influenzae* and *Salmonella* sp.

❍   **Fatality of hereditary angioedema can occur due to what condition?**

Edema of the larynx.

❍   **What is the definition of neutropenia?**

Absolute Neutrophil Count (ANC) < 1500 cell/ml.

❍   **Aside from chemotherapeutics which suppress bone marrow, what other agents are most commonly implicated?**

Phenothiazine, semisynthetic penicillin, NSAID's, aminopyrine derivatives, antithyroid medications.

❍   **What is the most common cause of transient neutropenia?**

Viral infections which most commonly include Hepatitis A, Hepatitis B, Influenza A and B, measles, rubella, and varicella.

❍   **How long would you expect the neutropenia to persist?**

It may persist the first three to six days of the acute viral syndrome.

❍   **Neutropenia and bacterial infection may herald the onset of what clinical entity?**

Overwhelming sepsis.

❍   **What effects of corticosteroids are likely after two hours?**

Fall in peripheral eosinophils and lymphocytes.

❍   **What effects of corticosteroids are likely after six to eight hours?**

Improvement in pulmonary function in asthmatics and hyperglycemia.

○ **Describe the clinical manifestation of urticaria?**

Well-circumscribed, erythematous raised skin lesions.

○ **What is most common form of urticaria caused by physical factors?**

Cold urticaria.

○ **What is the most effective treatment for control of urticaria?**

0.5 mg/kg Hydroxyzine (Atarax).

○ **When do most anaphylactic reactions occur?**

Within the first 30 minutes after initial exposure.

○ **What are typical initial symptoms of an anaphylactic reaction?**

A tingling sensation around the mouth, followed by a warm feeling and tightness in the chest or throat.

○ **What is the standard treatment for an anaphylactic reaction?**

Aqueous epinephrine 1:1000 at 0.1 ml/kg with maximum dosage of 0.3 ml for a child.

○ **What is the most common manifestation of an adverse drug reaction?**

Cutaneous eruption with urticarial, exanthematous, and eczematoid types occurring predominantly.

○ **What infectious agent is implicated in chronic blepharitis infection?**

Staphylococcal.

○ **An 8-year-old boy is complaining of lacrimation, itching, and burning of both eyes, with significant photophobia. The patient has a past medical history significant for asthma. What is your diagnosis?**

Vernal conjunctivitis.

○ **If you decide to treat the vernal conjunctivitis with topical steroids, what must be monitored?**

Intraocular pressure.

○ **Define Graft Versus Host Disease (GVHD)?**

Engraftment of immunocompetent donor cells into an immunocompromised host, resulting in cell mediated cytotoxic destruction of host cells if an immunologic incompatibility exists.

○ **When does acute GVHD present and what are the typical manifestations?**

Acute GVHD typically occurs about day 19 (median) just as the patient begins to engraft and is characterized by erythroderma, cholestatic hepatitis, and enteritis.

○   **What are the significant categories of toxic side effects of cyclosporine therapy?**

Neurotoxic:  Tremors, paraesthesia, headache, confusion, somnolence, seizures, and coma.
Hepatotoxic:  Cholestasis, cholelithiasis, and hemorrhagic necrosis.
Endocrine:  Ketosis, hyperprolactinemia, hypertestosteronemia, gynecomastia, and impaired spermatogenesis.
Metabolic:  Hypomagnesemia, hyperuricemia, hyperglycemia, hyperkalemia, and hypocholesterolemia.
Vascular:  Hypertension, vasculitic hemolytic-uremic syndrome, and atherogenesis.
Nephrotoxic:  Oliguria, acute tubular damage, fluid retention, interstitial fibrosis, and tubular atrophy.

○   **One month after renal transplant, what infectious agent most commonly causes a urinary tract infection?**

Pseudomonas aeruginosa.

○   **A renal transplant patient thirty days post-transplant presents with fever, oliguria, hypertension, and elevated serum creatinine. What two diagnostic tests would you perform next?**

Renal ultrasound and renal scan to evaluate renal blood flow.

○   **What are the most common manifestations of JRA?**

High intermittent fever, rheumatoid rash, arthralgia or myalgia (during febrile episodes), and persistent arthritis of greater than six weeks duration.

○   **What is the potentially irreversible sequelae of neonatal lupus?**

Congenital heart block.

○   **List the potentially fatal manifestations of Henoch-Schönlein syndrome.**

Acute renal failure; GI complications, such as hemorrhage, intussusception, and bowel infarction; and CNS involvement, which may precipitate seizures, paresis, or coma.

○   **What syndrome is the leading cause of acquired heart disease in the US, and what percent of cases are fatal?**

Kawasaki's disease. 1-2% or cases are fatal.

○   **What are the major Jones criteria used to diagnose rheumatic fever?**

Carditis, chorea (Sydenham), erythema marginatum, migratory polyarthritis, and subcutaneous nodules. The diagnosis requires either 2 major or 1 major and 2 minor with evidence of previous strep infection.

○   **What Jones criteria alone is sufficient for the diagnosis of rheumatic fever?**

Sydenham chorea. Deterioration in handwriting and increased clumsiness are commonly seen.

# GENITOURINARY AND RENAL

○ **What is the <u>most</u> <u>common</u> cause of acute renal failure?**

Acute tubular necrosis.

○ **What is the most important feature for distinguishing between testicular torsion and epididymitis?**

The rate of the onset of pain. Torsional pain begins instantaneously at maximum intensity, whereas epididymal pain grows steadily over hours or days. Clinically, elevation of the scrotum will relieve pain related to epididymitis, but is not effective with torsional pain.

○ **What is the <u>most</u> <u>common</u> cause of epididymitis?**

1) Prepubertal boys: Coliform bacteria.
2) In men younger than 35: *Chlamydia* or *Neisseria* gonorrhea.
3) Older than 35: Coliform bacteria.
4) Epididymitis is caused by urinary reflux, prostatitis, or urethral instrumentation.

○ **What does epididymitis in childhood suggest?**

Obstructive or fistulous urinary defects. Epididymitis is rare in children.

○ **What is the significance of the "blue dot" sign?**

This is pathognomonic for a torsion of the appendix testis or epididymis. With transillumination of the testis, a blue reflection occurs from the infracted tissue.

○ **How does the pain associated with epididymitis differ from that produced by prostatitis?**

1. <u>Epididymitis</u>: The pain begins in the scrotum or groin and radiates along the spermatic cord. It intensifies rapidly, is associated with dysuria, and is relieved with scrotal elevation (Prehn's sign).
2. <u>Prostatitis</u>: Patients will have frequency, dysuria, urgency, bladder outlet obstruction, and retention. They may have low back pain and perineal pain associated with fever, chills, arthralgias, and myalgias.

○ **What percentage of patients with epididymitis will also have pyuria?**

25%.

○ **What 4 clinical findings are indicative of acute glomerulonephritis (GN)?**

1. Oliguria.
2. Hypertension.
3. Pulmonary edema.
4. Urine sediment containing red blood cells, white blood cells, protein, and red blood cell casts.

○ **What is the <u>most</u> <u>common</u> cause of hematuria in children presenting to the ED?**

Infection.

○ **What are some causes of false-positive hematuria?**

Food coloring, beets, paprika, rifampin, phenothiazine, Dilantin, myoglobin, or menstruation.

○ **A urinalysis reveals red cell casts and dysmorphic RBCs in the urine. What is the probable origin of hematuria?**

Glomerulus.

○ **A 4-year-old boy presents with a painless mass in his scrotum that fluctuates in size with palpation. The mass transilluminates. What is the diagnosis?**

Hydrocele.

○ **What is the most common kidney stones?**

Calcium oxalate (65%), followed by magnesium ammonium phosphate (struvite) (20%), calcium phosphate (7.5%), uric acid (5%), and crystine (1%).

○ **What percent of urinary calculi are radiopaque?**

90%.

○ **What are the admission criteria for patients with renal calculi?**

Infection with obstruction, a solitary kidney, uncontrolled pain, intractable emesis, or large stones (because only 10% of stones > 6 mm pass spontaneously), renal insufficiency and complete obstruction or urinary extravasation.

○ **What percent of patients with urinary calculi will not have hematuria?**

10% - 25%.

○ **What percent of patients spontaneously pass kidney stones?**

80%. This is largely dependent on size. 75% of stones less than 4 mm pass spontaneously, while only 10% of those larger than 6 mm pass spontaneously.

○ **What is the most common cause of nephrotic syndrome in children?**

Minimal change disease.

○ **What is the definition of oliguria? Of anuria?**

Oliguria is as a urine output of less than 500 mL/day. Anuria is a urine output of less than 100 mL/day.

○ **What is the initial treatment for priapism?**

Ice packs and analgesia.

○ **What is the most common origin of proteinuria?**

Benign orthostatic Proteinuria.

○ **What are the risk factors for subclinical pyelonephritis?**

Multiple prior UTIs, longer duration of symptoms, recent pyelonephritis, diabetes, anatomic abnormalities, immunocompromised patients, and in indigents.

○ **What is the most common cause of intrinsic renal failure?**

Acute tubular necrosis (80-90%), resulting from an ischemic injury.

○ **If a urine dipstick is positive for blood yet the UA on the same urine is negative for RBCs, what is the probable disease?**

Rhabdomyolysis. Severe muscle damage can result in free myoglobin in the blood.

○ **What is the most common neoplasm in men under 30?**

Seminomas.

○ **Testicular torsion is most common in which age group?**

14-year-olds. Two-thirds of the cases occur in the second decade. The next most common group is newborns.

○ **T/F: Testicular torsion frequently follows a history of strenuous physical activity or occurs during sleep.**

True.

○ **T/F: Forty percent of patients with testicular torsion have a history of similar pain in the past that resolved spontaneously.**

True.

○ **What is the definitive diagnostic test for testicular torsion?**

Emergent surgical exploration.

○ **What is the definitive treatment for testicular torsion?**

Bilateral orchiopexy in which the testes are surgically attached to the scrotum.

○ **What is the most common cause of urinary tract infections (UTI)?**

*E. coli* (80%). *E. coli* is also the most common cause of pyelonephritis and pyelitis due to its ascension from the lower urinary tract. *Staphylococcus saprophyticus* accounts for 5-15% of the UTI cases.

○ **Varicoceles are most common in which part of the scrotum?**

The left. Varicoceles are a collection of veins in the scrotum.

○ **What is the most common renal tumor in children?**

Wilms tumor. This occurs in children under 5 years of age.

○ **What anatomic factors predispose a child to a urinary tract infection?**

Vesicoureteral reflux, obstruction, urinary stasis, and calculi.

○ **What is the most common cause of hypertension in children?**

Chronic pyelonephritis.

○ **What is the gold standard laboratory test for diagnosing a urinary tract infection?**

Urine culture.

○ **A newborn presents with a palpable abdominal mass. What is the most common cause?**

A hydronephrotic kidney.

○ **Were is the most common site of urinary tract obstruction in children?**

The ureteropelvic junction.

○ **A neonate presents with a renal mass, what is the differential diagnosis?**

Ureteropelvic junction obstruction, multicystic renal dysplasia, solid renal tumor, and renal vein thrombosis.

○ **What is the most common cause of a urethral stricture in a male child?**

Urethral trauma due to either iatrogenic causes (catheterization, endoscopic procedures, previous urethral reconstruction) or accidental such as straddling injuries or pelvic fractures.

○ **What is hypospadias?**

A congenital penile deformity resulting from incomplete development of the distal or anterior urethra.

○ **What is phimosis?**

An inability to retract the prepuce at an age when it should normally be retracted.

○ **What is a paraphimosis?**

A condition where a phimotic prepuce is retracted behind the coronal sulcus and this retraction cannot be reduced.

○ **What are the findings in a patient with testicular torsion?**

The scrotum is swollen, tender and difficult to examine. The cremasteric reflex is absent.

○ **What are the complications of circumcision?**

Hemorrhage, infection, dehiscence, denudation of the shaft, glandular injury, and urinary retention.

○ **What is balanitis?**

Infection of the prepuce most often due to mixed flora.

○   **Gross hematuria of renal origin has what characteristics?**

The color is generally brown or cola-colored and may contain red blood cells casts.

○   **How should a child presenting with gross hematuria be managed initially?**

The patient should be hospitalized for evaluation because of the increased likelihood of finding hypertension and renal failure.

○   **A 9-year-old male presents to your clinic with persistent microscopic hematuria detected on routine analysis brought on a febrile illness. Proteinuria is absent and the physical exam and laboratory evaluation are normal, what is the most likely diagnosis?**

Familial benign hematuria.

○   **A 5-year-old child presents with sudden onset of gross hematuria, edema, hypertension, and renal insufficiency two weeks after a sore throat, what is the most likely diagnosis?**

Acute post-streptococcal glomerulonephritis.

○   **What are the complications of acute post-streptococcal glomerulonephritis?**

Hyperkalemia, hypertension, hyperphosphatemia, hypocalcemia, acidosis, seizures, uremia, and volume overload.

○   **What is the prognosis for a patient with post-streptococcal glomerulonephritis?**

95% of children will completely recover within one month.

○   **What are the causes of nephrotic syndrome during the first six months of life?**

Congenital infection, (syphilis toxoplasmosis cytomegalovirus), congenital nephrotic syndrome, and diffuse mesangial sclerosis of unknown etiology.

○   **What are the most common causes of nephrotic syndrome between six months and one year of age?**

Idiopathic nephrotic syndrome or drug-induced nephrosis.

○   **An 11-year-old female presents with a purpuric rash on the buttocks and lower extremities, arthralgias, and abdominal pain. What is the most likely diagnosis?**

Henoch-Schönlein purpura.

○   **A 4-year-old presents with irritability, weakness, lethargy, dehydration, edema, petechiae, and a hepatosplenomegaly ten days after an episode of gastroenteritis. Laboratory results reveal a low platelet count and hemoglobulin level, what is the most likely diagnosis?**

Hemolytic-uremic syndrome.

○   **What are the complications of hemolytic uremic syndrome?**

Fluid overload, anemia, acidosis, hyperkalemia, congestive heart failure, hypertension, and uremia.

○ **What is the treatment for hemolytic uremic syndrome?**

Control of fluid and electrolyte balance, control of hypertension, careful use of red cell transfusions, and early initiation of dialysis for the correction of hyperkalemia, metabolic acidosis, severe uremia, or volume overload.

○ **A patient presents with proteinuria on routine urinalysis, which is absent, after obtaining a voiding specimen from the same patient upon awakening in the morning, what is the most likely diagnosis?**

Postural (orthostatic) proteinuria.

○ **What is a major complication of nephrotic syndrome?**

Infection.

○ **What is the most common type of infection in a patient with nephrotic syndrome?**

Peritonitis with strep pneumoniae.

○ **What is most common cause of interstitial nephritis in a hospitalized child?**

Medications.

○ **What are the causes of acute renal failure in the newborn?**

Sepsis, shock, hemorrhage, renal vein thrombosis, dehydration, congenital heart disease, obstructive uropathy, renal dysgenesis, and renovascular accidents.

○ **What are the most common causes of chronic renal failure in a child under 5 years of age?**

Anatomic abnormalities of the kidneys.

○ **What are the most common causes of chronic renal failure in children greater than 5 years of age.**

Glomerulonephritis, hemolytic uremic syndrome, or hereditary disorders (Alport syndrome, cystic disease).

○ **What are the causes of hypertension in a patient with chronic renal failure?**

Sodium and water overload and excessive renin production.

○ **Which initial study should be used to differentiate obstructive from intrinsic renal causes of acute renal failure?**

Renal ultrasound.

○ **What is the treatment for acute renal failure resulting from a pre-renal cause?**

Fluid resuscitation is the treatment of choice with an initial bolus of 20 ml/kg of crystalloid solution until vital signs become stable and urine flow is established.

○   **What are the indications for dialysis in a patient with acute renal failure?**

BUN greater than 100 mg/dl, persistent hyperkalemia, persistent metabolic acidosis, uremic syndrome, persistent congestive heart failure, and acute renal failure with oliguria due to rhabdomyolysis.

○   **A 6-year-old child presents with the following urine indices. Urine plasma urea nitrogen ratio greater than 8; urine: plasma creatinine ratio greater than 40; urine: plasma osmolality ratio greater than 500 mOsm/kg or greater than 1.5; and fractional excretion of sodium less than 1. What is the most likely cause of the renal failure?**

Prerenal cause such as decreased cardiac output or decreased intravascular volume due to hemorrhagic shock, dehydration, or third spacing of fluid.

○   **A child complains of "red urine". What foods can cause this?**

Beets, blackberries and red food coloring.

○   **What is the recommended course of action for a child with gross hematuria?**

Hospitalize and run the following tests: CBC, BUN/Cr, 24 hr creatine/protein/calcium, urine culture, serum C3, and anti-DNAse B titer. If these do not lead to a diagnosis then get an ultrasound or IVP to look for structural abnormalities.

○   **What is the most common cause of gross hematuria in children?**

IgA nephropathy.

○   **What is the classic presentation of post-streptococcal glomerulonephritis(PSG)?**

Sudden development of gross hematuria, hypertension, edema and renal insufficiency following a throat or skin infection with group A B-hemolytic streptococcus. Patients frequently also have generalized complaints of fever, malaise, lethargy, abdominal pain, etc.

○   **HUS most commonly follows infection with what organism?**

*E. coli* (O157:H7). The disease is usually a sequelae to a bout of gastroenteritis caused by this organism. Pneumococcal pneumonia has also been associated with HUS, though this is much less common.

○   **What is the prognosis for patients with acute renal failure secondary to HUS?**

Over 90% survival with many patients eventually recovering normal renal function.

○   **The mother of a 2 month old male infant is concerned that she cannot retract the foreskin. Should you circumcise at this point?**

No. More than 85% of uncircumcised males can retract the foreskin by the 3rd year. Before this time it is not a concern.

○   **What is the most common cause of acute scrotal pain in patients less than 6 years old?**

Testicular torsion.

○   **What is the most common presentation of idiopathic nephrotic syndrome?**

Edema, frequently in conjunction with anorexia, diarrhea and abdominal pain.

○ **Are circumcised males more, less, or equally likely to develop urinary tract infection when compared to their uncut counterparts?**

Less.

○ **What is the most common cause of acute hemorrhagic cystitis in males?**

Adenovirus. In females, *E. coli* is more common, followed by adenovirus.

○ **What are the two most severe sequelae for congenital neurogenic bladder?**

Urinary incontinence and renal damage, from high intravesical pressures caused by lack of coordination of the sphincters and detrusor muscles.

○ **What is the treatment for paraphimosis?**

As the glans edema and venous engorgement can lead to arterial compromise, this is a true emergency. First, try to manually compress the edema, after which the foreskin may be successfully reduced. If this does not work, a superficial vertical incision of the constricting band (after local anesthetic) will decompress the gland. Obviously, this procedure should be performed by a urologist or emergency medicine physician.

○ **How long after the onset of testicular torsion do irreversible changes develop?**

About 4.5-5 hours.

○ **During a routine examination of a 12-year-old male you encounter, in the upper scrotum, a boggy enlargement. Should you(and he) be concerned?**

No. This is most likely a varicocele, which is very common. About 15-17% of adolescent males have an asymptomatic varicocele.

○ **How do you treat the first episode of genital herpes?**

Oral acyclovir (200 mg 5 times/day for 10 days).

○ **What is the most common STD in sexually active teenage males?**

Non-gonococcal urethritis due to *Chlamydia trachomatis*.

# HEMATOLOGY AND ONCOLOGY

○ **Which types of blood loss are indicative of a bleeding disorder?**

1) Spontaneous bleeding from many sites.
2) Bleeding from non-traumatic sites.
3) Delayed bleeding several hours after trauma.
4) Bleeding into deep tissues or joints.

○ **What common drugs have been implicated in predisposing to acquired bleeding disorders?**

Ethanol, ASA, NSAIDs, warfarin, and antibiotics.

○ **Bleeding into joints or potential spaces (i.e., retroperitoneum), as well as delayed bleeding, suggests what type of bleeding disorder?**

Coagulation Factor Deficiency.

○ **Below what platelet count is spontaneous hemorrhage likely to occur?**

< 10,000/mm$^3$.

○ **It is generally agreed that most patients with active bleeding and platelet counts < 50,000/mm$^3$ should receive platelet transfusion. How much will the platelet count be raised for each unit of platelets infused?**

10,000/mm$^3$.

○ **What groups of patients with thrombocytopenia would be unlikely to respond to platelet infusions?**

Those with platelet antibodies (ITP or hypersplenism). Also HUS may make hemolysis worse.

○ **What 5 treatment options are available for patients who are bleeding and have liver disease?**

1. Transfusion with PRBCS (maintains hemodynamic stability).
2. Vitamin K.
3. Fresh frozen plasma.
4. Platelet transfusion.
5. DDAVP (Desmopressin).

○ **What are the clinical complications of DIC?**

Bleeding, thrombosis, and purpura fulminans.

○ **What three laboratory studies would be most helpful in establishing the diagnosis of DIC?**

1. Prothrombin time—prolonged.
2. Platelet count—usually low.
3. Fibrinogen level—low.

O   **What are the <u>most</u> <u>common</u> hemostatic abnormalities in patients infected with HIV?**

Thrombocytopenia and acquired circulating anticoagulants (causes prolongation of aPTT).

O   **How much will one unit of Factor VIII concentrate raise the circulating Factor VIII level?**

2%.

O   **What is the <u>most</u> <u>common</u> inherited bleeding disorder?**

von Willebrand Disease.

O   **70-80% of patients with von Willebrand disease have Type I. What is currently the approved mode of therapy for bleeding in these patients? What is the dose?**

DDAVP (0.3 µg/kg IV or sc q 12h for 3–4 doses).

O   **What is the <u>most</u> <u>common</u> hemoglobin variant?**

Hemoglobin S (Valine substituted for glutamic acid in the sixth position on the ß-chain).

O   **What types of clinical crises are seen in patients with sickle-cell disease?**

1) Vasoocclusive (thrombotic).
2) Hematologic (sequestration and aplastic).
3) Infectious.

O   **What is the <u>most</u> <u>common</u> type of sickle-cell crisis?**

Vasoocclusive.

O   **What percentage of patients with sickle-cell disease have gallstones?**

75% (only 10% are symptomatic).

O   **What are the mainstays of therapy for a patient in sickle-cell crisis?**

1. Hydration.
2. Analgesia.
3. Oxygen (only beneficial if patient is hypoxic).
4. Cardiac monitoring (if patient has history of cardiac disease or is having chest pain).

O   **What is the <u>most</u> <u>commonly</u> encountered sickle hemoglobin variant?**

Sickle-cell trait.

O   **What is the <u>most</u> <u>common</u> human enzyme defect?**

Glucose-6-phosphate Dehydrogenase Deficiency (G-6-PD).

O   **What is the single most useful test in ascertaining the presence of hemolysis and a normal marrow response?**

The reticulocyte count.

○   **What is the most common morphologic abnormality of red cells in hemolytic states?**

Spherocytes.

○   **In a child 6 months to 4 year of age with an antecedent URI, the findings of fever, acute renal failure, microangiopathic hemolytic anemia, and thrombocytopenia are suggestive of what disorder?**

Hemolytic Uremic Syndrome.

○   **What is the most common worldwide cause of hemolytic anemia?**

Malaria.

○   **By how much will the infusion of one unit of PRBcs raise the hemoglobin and hematocrit in a 30 kg patient?**

Hemoglobin: 1 g/dL.
Hematocrit: 3%.

○   **What is the first step in treating all immediate transfusion reactions?**

Stop the transfusion.

○   **What type of immediate transfusion reaction is not dose-related and can often be completed following patient evaluation and treatment with diphenhydramine?**

Allergic transfusion reaction.

○   **What infection carries the highest risk of transmission by blood transfusion?**

Hepatitis C (1:3,300 units).

○   **What is von Willebrand's disease?**

It is an autosomal dominant disorder of platelet function. It causes bleeding from mucous membranes, menorrhagia, and increased bleeding from wounds. Patients with von Willebrand's disease have less (or dysfunctional) von Willebrand's factor.

○   **What lab abnormalities does DIC cause?**

Increased PT, elevated fibrin split products, decreased fibrinogen and thrombocytopenia.

○   **What factors are deficient in Classic hemophilia, Christmas disease, and von Willebrand's disease, respectively?**

Classic hemophilia:      Factor VIII.
Christmas disease:       Factor IX.
von Willebrand's disease: Factor VIIIc + von Willebrand's cofactor.

○   **Which blood product is given when the coagulation abnormality is unknown?**

FFP.

○ **The most frequently encountered platelet disorder of childhood is:**

Idiopathic thrombocytopenic purpura.

○ **How do gamma globulin and steroids work in the treatment of ITP?**

They block the uptake of antibody-coated platelets by splenic macrophages.

○ **Which patients with ITP and mild head trauma without neurological findings should be treated with gamma globulin?**

Patients whose platelet count < 20,000/mm3, with signs of easy or spontaneous bleeding within one week of diagnosis, and whose follow-up is uncertain.

○ **Typical lab findings in von Willebrand's Disease include:**

1) Normal platelet count.
2) Normal pro-time.
3) Normal or increase partial thromboplastin time.
4) Increased bleeding time.

○ **At what age is a sickle cell patient at greatest risk for sepsis?**

Six months to 3 years.

○ **Why is the patient from the previous question considered at high risk during this age?**

Because there is limited protective antibody, and splenic function is decreased or completely absent.

○ **How should you treat hypoxia in a sickle cell patient who has acute chest syndrome?**

Red cell transfusion (simple or exchange).

○ **What two processes are involved in the pathophysiology of a sickle cell patient with acute chest syndrome?**

Pulmonary infarction and/or pneumonia.

○ **How does renal papillary necrosis that is secondary to sickle cell vaso-occlusion commonly present?**

Painless hematuria that may worsen the anemia, and red blood cells without casts in urine sediment.

○ **Name some options for the treatment of priapism arising secondary to sickle cell vaso-occlusive crisis.**

Intravenous hydration, analgesics, red cell or exchange transfusion, and aspiration of the penile corpora.

○ **What are some of the signs and symptoms of central nervous system infarction secondary to sickle cell vaso-occlusion?**

Mild, fleeting TIA-like symptoms, seizures, hemiparesis, coma, death.

○ **What are the signs and symptoms of splenic sequestration crisis?**

Pallor, weakness, lethargy, disorientation, shock, decreased level of consciousness, and an enlarged spleen.

○ **How do you treat splenic sequestration crisis?**

Rapid infusion of saline, and transfusion of red cells or whole blood.

○ **Which factors contribute to physiologic anemia during infancy?**

Abrupt cessation of erythropoiesis with onset of respiration, low erythropoietin levels (made in the liver during the neonatal period), decreased half life and increased volume of distribution of erythropoietin, shortened survival of fetal RBCs, and expansion of the infant's blood volume with rapid weight gain during the first three months.

○ **What are the most common sites for bleeding in patients who are hemophiliacs?**

Joints, muscles, subcutaneous tissue.

○ **What serious sequela of hip hemarthrosis is common among hemophiliacs?**

Aseptic necrosis of the femoral head.

○ **A hemophiliac presents with pain in the abdomen and groin, flexion of the thigh, and paresthesia of the lower thigh. What condition do you suspect?**

Iliopsoas hemorrhage.

○ **A hemophiliac presents with a headache after minor head trauma. What should your management include?**

CT of the brain, and factor replacement.

○ **How may an oncologic patient with a serum calcium concentration of 13 mgs/dl may be treated?**

Furosemide and forced saline diuresis. Extreme hypercalcemia may require mithramycin.

○ **The most common form of childhood malignancy is?**

Leukemia.

○ **What is the best treatment for superior vena cava syndrome?**

Emergent radiation therapy to shrink the tumor.

○ **The treatment for a neutropenic febrile leukemic patient includes what?**

A semisynthetic antipseudomonal penicillin, an aminoglycoside, plus a first generation cephalosporin for gram positive coverage. Ceftazidime may be used by itself, as can cefepime.

○ **A 2-year-old male is brought in by his mother because he has a flank mass. He is hypertensive and polycythemic. Urinalysis reveals hematuria. What is your diagnosis?**

Wilms tumor.

○ **A 15-year-old male complains of tibial pain after playing football. X-ray shows an "onion skin" appearance of the tibia. What condition is the patient likely to have?**

Ewing Sarcoma. The onion skin appearance is characteristic of this tumor.

○ **What is the leading cause of death from leukemia?**

Infection. The second leading cause is hemorrhage.

○ **What are the most common malignancies to cause tumor lysis syndrome?**

Advanced leukemia and non-Hodgkin's lymphoma. Large tumor burdens with aggressive chemotherapy are risk factors.

○ **Acute renal failure, Coomb's negative hemolytic anemia, and thrombocytopenia comprise the triad for which syndrome?**

Hemolytic-Uremic Syndrome (HUS).

○ **Aplastic crisis in sickle cell disease is associated with what condition?**

Parvo virus. Primary erythropoietic failure can result in life-threatening anemia in a patient with a significantly decreased RBC life span.

○ **Primary or spontaneous bacterial peritonitis is more frequently seen with patients who have which underlying conditions?**

Nephrotic syndrome, chronic liver disease, and systemic lupus erythematosus.

○ **What symptoms characterize tumor lysis syndrome?**

Hyperuricemia, hyperkalemia, and hyperphosphatemia.

○ **The major goal of therapy for tumor lysis syndrome is to prevent?**

Acute renal failure. The principles for treatment include alkalinization of the urine, vigorous hydration and diuresis, and prevention of the formation of toxic metabolites.

○ **What is the treatment of choice for a brain tumor edema?**

Dexamethasone.

○ **A four-year-old sickle cell patient presents with pallor, weakness, tachycardia and abdominal fullness. What should you suspect?**

Acute splenic sequestration.

○ **How should you treat the patient characterized in the previous question?**

Colloid and whole blood transfusion for correction of hypovolemia, anemia and prevention of circulatory failure.

○ **How many subsequent episodes of acute splenic sequestration be avoided?**

Splenectomy or chronic transfusions.

# DERMATOLOGY

○ **Are the nodules of erythema nodosum most often symmetrically or asymmetrically distributed?**

Erythema nodosum produces distinctive bilateral tender nodules with underlying red or purple shiny patches of skin that develop in a symmetric distribution along the shins, arms, thighs, calves, and buttocks.

○ **What therapy is effective for treating erythema nodosum?**

There is no therapy known to alter the course of the disease. The disease usually lasts several weeks but the pain associated with the tender lesions can be relieved with non-steroidal anti-inflammatory agents.

○ *Candida albicans* **infections of the skin are most commonly located where?**

In the intertriginous areas (i.e., in the folds of the skin, axilla, groin, under the breasts, etc.) *Candida albicans* appears as a beefy red rash with satellite lesions.

○ **What is a carbuncle?**

A deep abscess that interconnects and extends into the subcutaneous tissue. Commonly seen in patients with diabetes, folliculitis, steroid use, obesity, heavy perspiration, and in areas of friction.

○ **A mother is worried that her 5-year-old will get chicken pox because she was playing with her neighbor who was diagnosed with chicken pox and had crusty lesions all over his body. If this was the only day she played with the neighbor will she develop chicken pox too?**

No. Chicken pox is only contagious 48 hours before the rash breaks out and until the vesicles have crusted over.

○ **A mother brings her 14-year-old boy to you a week after you prescribed ampicillin for his pharyngitis. Mom says he developed a rash over his torso, arms, legs, and even the palms of his hands. On examination the patient has a erythematous, maculopapular rash in the places described. What might the child have other than pharyngitis?**

Infectious mononucleosis.

○ **Ecthyma most commonly presents on what body parts?**

The lower legs. Ecthyma is similar to impetigo but can also be associated with a fever and lymphadenopathy and is caused by *Staphylococcus aureus*.

○ **What is the most common bullous disease?**

Erythema multiforme. Patients may also have plaques, papules, and bullous lesions.

○ **What is the most common cause of erythema multiforme?**

Herpes simplex infections (90%).

○ **What is the most common location of erythema nodosum?**

The shins. They can also be found on the extensor surfaces of the forearms.

○ **A patient presents with a raised, red, small, and painful plaque on the face. On exam, a distinct, sharp, advancing edge is noted. What is the disorder and cause?**

Erysipelas is caused by group A streptococci.

○ **What are the causes of exfoliative dermatitis?**

Chemicals, drugs, and cutaneous or systemic diseases.

○ **What is a furuncle?**

A deep-inflammatory nodule which grows out of superficial folliculitis.

○ **What is hidradenitis suppurativa?**

Chronic suppurative abscesses found in the apocrine sweat glands of the groin and/or axilla.

○ **Your neighbor brings her 4-year-old little girl to you because she has a "disgusting" rash. The child's face is patched with vesiculopustular lesions covered in a thick, honey-colored crust. Just two days ago, these lesions were small red papules. Diagnosis?**

Impetigo contagiosa.

○ **What is the most common organism responsible for the above child's infection?**

*Staphylococcus aureus*. *β-Hemolytic Streptococcus* is the second most common infecting agent.

○ **What is the Koebner phenomenon?**

The development of plaques in areas where trauma has occurred. This is most common in patients with psoriasis and lichen planus.

○ **What is a pilonidal abscess?**

An abscess which occurs in the gluteal fold as a result of disruption of the epithelial surface.

○ **Where does a perirectal abscess originate?**

Anal crypts and burrows through the ischiorectal space.

○ **A 12-year-old female comes to your office complaining of intense itching in the webs between her fingers that worsens at night. On close examination you see a few small squiggly lines 1 cm x 1 mm where the patient has been scratching herself. Diagnosis?**

Scabies. Scabies are due to the mite *Sarcoptes scabiei* var. *hominis*. Scabies are spread by close contact; therefore, all household contacts should also be treated.

○ **Where is the most common site of eruption of herpes zoster?**

The thorax.

# DERMATOLOGY

○ **A 14-year-old female comes to your office complaining of a painful red rash with crops of blisters on erythematous bases in a band-like distribution on the right side of her lower back spreading down and out towards her hip. Diagnosis?**

Shingles or herpes zoster disease.

○ **A patient with shingles extending to the tip of his nose is at risk for what?**

Corneal ulceration and scarring. Lesions on the tip of the nose indicate that the nasociliary branch of the ophthalmic nerve is affected and the cornea is at risk. This is a medical emergency and needs immediate referral.

○ **What are the 2 distinct causes of toxic epidermal necrolysis (scalded skin syndrome)?**

(1) Staphylococcal and (2) drugs or chemicals.

○ **What areas does staphylococcal scalded skin syndrome (SSSS) usually affect?**

The face around nose and mouth, neck, axillae, and groin.

○ **What is the treatment of SSSS?**

Oral or IV penicillinase-resistant penicillin, baths of potassium permanganate or dressings soaked in 0.5% silver nitrate, and fluids.

○ **What is the most common cause of Stevens-Johnson syndrome?**

Drugs, most commonly sulfa drugs.

○ **What is the treatment of a tetanus prone wound?**

Surgical debridement, 3,000–10,000 units of human tetanus immune globulin [TIG (hours), (Hyper-tet)], IM (do not inject into wound), penicillin G, or metronidazole.

○ **Tinea capitis is most commonly seen in what age group?**

Children aged 4–14. This is a fungal infection of the scalp that begins as a papule around one hair shaft and then spreads to other follicles. *Trichophyton tonsurans* is responsible for 90% of the cases.

○ **What organism is the most common cause of bullous impetigo?**

Coagulase positive *Staph. aureus*.

○ **What is the best treatment for impetigo?**

Oral erythromycin mupirocin (Bactroban) topical lotion.

○ **What is the treatment for atopic dermatitis?**

Oral antihistamines, topical steroids, emollients, and avoidance of irritants.

○ **What is the recommended therapy for tinea capitis?**

Oral Griseofulvin (15-20 mg/kg/day) and shampooing twice a week with 2.5% Selenium Sulfide.

○ **If you want to sound more sophisticated while writing your H&P on a child with tinea capitis and a tender, fluctuant mass, what would you call it?**

A kerion.

○ **What is the causative agent of tinea versicolor?**

*Pityrosporum orbiculare* (malassezia furfur), a fungus.

○ **What is the drug of choice for head lice?**

Permethrin (Nix).

○ **What is the treatment of choice for scabies?**

5% Permethrin cream.

○ **What is the life expectancy of the newborn that develops erythema toxicum three days after his birth?**

Normal. This is a benign and self-limited disease that is extremely common in the neonate.

○ **An 11-year-old female presents with a maculopapular rash on trunk and upper legs. The rash is in lines along the long axis of the ovoid lesions. The patient states that 1 week ago, she had only 1 lesion which was round and "about as wide as a golf ball". What is your diagnosis?**

Pityriasis rosea.

○ **What is the distribution of the rash in pityriasis rosea?**

"Christmas tree" pattern with parallel rows of lesions on the trunk.

○ **Is there a role for topical steroids in acute severe sunburn?**

Yes. It may relieve pain and inflammation.

○ **Patients on which antibiotic are most likely to have photoallergic drug reaction?**

Tetracycline and sulfonamides.

○ **A 17-year-old girl complains that she can't wear gold earring without developing a localized rash. This is true not only in her earlobes, but also in all the pierced body parts (nose, navel, and eyebrows). What is her allergy to?**

Nickel, which is commonly found in some jewelry. She would have to wear either stainless steel or pure gold to avoid the allergy.

○ **In a child with scalded skin syndrome (SSS), you notice that pressing on the blister enlarges it laterally. What is the name of this phenomenon?**

Nikolsky sign-A sign of epidermal fragility.

○ **What is the treatment for scalp lesions of seborrheic dermatitis?**

Antiseborrheic shampoo (i.e. tar, selenium sulfide).

○ **Can you develop Rhus dermatitis from physical contact with someone who already has the condition?**

Not unless they have not yet washed off the resin which contains the allergen.

# SURGICAL EMERGENCIES

○ **How many days should sutures remain in the following areas: face, scalp, trunk, hands and back, and the extremities?**

Face: 3-5; scalp: 5-7; trunk: 7-10; hands and back: 10-14; extremities: 10-21.

○ **Why is epinephrine added to local anesthesia?**

To increase the duration of the anesthesia. However, epinephrine also causes vasoconstriction and decreased bleeding, which weakens tissue defenses and increases the incidence of wound infection.

○ **How should hair be removed prior to wound repair?**

Clip the hair around the wound. Do not use a razor during the preparation, as it will increase the infection rate.

○ **Lidocaine with epinephrine is a useful combination for anesthesia and the cessation of bleeding. On which parts of the body is this mixture contraindicated?**

The nose, ears, digits, and penis. Epinephrine causes local constriction of the blood vessels, which can also increase infection.

○ **What is the rate of wound infection in the average surgical service?**

4–7%. Clean wound infection rate is 2%, clean-contaminated wounds 3–4%, contaminated wounds 10–15%, and dirty wounds 25–40%. Wound infection is dependent on the degree of contamination, viability of tissue, blood supply to the tissue, dead space, amount of foreign material, age, concomitant infections, nutrition, and immunocompromised status.

○ **What mechanisms of injury create wounds that are most susceptible to infection?**

Compression or tension injuries. They are 100 times more susceptible to infection.

○ **A 15-year-old stepped on a nail that went right through her shoe and into her foot. Aside from normal skin flora, what organism might infect her puncture wound?**

*Pseudomonas aeruginosa.*

○ **Which has a greater resistance to infection, sutures or staples?**

Staples.

○ **What is the amount of bacteria necessary to cause wound infection, with and without a foreign body?**

With foreign body: 100 bacteria.
Without foreign body: > 1 million bacteria.

○ **Which two factors determine the ultimate appearance of a scar?**

Static and dynamic skin tension on surrounding skin.

○ **What are the characteristics of tetanus prone wounds?**

| | |
|---|---|
| Age of wound: | > 6 hours |
| Configuration: | Stellate wound |
| Depth: | > 1 cm |
| Mechanism of injury: | Missile, crush, burn, frostbites |
| Signs of infection: | Present |
| Devitalized tissue: | Present |
| Contaminants: | Present |
| Denervated and/or ischemic tissue: | Present |

○ **How long should one wait before delayed primary closure?**

4 days. This will decrease the infection rate; it is used for severely contaminated wounds.

○ **How long should an area of abraded skin or a laceration be kept out of the sun?**

6 months. Abraded skin will develop permanent hyperpigmentation after exposure to the sun.

○ **What is the most common organism in wound infections?**

*Staphylococcus*.

○ **How much fluid needs to collect in the chest if it is to be seen on a decubitus or upright chest x-ray?**

200–300 ml; if supine, greater than 1 L may be necessary to be seen on AP CXR.

○ **What is Kehr's sign?**

A pain in the left shoulder made worse in Trendelenburg. This is a sign of splenic injury or inflammation.

○ **Which organisms are most commonly responsible for overwhelming postsplenectomy sepsis?**

Encapsulated organisms: *Pneumococcus* (50%); *Meningococcus* (12%); *E. Coli* (11%); *H. Influenzae* (8%); *Staphylococcus* (8%); and *Streptococcus* (7%).

○ **What is the most common acute surgical condition of the abdomen?**

Acute appendicitis.

○ **Why would you order a chest x-ray in a case of acute abdomen?**

An upright chest x-ray can more easily show air under the diaphragm, an indication of a ruptured viscous.

○ **What might the abdominal films reveal on a patient with appendicitis?**

Sentinel loops with air fluid levels in the RLQ, a gas filled appendix or a fecalith (pathognomonic).

○ **What is the most common cause of appendicitis?**

Fecaliths. Fecaliths are found in 40% of uncomplicated appendicitis cases, 65% of cases involving gangrenous appendices that have not ruptured, and in 90% of cases involving ruptured appendices.

○   **How does retrocecal appendicitis most commonly present?**

Dysuria and hematuria (due to the proximity of the appendix to the right ureter). Poorly localized abdominal pain, anorexia, nausea, vomiting, diarrhea, mild fever, and peritoneal signs are also frequently common.

○   **What is the characteristic temporal sequence of the following signs and symptoms of appendicitis?**

Anorexia, abdominal pain, and vomiting are the order of occurrence in 95% of patients with acute appendicitis.

○   **Differentiate between McBurney's point, Rovsing's sign, the obturator sign, and the psoas sign.**

McBurney's point — Point of maximal tenderness in a patient with appendicitis. Location is 2/3 of the way between the umbilicus and the iliac crest on the right side of the abdomen.
Rovsing's sign — Palpation of LLQ causes pain in the RLQ.
Obturator sign — Internal rotation of a flexed hip causes pain.
Psoas sign — Extension of the right thigh causes pain. This is also indicative of an inflamed appendix.

○   **What is the higher rupture rate in appendicitis?**

The pediatric population has a rupture rate of 15–50%, and an associated mortality rate of 3%.

○   **What are Grey-Turner's and Cullen's signs?**

Grey-Turner's sign–flank ecchymosis indicative of pancreatic disease.

Cullen's sign- periumbilical ecchymosis indicative of pancreatic disease. Both are caused by dissection of blood retroperitoneally.

○   **Serum amylase is frequently elevated in acute pancreatitis. What other conditions can cause a similar rise in amylase?**

Bowel infarct, cholecystitis, mumps, perforated ulcer, and renal failure. A lipase level is more specific for pancreatitis.

○   **What is the most common cause of pancreatic pseudocysts in children ?**

Trauma. Pseudocysts are generally filled with pancreatic enzymes and are sterile. They appear as upper abdominal pain with anorexia and weight loss, about one week after a bout of acute pancreatitis. 40% of them regress on their own.

○   **What is the treatment for pancreatic pseudocysts?**

Initial therapy is to wait 4-6 weeks for regression. If there is no improvement, or if superinfection occurs, surgical drainage or excision is required.

○   **What clinical sign can help in the diagnosis of cholecystitis?**

Pain on inspiration with palpation in RUQ. This is called Murphy's sign. As the patient breaths in, the gallbladder is lowered in the abdomen and comes in contact with peritoneum just below the examiner's hand. An inflamed gallbladder will be greatly aggravated by this event, and the patient will discontinue her deep breath.

○ **What is the difference between cholelithiasis, cholecystitis, choledocholithiasis, and cholangitis?**

Cholelithiasis: The existence of gallstones in the gallbladder.
Cholecystitis: The inflammation of the gallbladder secondary to gallstones.
Choledocholithiasis: The existence of gallstones in the common bile duct that have migrated from the gallbladder.
Cholangitis: The inflammation of the common bile duct often secondary to bacterial infection or choledocholithiasis.

○ **Where do most hernias occur?**

In the groin (75%). Incisional and ventral hernias account for 10%, and umbilical hernias account for 3%.

○ **The majority of inguinal hernias in infants and children are what kind of hernias?**

Indirect inguinal hernias.

○ **Differentiate between reducible, incarcerated, and strangulated.**

Reducible: The contents of the hernia sac return to the abdomen spontaneously, or with slight pressure, when the patient is in a recumbent position.

Incarcerated: The contents of the hernia sac are irreducible and cannot be returned to the abdomen.

Strangulated: The sac has compromised blood flow.

○ **What is the most common hernia in females?**

Direct hernias.

○ **Of all the hernias in the groin area, which type will most likely strangulate?**

A femoral hernia.

○ **What is the most common site for duodenal ulcers?**

The duodenal bulb (95%).

○ **What are the common causes of neonatal bowel obstruction?**

Annular pancreas, Hirschsprung's disease, intestinal atresia, malrotation and volvulus or peritoneal bands, meconium plug, small left colon syndrome, and stenosis.

○ **Where does atresia of bowel most commonly occur?**

The duodenum (40%), jejunum (20%), ileum (20%), and colon (10%).

○ **What is the double bubble sign?**

The appearance of the distended stomach and duodenum on x-ray in a patient with duodenal obstruction. This is classically seen in duodenal atresia of the newborn.

○ **What is the most common cause of bowel obstruction in children?**

Hernia.

○ **Volvulus of the colon most frequently involves which segment?**

Sigmoid (65%), cecum (30%), transverse colon (3%) and splenic flexure (2%). Volvulus is the cause of 5–10% of all large bowel obstructions.

○ **What is the major cause of death in patients with Hirschsprung's disease?**

Enterocolitis.

○ **What is the Meckel's diverticulum rule of 2's?**

2% of the population has it, it is 2 inches long, it is 2 feet from the ileocecal valve, it most commonly occurs in children under 2, and is symptomatic in 2%.

○ **Rectal bleeding in a patient with Meckel's diverticulum is most likely due to what condition?**

Ulceration of ectopic gastric mucosa.

○ **A patient complains of severe pain with defecation, constipation, and blood streaked stools, which contain bloody discharge, following bowel movements?**

Anal fissure. 90% of anal fissures are found in the posterior midline.

○ **What is the treatment for an ingrown toenail?**

Wedge resection in which the ingrown part of the nail is cut at a 30° angle. This treatment is recommended only after a conservative approach of soaking in warm water and hydrogen peroxide, wide shoes, good hygiene, and a course of antibiotics has been tried.

○ **A felon is a subcutaneous infection of the pulp space of the fingertip, usually *Staphylococcus aureus*. What is the treatment for this disorder?**

Treat by incising the pulp space.

# TRAUMA

○ **A patient opens his eyes to voice, makes incomprehensible sounds, and withdraws to painful stimulus. What is his GCS?**

9.
Glasgow coma scale:

| Eye opening | Best verbal response | Best motor response |
|---|---|---|
| 4 spontaneously | 5 oriented x 3 | 5 obeys command |
| 3 on request | 4 confused conversation | localizes pain stimulus |
| 2 to pain | 3 words spoken | 3 flexes either arm |
| 1 no opening | 2 groans to pain | 2 extends arm to pain |
|  | 1 no response | 1 no response |

○ **Can significant head trauma, causing intracranial bleeding, lead to hypovolemic shock in a child?**

As a general rule, closed head trauma, not matter how significant, rarely causes hypovolemic shock in children. However, children less than 12 months of age who have large epidural hematomas with overlying skull fractures may decompress the hematoma into the scalp to a degree that significant blood loss can occur. This is the one rare exception to the rule.

○ **A 15-year-old fire victim is burned over both legs, his entire back, and his right arm. What percentage of his body is burned?**

63%. Follow the adult rule of 9s. Face = 9%. Arms = 9% each. Front = 18%. Back = 18%. Legs = 18% each.

○ **A 14-year-old patient who has been burned over the entire top of his body (arms and torso, front and back) develops severe difficulty breathing and appears to be going into respiratory arrest. What should you do?**

Perform an escharotomy. The patient is most likely suffering ventilatory restriction due to the circumferential eschar about his chest that is constricting the chest cavity. Escharotomies need not be performed with anesthesia, not even local anesthesia, because third degree burns involve the nervous tissue and are thus insensitive to pain.

○ **What is the initial treatment of tension pneumothorax?**

Large bore IV catheter placed in the second intercostal space (not a chest tube).

○ **How much fluid needs to collect in the chest if it is to be seen on a decubitus or upright chest x-ray?**

200–300 ml; if supine, greater than 1 L may be necessary to be seen on AP CXR.

○ **What should be checked prior to inserting a chest tube in an intubated patient with respiratory distress and decreased breath sounds on one side?**

Position of the ET tube.

○ **When does a subdural hematoma become isodense?**

Between 1–3 weeks after the bleed. At that time, it may not show up on a CT unless you use contrast.

○ **What percentage of C-spine fractures will be identified on a lateral x-ray?**

90%.

○ **Describe the key features of spinal shock.**

Sudden areflexia which is transient and distal and lasts hours to weeks. BP is usually 80–100 mmHg with paradoxical bradycardia.

○ **The corneal reflex tests:**

Ophthalmic branch ($V_1$) of the trigeminal (fifth) nerve afferent and the facial (seventh) nerve efferent.

○ **Define increased intracranial pressure.**

ICP > 15 mmHg.

○ **What is the most sensitive indicator of shock in children?**

Tachycardia.

○ **What is the initial fluid bolus that should be given to children in shock?**

20 ml/kg.

○ **Do post-traumatic seizures occur more frequently in children or young adults?**

Children.

○ **Where is the most common site of compartment syndrome?**

Anterior compartment of the leg.

○ **What are the most common lower extremity injuries to bone in children?**

Tibial and fibular shaft fractures, usually secondary to twist forces.

○ **What is the basic disorder contributing to the pathophysiology of compartment syndrome?**

Increased pressure within closed tissue spaces compromising blood flow to muscle and nerve tissue. There are three prerequisites to the development of compartment syndrome:

1) Limiting space.
2) Increased tissue pressure.
3) Decreased tissue perfusion.

○ **What are the two basic mechanisms for elevated compartment pressure?**

1) External compression—by burn eschar, circumferential casts, dressings, or pneumatic pressure garments.
2) Volume increase within the compartment—hemorrhage into the compartment, IV infiltration, or edema due to post-ischemic (postischial) swelling or secondary to injury.

○ **Which two fractures are most commonly associated with compartment syndrome?**

Tibia (resulting most often in anterior compartment involvement), and supracondylar humerus fractures.

○ **What are the early signs and symptoms of compartment syndrome?**

1) Tenderness and pain out of proportion to the injury.
2) Pain with active and passive motion.
3) Hypesthesia (paresthesia)—abnormal two point discrimination.

○ **What are the late signs and symptoms of compartment syndrome?**

1) Compartment is tense, indurated, and erythematous.
2) Slow capillary refill.
3) Pallor and pulselessness.

○ **How long does it take to prepare fully crossmatched blood?**

30–60 minutes.

○ **What is the risk associated with not treating a septal hematoma of the nose?**

Aseptic necrosis followed by absorption of the septal cartilage, resulting in septal perforation.

○ **What are the important structures to be considered when repairing lacerations of the cheek?**

Facial nerve, parotid duct, and gland.

○ **What procedure should be considered as an alternative to cricothyroidotomy in children?**

Needle cricothyroidotomy with jet insufflation.

○ **What are the features of central cord syndrome?**

There is a loss of motor function, worse in the upper extremities than the lower extremities. There is often sparing of perianal sensation. It is usually caused by hyperextension of the neck.

○ **What are the features of the Brown-Sequard syndrome?**

Caused by penetrating injury to one side of the spinal cord, it presents with ipsilateral motor deficit and contralateral loss of pain and temperature sensation. Light touch is usually absent on the side of the lesion.

○ **Which pattern of partial cord injury has the worst rate of functional recovery?**

Anterior cord syndrome.

○ **At what level of the cervical vertebrae is *pseudosubluxation* most commonly seen in children?**

C2 on C3, and C3 on C4.

○ **What is the upper limit for the normal Atlas-dens interval on a pediatric C-spine x-ray?**

4 mm. In an adult the space should be no wider than 2-3 mm.

○ **How is Cerebral Perfusion Pressure calculated?**

CPP=MAP-ICP. Ideal CPP is 50-60 mm Hg.

○ **What is the most likely cause of a subdural hematoma with retinal hemorrhages in a child?**

Child abuse.

○ **A child is intubated following a closed head injury. Hyperventilation should be instituted with what target arterial $PCO_2$?**

22-30 mm Hg.

○ **What is SCIWORA?**

Spinal Cord Injury Without Radiographic Abnormality. This can be seen at any age, but more commonly in children under 8. Thought to be related to the deformability and elasticity of the pediatric spine.

○ **What percent of pediatric burns are inflicted?**

16-20%.

○ **A child sustains an electrical burn to the corner of his mouth from chewing an electrical cord. What complication should be anticipated?**

Delayed hemorrhage from the labial artery in 5-15 days.

○ **What clinical features differentiate partial thickness from full thickness burns?**

Partial thickness: Pink to mottled red, blisters, bullae or moist weeping surface, painful.
Full thickness: Waxy white, charred or dark red, dry leathery, insensate.

○ **In estimating the size of a burn, which body part varies most as a percent body surface area with age?**

The head. At birth the head accounts for 19% BSA. At age 1 it is 17%, age 5=13%, age 10=11%, age 15=9%, adult =7%.

○ **Which fractures are thought to be specific for child abuse?**

Metaphyseal fractures (chip fractures in a corner), posterior rib fractures, acromioclavicular fractures, and multiple fractures of different ages.

○ **Which bony lesions suggest possible child abuse?**

Spinal fractures, digital fractures, complex skull fractures, spiral long bone fractures, scapular fractures, sternal fractures, metaphyseal fractures, and periosteal separation.

❍ **What findings comprise the shaken baby syndrome?**

Retinal hemorrhage, subdural hematoma, and rib fractures.

❍ **What is Volkmann's ischemia?**

It is pain worsened by passive motion of a muscle and associated neurologic deficits secondary to ischemia of the muscles and nerves; it is usually associated with a compartment syndrome.

❍ **What is Volkmann's contracture?**

It is the result of untreated Volkmann's ischemia, a contracture deformity secondary to muscle necrosis.

❍ **What is the leading cause of death and disability in the pediatric age group?**

Trauma.

❍ **What are the three most common failures in pediatric trauma resuscitation?**

Failure to open and maintain an airway.
Failure to provide appropriate fluid resuscitation.
Failure to recognize and treat internal hemorrhage.

❍ **At what point should a qualified surgeon be involved in pediatric trauma care?**

As early as possible in the course of resuscitation.

❍ **How can significant mortality risk be defined?**

Pediatric Trauma Score of 8 or less or Revised Trauma Score of 11 or less.

❍ **What special consideration must be taken in opening the airway of a multisystem trauma victim?**

Control of the cervical spine.

❍ **Why is the pediatric airway difficult to control?**

It is narrow and easily obstructed by foreign matter such as blood, mucus, and dental fragments.

❍ **T/F: Cervical spine injury is less common in pediatric than adult trauma.**

True, because the child's spine is more elastic and mobile than that of the adult, and the softer pediatric vertebrae are less likely to fracture with minor stress.

❍ **Spinal cord damage secondary to acceleration-deceleration injury is usually secondary to what spinal injury?**

Subluxation, most often at the atlantooccipital base (base of skull-C1) or atlantoaxial (C1-C2) joints in infants and toddlers or the lower (C5-C7) cervical spine in school-age children.

❍ **What is it about the pediatric spine that permits SCIWORA?**

Its increased elasticity and mobility caused by relative laxity of the cervical spine ligaments, incomplete development of the cervical musculature, and the shallow orientation of facet joints in young children.

○ **Because of the recognition of SCIWORA as an important cause of pediatric spinal cord injury, what test used in adults to rule out injury in the cervical spine in adult blunt trauma victims cannot rule out such injury in children?**

The lateral cervical spine x-ray.

○ **As a result of the recognition of SCIWORA, what special precautions must be taken in all children with multiple injuries, especially those who are apneic?**

Precautions to avoid potential exacerbation of cervical spine injury in each phase of airway management and control.

○ **T/F: Traction must be maintained on the neck at all times.**

False. Neutral stabilization, never traction.

○ **At what point may an oral airway be used?**

After the airway has been effectively opened and the cervical spine has been simultaneously stabilized, an oral airway may be placed in an unconscious patient.

○ **Why is correct semirigid extrication collar sizing important?**

Because excessively large collars may allow neck flexion or hyperextension.

○ **Why should soft collars be avoided?**

They do not immobilize the cervical spine effectively and have no role in initial stabilization of the child with potential cervical spine injuries.

○ **What are the five indications for endotracheal intubation of the child trauma victim?**

1) Respiratory failure/arrest.
2) Airway protection.
3) Airway obstruction.
4) Coma.
5) Need for prolonged ventilatory support or neurological resuscitation.

○ **How is coma defined in children?**

Glasgow Coma or modified Pediatric Coma Score of 8 or less.

○ **Why is the nasotracheal route contraindicated in children less than 8 years of age?**

Because it is extremely difficult to direct the tube anteriorly through the vocal cords in young children without direct visualization. In addition, adenoid tissue is much more prominent and susceptible to injury during emergency intubation.

○ **If the child is conscious, what should be done prior to intubation to avoid increasing intracranial pressure?**

Administer a sedative, Lidocaine, and a defasciculating dose of a neuromuscular blocker before giving succinylcholine.

○ **T/F: Cricothyrotomy is commonly used to control the pediatric airway.**

False. It is rarely necessary.

○ **When may cricothyrotomy be required?**

In the presence of orofacial trauma.

○ **How should an injured child with adequate ventilation receive supplemental oxygen?**

In the highest available concentration through a nonrebreathing mask.

○ **What should you do if respiratory effort is ineffective?**

Assist ventilations with a bag-valve-mask device and reservoir delivering 100% oxygen.

○ **What is associated with respiratory acidosis secondary to injury?**

Alveolar hypoventilation.

○ **What type of acidosis is caused by hypovolemia and shock?**

Metabolic.

○ **Why should extreme hyperventilation be avoided?**

It may reduce cerebral blood flow to levels associated with ischemia.

○ **What factors can compromise ventilation of the injured child?**

Gastric distention and leak around an uncuffed endotracheal tube.

○ **What is thought to be the leading cause of preventable death in children with multiple injuries?**

Failure to recognize and control internal bleeding.

○ **Why is blood transfusion of paramount importance in the initial stabilization of the pediatric trauma patient who has sustained significant blood loss?**

To restore oxygen delivery to tissues as well as intravascular volume.

○ **Bicycle helmets appear to reduce the risk of bicycle-related head injury by about how much?**

80%.

○ **What is the leading cause of death among children aged 1 - 14 years in the United States?**

Motor vehicle traffic injuries.

○ **How do you accomplish the immediate control of external hemorrhage?**

Direct pressure with a gloved hand over the wound using sterile gauze dressings.

○ **When should tourniquets be used?**

Only in cases of traumatic amputation associated with uncontrolled bleeding from a major vessel.

○ **Above what percentage of blood volume loss will signs of shock be observed?**

20%.

○ **After what percentage of blood loss will hypotension be present?**

After 25%-30% or more of the child's blood volume has been lost acutely.

○ **What class of hemorrhage is present in compensated shock?**

Class I-II, mild to moderate hypovolemia.

○ **How should compensated shock be treated?**

With rapid volume replacement with a bolus of 20 ml/kg of isotonic crystalloid solution.

○ **What two isotonic crystalloids are used in resuscitation?**

Normal saline and lactated ringers.

○ **What class of hemorrhage is uncompensated shock?**

Class III-IV.

○ **What percentage of blood loss results in uncompensated shock?**

25%-30%.

○ **What is the immediate treatment for uncompensated shock?**

Immediate volume replacement and blood transfusion.

○ **How should these fluids be administered?**

Using a pressure infusion system or "wide open" intravenous system may be necessary.

○ **When should urgent transfusion and possibly surgery be considered?**

If the child fails to respond to the administration of two or three boluses of crystalloid solution (approximately 40-60 ml/kg).

○ **What type of blood transfusion should be given in shock?**

Packed red blood cells mixed with normal saline warmed to body temperature.

○ **How many times should you repeat these doses?**

Until systemic perfusion is adequate.

○ **T/F: Administered blood should always be type specific and crossmatched.**

False. Transfusions must not be delayed to await compatibility studies if shock continues despite crystalloid therapy. Instead, O-negative blood should be administered immediately.

○ **What is indicated if shock persists despite control of external hemorrhage and volume resuscitation?**

Internal bleeding.

○ **T/F: Volume resuscitation should be limited in a child with head injury.**

False. Volume resuscitation and blood transfusion should continue as long as signs of shock are present in a child with head injury.

○ **Won't volume resuscitation increase the likelihood of cerebral injury in head trauma?**

No, ischemia may complicate traumatic brain injury unless intravascular volume is effectively restored.

○ **T/F: Isolated head injury can cause sufficient blood loss to produce shock in a child.**

True, isolated head injury rarely causes shock but may if bleeding scalp lacerations are not appropriately managed.

○ **What nasogastric findings support the diagnosis of organ rupture?**

Blood from the NG tube.

○ **T/F: Serious chest injuries are common in pediatric trauma.**

False, they are uncommon.

○ **What types of intrathoracic injuries constitute an immediate threat to life.**

Tension pneumothorax.
Open pneumothorax.
Massive hemothorax.
Cardiac tamponade.
Flail chest.

○ **Why is it more likely to find severe intrathoracic injury without chest wall or rib injury in children than in adults?**

Because the pediatric chest wall is extremely compliant, kinetic energy is transmitted to internal organs with minimal dissipation of the energy occurring.

○ **What is indicated by the presence of rib fractures?**

That severe chest trauma has occurred, and injury to underlying organs, such as the liver, spleen, and lungs is likely to be present.

○ **Which two injuries are most likely to impede initial stabilization of the pediatric trauma victim?**

Tension pneumothorax and open pneumothorax.

○ **How are flail chest and massive hemothorax best managed?**

Initially by aggressive treatment of the respiratory failure and shock they produce.

○ **How is flail chest best managed?**

Positive-pressure ventilation.

○ **How is a hemothorax managed?**

Chest tube.

○ **T/F: Cardiac tamponade is common in childhood blunt trauma.**

False.

○ **What causes a tension pneumothorax?**

The trapping of air behind a one-way "flap-valve" or defect in the lung that results from penetrating chest trauma or acute barotrauma sustained at the moment of blunt injury.

○ **What are the signs of a child with tension pneumothorax?**

Severe respiratory distress.
Distended neck veins.
Contralateral tracheal deviation.
Hyperresonance, decreased chest expansion and diminished breath sounds on the side of injury.
All of these may be difficult to assess in children.

○ **As tension pneumothorax progresses, what are the effects on systemic circulation?**

Systemic perfusion will be severely compromised as the mediastinum shifts to the contralateral side, twisting the superior and inferior vena cavae and obstructing venous return.

○ **What is the treatment for tension pneumothorax?**

Needle decompression followed by placement of a chest tube.

○ **T/F: Tension pneumothorax should be confirmed by chest x-ray prior to decompression.**

False. Decompression must precede confirmatory chest x-ray if signs of respiratory distress or shock are present.

○ **What type of needle is used for chest decompression?**

An over-the-needle catheter.

○ **Where is the needle inserted?**

Second intercostal space, midclavicular line, just above the third rib.

○ **What is another name for open pneumothorax?**

Sucking chest wound.

○ **What causes open pneumothorax?**

A penetrating chest wound that allows free, bi-directional flow of air between the affected hemithorax and the surrounding atmosphere.

○ **How does an open pneumothorax prevent effective ventilation?**

By causing equilibration of intrathoracic and extrathoracic pressure. This results in a paradoxical shifting of the mediastinum to the contralateral side with each spontaneous breath. Also, if the defect is 2/3 the diameter of the trachea, air will go through the defect instead of down the trachea.

○ **Why are sucking chest wounds more lethal in children than adults?**

Because the mediastinum is particularly mobile during childhood.

○ **What is the primary treatment for respiratory decompensation associated with an open pneumothorax?**

Positive pressure ventilation.

○ **What else should be done?**

The wound should be covered using an occlusive dressing such as Vaseline® gauze. This dressing should be taped on three sides to allow egress of entrapped air during exhalation. Dressing application should be followed by insertion of a chest tube, unless the defect is so large that it requires immediate surgical repair.

○ **What is the number one cause of death for African-American males between the ages of 10 and 24?**

Firearm injury.

○ **Do intentional or unintentional causes account for more firearm-related deaths?**

Intentional, which account for 94% wereas unintentional firearm injuries account for about 5%.

○ **What are the relative risks for suicide and homicide if a gun is kept in the home?**

Suicide is 5 times more likely to occur while homicide is 3 times more likely to occur.

○ **What is the clinical significance of the increased availability of semi-automatic weapons?**

Between 1982 and 1992, the percentage of gunshot victims with multiple gunshot wounds increased from 5% to 20%.

○ **What is the order of recruitment of accessory muscles of respiration in distress?**

Subcostal < intercostals < substernal < supraclavicular < nasal flaring < head bobbing.

○ **What injuries are associated with lap belt or bicycle handlebar injury?**

Perforations of the duodenum and proximal jejunum.

○ **Facial trauma in children is associated with?**

55 percent of children with facial trauma have associated intracranial injury.

○ **What bone is most commonly associated with posttraumatic developmental deformities?**

Mandible.

○ **What is the most common cause of death during the first hour after a burn injury?**

Inhalation injury produces upper airway edema leading to respiratory impairment.

# ORTHOPEDIC EMERGENCIES

○ **A child has posttraumatic tenderness at the end of a long bone. A joint effusion is the only radiographic finding. What is the appropriate management?**

Immobilization and subsequent orthopedic evaluation for possible separation of the epiphysis from the metaphysis (i.e., Salter-Harris type I fracture).

○ **Describe a common patient with a slipped capital femoral epiphysis.**

Obese boy, 10–16 years old. Groin or knee discomfort increases with activity; they may have a limp. Often bilateral. The slip is best seen on a lateral view.

○ **What is the most common ankle injury?**

75% of ankle injuries are sprains with 90% of these involving the lateral complex. 90% of lateral ligament injuries are anterior talofibular.

○ **What is the most helpful physical exam test for anterior talofibular ligament injury?**

Anterior drawer test. > 3 mm of excursion might be significant (compare sides); > 1 cm is always significant.

○ **How are sprains classified?**

1°—stretching of ligament, normal x-ray.
2°—severe stretching with partial tear, marked tenderness, swelling, pain, normal x-ray (now stressed).
3°—complete ligament rupture, marked tenderness, swollen and/or obviously deformed joint. x-ray may show an abnormal joint.

○ **Which bone is most commonly fractured at birth?**

The clavicle.

○ **A patient cannot actively abduct her shoulder. What injury does this suggest?**

Rotator cuff tear.

○ **Why is a displaced supracondylar fracture (of distal humerus) in a child considered a true emergency?**

The injury often results in injury to brachial artery or median nerve and possible compartment syndrome.

○ **What is the significance of the fat pad sign with an elbow injury?**

Fat pad sign is a radiolucency just anterior to the distal humerus and is indicative of effusion or hemarthrosis of the elbow joint; this suggests an occult fracture of the radial head.

○ **What type of Salter-Harris fracture has the worst prognosis?**

Type V—compression injury of the epiphyseal plate.

O    Which is the more sensitive test used to determine an anterior cruciate ligament tear in the knee: the anterior drawer test or the Lachman test?

Lachman test. While the knee is held at 20° flexion and the distal femur is stabilized, the lower leg is pulled forward. Greater than 5 mm anterior laxity compared to the other knee is evidence of an anterior cruciate ligament tear.

O    What is a stress fracture?

A fracture is caused by small, repetitive forces usually involving the metatarsal shafts, the distal tibia, and the femoral neck.

O    What is "nursemaid's elbow"?

Subluxation of the radial head. During forceful retraction, some fibers of the annular ligament that encircle the radial neck become trapped between the radial head and the capitellum. On presentation, the arm is held in slight flexion and pronation.

O    A patient presents with pain along the radial aspect of the wrist extending into the forearm. What is the diagnostic test of choice?

Finkelstein's test confirms the diagnosis of deQuervain's tenosynovitis, an overuse inflammation of the extensor pollicis brevis and the abductor pollicis where they pass along the groove of the radial styloid. The patient makes a fist with the thumb tucked inside the other fingers. The test is positive if pain is reproduced when the examiner gently deviates the fist in the ulnar direction.

O    In carpal tunnel syndrome, Tinel's sign is produced by tapping the volar wrist over the median nerve. If the test is positive, what does the patient experience?

Paresthesias extending into the index and long fingers.

O    Where is the most common site of compartment syndrome?

Anterior compartment of the leg.

O    What are the most common lower extremity injuries to bone in children?

Tibial and fibular shaft fractures, usually secondary to twist forces.

O    What radiograph would one order with suspected patellar fracture in a child?

Standard radiographs including patellar or "sunrise" views, plus comparison radiographs of uninvolved knee.

O    What are the differences between avulsion of tibial tubercle and Osgood-Schlatter disease?

Both occur at tibial tubercle. Avulsion presents with acute inability to walk, lateral view of the knee is most diagnostic; treatment is surgical. Osgood-Schlatter's has vague history of intermittent pain, is bilateral in 25% of cases, has pain with range of motion but not with rest; treatment is symptomatic and not surgical.

O    What is a toddler fracture?

A spiral fracture of the distal 1/3 of the tibia, without fibular involvement.

○ **What is the most common Salter-Harris class fracture?**

Type II. A triangular fracture involving the metaphysis (Thurston-Holland fragment) and an epiphyseal separation.

○ **What is the basic disorder contributing to the pathophysiology of compartment syndrome?**

Increased pressure within closed tissue spaces compromising blood flow to muscle and nerve tissue. There are three prerequisites to the development of compartment syndrome:

1) Limiting space.
2) Increased tissue pressure.
3) Decreased tissue perfusion.

○ **What are the two basic mechanisms for elevated compartment pressure?**

1) External compression—by burn eschar, circumferential casts, dressings, or pneumatic pressure garments.
2) Volume increase within the compartment—hemorrhage into the compartment, IV infiltration, or edema due to post-ischemic (postischial) swelling or secondary to injury.

○ **What is the most common ligamentous injury to the knee?**

Anterior cruciate ligament.

○ **What is the weakest portion of a child's bone?**

The physis (epiphyseal plate).

○ **What is the major concern with injury to the physis?**

The potential for subsequent growth arrest.

○ **What is a Type I Salter-Harris fracture?**

A separation of the epiphysis from the metaphysis. Usually caused by avulsion or shearing forces. Prognosis is good.

○ **What is a Type II Salter-Harris fracture?**

A fracture through the physis which exits the metaphysis. Prognosis is good.

○ **What is a Type III Salter-Harris fracture?**

A fracture through the physis which exits the epiphysis into the articular surface. Much worse prognosis than Types I & II. ORIF is often required.

○ **What is a Type IV Salter-Harris fracture?**

A fracture extending through the metaphysis, physis and epiphysis. Carries a high rate of premature physeal arrest.

○ **What is the most common cause of painful hip in older children?**

Transient synovitis.

○ **What is a Type V Salter-Harris fracture?**

A crushing injury of the physis. Often difficult to pick up radiographically. Usually diagnosed retrospectively after growth arrest occurs.

○ **What is the resultant deformity if an auricular hematoma is not properly treated?**

Cauliflower ear.

○ **What is a "green stick" fracture?**

A cortical disruption on one side of the bone without a disruption on the other side.

○ **What are some of the proposed etiologies of acute osteomyelitis in children?**

Bacteremia, trauma, malnutrition, and recent illness.

○ **What are some possible findings in a child with a septic hip joint?**

The hip may be held in external rotation and flexed. Any motion of the joint will be very painful.

○ **What bacterial pathogens are associated with osteomyelitis in children?**

Staph aureus is the most common (40-80% of cases).

○ **Are x-rays helpful in diagnosing osteomyelitis?**

Periosteal reaction and bony destruction take about 10-14 days to become radiographically evident.

○ **What is the treatment of osteomyelitis in children? Of a septic joint?**

Treat with broad-spectrum antibiotics including coverage for S. aureus; neonates should also be covered for group B strep, and gram negative coliforms; treatment for osteomyelitis associated with puncture wounds should provide coverage for *Pseudomonas*.

○ **What is the treatment of a septic joint?**

Treatment should provide coverage for *S. aureus*. Primary treatment for a septic joint is irrigation and drainage of the joint in the operating room, obtaining cultures prior to starting antibiotics. Sexually active patients should be covered for *N. gonorrhoeae*.

○ **What is Köhler disease?**

It is an idiopathic avascular necrosis (osteochondrosis) of the tarsal navicular bone. It is unique among the osteochondroses in that it occurs more commonly in school-aged rather than adolescent children.

○ **Are dislocations and sprains more common in children or adults?**

Dislocations and ligamentous injuries are uncommon in prepubertal children as the ligaments and joints are quite strong as compared to the adjoining growth plates. Excessive force applied to a child's joint is more likely to cause a fracture through the growth plate than a dislocation or sprain.

○ **Which type of fracture deformity can be particularly difficult to correct?**

Rotational deformities do not correct spontaneously and require meticulous realignment.

❍ **What is a torus fracture?**

A torus, or buckle, fracture is unique to children secondary to compressive forces causing buckling of the bone, leaving the cortices intact.

❍ **What is Volkmann's ischemia?**

It is pain worsened by passive motion of a muscle and associated neurologic deficits secondary to ischemia of the muscles and nerves; it is usually associated with a compartment syndrome.

❍ **What is Volkmann's contracture?**

It is the result of untreated Volkmann's ischemia, a contracture deformity secondary to muscle necrosis.

❍ **What is an antalgic limp?**

It is a painful limp characterized by a shortened stance phase to decrease time on the affected extremity.

❍ **What is a Trendelenburg gait?**

It is a non-painful limp, indicative of underling hip instability or muscle weakness, characterized by an equal stance phase between the involved and uninvolved side. The child will attempt to shift the center of gravity over the involved side for improved balance.

❍ **What are some causes (according to age) of painful limping?**

Antalgic gait may be caused by: (1-3-year-old): infection, occult trauma, or neoplasm; (4-10-year-old): infection, transient synovitis of the hip, Legg-Calve-Perthes disease, rheumatologic disorder, trauma, or neoplasm; (11+-year-old): slipped capital femoral epiphysis, rheumatologic disorder, trauma. It may also be seen in sickle cell disease.

❍ **What are some causes of Trendelenburg gait?**

1-3-year-old: hip dislocation, neuromuscular disease.
4-10-year-old: hip dislocation, neuromuscular disorder.

❍ **What is the Ortolani maneuver?**

Gentle abduction with the hip in flexion while lifting up on the greater trochanter which results in reduction of a dislocated hip with an palpable "clunk" as the femoral head slips over the posterior rim of the acetabulum.

❍ **What is the Barlow maneuver?**

Adduction of the hip in flexion while pushing down gently on the on the femoral head, in a dislocatable hip, will cause dislocation as the femoral head slips out of the acetabulum.

❍ **What is the most sensitive indicator of hip disease?**

Decreased internal rotation of the hip.

❍ **What makes the blood supply to the capital femoral epiphysis vulnerable?**

The retinacular vessels lie on the surface of the femoral neck and are intracapsular; they enter the epiphysis from the periphery and are subject to damage from trauma, joint infection, and other vascular insults.

○ **What is Legg-Calve-Perthes disease (LCPD)?**

It is an idiopathic avascular necrosis of the capital femoral epiphysis in a child (usually male) aged 2-12 years (mean: 7 years).

○ **What are some clinical manifestations of LCPD?**

Antalgic gait, muscle spasm (with restricted abduction and internal rotation), proximal thigh atrophy, thigh pain, and mild shortness of stature.

○ **What is the most common adolescent hip disorder?**

Slipped capital femoral epiphysis (SCFE).

○ **What is SCFE?**

It is an inferior and posterior slippage of the head of the femur off the femoral neck. Slips can be either chronic or acute.

○ **SCFE typically occurs in which individuals?**

Obese adolescents with delayed skeletal maturation or in tall, thin children after a recent growth spurt.

○ **Is SCFE bilateral or unilateral?**

The disease usually presents unilaterally with thigh, knee, or groin pain and a limp. Up to 30-40% of children with one slip will develop bilateral disease eventually and must be followed for this possibility.

○ **What radiographic views may be helpful in diagnosing SCFE or LCPD?**

Anteroposterior and Lauenstein (frog-leg) radiographs.

○ **What is the treatment of SCFE?**

SCFE is one of the few pediatric orthopedic emergencies. Weight bearing must cease to prevent a partial slip from becoming complete (complete slips carry an increased risk of vascular compromise and aseptic necrosis). The treatment is surgical.

○ **What are the two major complications of SCFE?**

Osteonecrosis (secondary to damage to the retinacular vessels) and chondrolysis (degeneration of the articular cartilage) of the hip.

○ **What are growing pains?**

They are nighttime thigh and calf pains most commonly seen in 4-10 year olds with symmetric limb pains unaccompanied by systemic symptoms such as fever or weight loss. Although termed growing pains, they are usually not seen in adolescents who undergo a faster rate of growth than younger children.

○ **Is back pain in children common?**

No, it is unusual and frequently due to organic causes. Etiologies include inflammatory diseases, rheumatologic diseases, developmental diseases, mechanical trauma, and neoplastic diseases.

○ **What is torticollis?**

Twisted or wry, neck, where the head is tipped to one side, with the occiput rotated toward the shoulder. Etiologies include soft tissue trauma, rotary subluxation of the cervical spine, dystonic reactions, and muscular causes (e.g. viral myositis).

O    **What is "Little League elbow"?**

Medial epicondylitis or osteochondritis desiccans of the capitellum and/or radial head laterally. Children usually present with pain after throwing or after gymnastics.

O    **What is osteochondritis desiccans?**

Degenerative process localized to an area of bone and its articular surface that may be due to ischemia or repeated trauma; the exact cause is unknown. The bone becomes avascular and ultimately separates from the underlying proximal bone.

O    **What is the most common site of osteochondritis desiccans?**

The lateral aspect of the medial femoral condyle; it may also be seen in the ankle and the elbow.

O    **What is a ganglion?**

It is a fluid-filled cyst at the wrist where a defect in the joint capsule allows herniation of the synovium.

O    **An adolescent boy presents with pain over the tibial tubercle after athletic activity and presents with a tender prominent tibial tubercle. What is the diagnosis?**

Osgood-Schlatter disease; complete resolution of symptoms over 1-2 years is expected as physeal closure of the tubercle occurs. Symptomatic care with rest, anti-inflammatories, and non-steroidal medication is the usual treatment.

O    **What is the apprehension test?**

Attempts to displace the patella laterally gives a subjective feeling of imminent patellar subluxation in patients with maltracking patellas who are predisposed to dislocation. The apprehension test refers to the patient's anxiety over this imminent subluxation during the above described maneuver.

O    **What is the most common carpal bone fractured?**

Scaphoid (navicular).

O    **What is osteogenesis imperfecta?**

It is the most prevalent of the osteoporotic syndromes in children. It is the result of a variety of defects in the production of type I collagen, with mutations in one of the two genes for type I procollagen. It is divided into four types. Type II is usually lethal in the perinatal period and characterized by "crumpled bone" syndrome and beaded ribs. Approximately 50% are stillborn and most die of respiratory insufficiency. Type III and IV are rare.

O    **What are some of the characteristics of Osteogenesis Imperfecta Type I?**

Thin bone cortices, osteoporosis, multiple bone fractures usually occurring between ages 2 and 3 years and continuing through early adolescence. Patients may present with hypermobile joints, kyphoscoliosis, joint dislocations, bowed limbs, increased capillary fragility, thin skin, and blue scleras.

O    **What is spondylolysis?**

It refers to a defect, lysis, or stress fracture of the pars interarticularis; the pars interarticularis is the bony connection between the superior facet of one vertebra and the posterior elements of the vertebra above it. Symptomatic children may experience low back pain worsened with activity and hamstring tightness.

○ **What is spondylolisthesis?**

Slippage of the superior vertebra on the lower one. Symptoms of nerve root compression (usually L-5) such as muscle weakness, sphincter problems, and sensory loss may be present.

# EYES, EARS, NOSE, THROAT & NECK

○ **What is the range of normal intraocular pressure?**

10–23 mmHg. Patients with acute angle closure glaucoma generally have pressures elevated to 40–80 mmHg.

○ **Topical steroids for the eyes are absolutely contraindicated in what cases?**

When the patient has a herpetic lesion in the eye (often seen as dendritic lesions on slit lamp) or a herpetic infection elsewhere.

○ **What is the most common finding on funduscopic examination of the AIDS patient?**

Cotton wool spots due to disease of the microvasculature. Other findings are hemorrhage, exudate, or retinal necrosis.

○ **If you suspect rupture of the round or oval window in a patient that comes to you for acute hearing loss what test might you perform?**

Applying positive pressure to the tympanic membrane will cause the patient to have ipsilateral nystagmus if there is a rupture.

○ **Acute tinnitus is associated with toxicity of what medication?**

Salicylates.

○ **Hairy leukoplakia is characteristic of what two viruses?**

HIV and Epstein-Barr virus. Hairy leukoplakia is usually found on the lateral aspect of the tongue. Oral thrush may also be associated with patients with HIV.

○ **What is the most common cause of odontogenic pain?**

Carious tooth.

○ **A child falls and knocks out his front tooth. How would treatment differ if the child was age 3 versus age 13?**

With primary teeth, no reimplantation should be attempted because of the risk of ankylosis or fusion to the bone. However, with permanent teeth reimplantation should occur as soon as possible. Remaining periodontal fibers are a key to success. Thus, the tooth should not be wiped dry as this may disrupt the periodontal ligament fibers still attached.

○ **What is the best transport medium for an avulsed tooth?**

Hank's solution, a pH balanced cell culture medium, which can even help restore cell viability if the tooth has been avulsed for more than 30 minutes. Milk is an alternative, or the patient, if able to keep from aspiration, may place the tooth underneath his/her tongue.

○  **A patient complains of a tongue irritation from a slightly chipped tooth after a fall. No dentin is exposed. What treatment can be offered to this patient?**

Tooth fractures only involving the enamel are called Ellis Class I fractures. The sharp edges can be filed with an emery board for immediate relief and the patient can be referred to a dentist for cosmetic repair.

○  **How can one differentiate Ellis class II and III fractures?**

Class II:   Fractures involving the dentin and enamel. The exposed dentin will be pinkish.
Class III:  Fractures involving the enamel, dentin, and pulp. A drop of blood is frequently noted in the center of the pink dentin.

○  **Why should topical analgesics not be used in Ellis class III tooth fractures?**

Severe tissue irritation or sterile abscesses may occur with their use. Treatment includes application of tinfoil, analgesics, and immediate dental referral.

○  **A patient presents with gingival pain and a foul mouth odor and taste. On exam, fever and lymphadenopathy are present. The gingiva is bright red and the papillae are ulcerated and covered with a gray membrane. What is the diagnosis and treatment?**

Acute necrotizing ulcerative gingivitis. Antibiotics (tetracycline or penicillin) and topical anesthetic. A possible complication of this disease is destruction of alveolar bone.

○  **What is the most common oral manifestation of AIDS?**

Oropharyngeal thrush.

○  **A 17-year-old female presents complaining of excruciating waxing and waning "electric shock type" pain in the right cheek. What is the diagnosis and treatment?**

Tic douloureux. The most significant finding is that the pain follows the distribution of the trigeminal nerve. Carbamazepine (100 mg bid starting dose and increasing to 1200 mg daily if needed).

○  **A three-year-old child presents with a unilateral purulent rhinorrhea. What is the most likely diagnosis?**

Nasal foreign body.

○  **What potential complications of nasal fractures should always be considered on physical examination?**

Septal hematoma and cribriform plate fractures. A septal hematoma appears as a bluish mass on the nasal septum and if not drained aseptic necrosis of the septal cartilage and septal abnormalities may occur. A cribriform plate fracture should be considered in a patient who has a clear rhinorrhea after trauma.

○  **What physical exam findings would make posterior epistaxis more likely than anterior epistaxis?**

1) Inability to see the site of bleeding. Anterior nosebleeds usually originate at Kiesselbach's plexus, an area easily visualized on the nasal septum.
2) Blood from both sides of the nose. In a posterior nosebleed the blood can more easily pass to the other side because of the proximity of the choanae.
3) Blood trickling down the oropharynx.
4) Inability to control bleeding by direct pressure.

○ **What is the most common site of bleeding in posterior nosebleeds?**

The sphenopalatine artery's lateral nasal branch.

○ **A patient returns to the emergency department with fever, nausea, vomiting and hypotension, two days after having nasal packing placed for an anterior nosebleed. What potential complication of nasal packing should be considered?**

Toxic shock syndrome.

○ **A child with a sinus infection presents with proptosis, a red swollen eyelid and a inferolaterally displaced globe. What is the diagnosis?**

Orbital cellulitis and abscess associated with ethmoid sinusitis.

○ **A patient with a frontal sinusitis presents with a large forehead abscess. What is the diagnosis?**

Pott's puffy tumor. This is a complication of frontal sinusitis where the anterior table of the skull is destroyed allowing the formation of the abscess.

○ **An ill-appearing patient presents with a fever of 103°F, bilateral chemosis, third nerve palsies, and untreated sinusitis. What is the diagnosis?**

Cavernous sinus thrombosis. This life-threatening complication occurs from direct extension through the valveless veins. Complication of sinusitis may be local (osteomyelitis), orbital (cellulitis), or within the central nervous system (meningitis or brain abscess).

○ **Retropharyngeal abscess is most common in what age group, and why?**

Six months to three years. This is due to size regression of the retropharyngeal lymph nodes after the age of three.

○ **How do patients with retropharyngeal abscesses appear?**

Febrile, ill-appearing, stridorous, drooling, and in an opisthotonic position. These children may complain of difficulty swallowing, or may refuse to feed.

○ **What radiographic sign can be used to make the diagnosis of a retropharyngeal abscess?**

A widening of the retropharyngeal space (normal 3-4 mm or less than half the width of the vertebral bodies). False widening may occur if the x-ray is not done during inspiration with the patient's neck extended (occasionally, an air fluid level may be noted in the retropharyngeal space).

○ **What is the most common organism to cause a retropharyngeal abscess?**

*β-hemolytic Streptococcus.*

○ **A 15-year-old male presents with a high fever, trismus, dysphagia, and swelling inferior to the mandible in the lateral neck. What is the diagnosis?**

Parapharyngeal abscess.

○ **What is the most common origin of Ludwig's angina?**

Lower second and third molar. It is a swelling in the region of the submandibular, sublingual, and submental spaces. This soft tissue swelling may cause displacement of the tongue upward and posteriorly. The most common organisms are hemolytic streptococci, *Staphylococcus*, and mixed anaerobes and aerobes.

○ **A 16-year-old female presents with dull right ear and jaw pain and a burning sensation in the roof of her mouth, which is worse in the evening. She also hears a "popping" sound when she opens and closes her mouth. Exam reveals tenderness of the joint capsule. What is the diagnosis and treatment?**

TMJ syndrome. Treat with physiotherapy, analgesia, soft diet, muscle relaxants and occlusive therapy. Apply warm moist compresses 4–5 times daily for 15 minutes for 7–10 days.

○ **A 14-year-old diabetic male presents with pain, itching, and discharge from the right ear. The tympanic membrane is intact. What is the diagnosis?**

Otitis externa. Treat by suctioning ear and 1 week of antibiotic steroid otic solution. An ear wick may improve delivery of the antibiotic. Suspect malignant otitis externa in the diabetic patient.

○ **A patient presents with ear pain and fluid-filled blisters on the tympanic membrane. What is the diagnosis?**

Bullous myringitis, commonly caused by Mycoplasma or viruses. Treat with erythromycin.

○ **A patient presents with a swollen, tender, red left auricle. What is the diagnosis?**

Perichondritis caused by *Pseudomonas*.

○ **What is the most frequent cause of hearing loss?**

Cerumen impaction.

○ **If a patient has bilateral sensory hearing loss, what causes should be suspected?**

Noise or ototoxics, such as certain antibiotics, loop diuretics, or antineoplastics.

○ **Name some causes of tympanic membrane perforation.**

Blast injuries (water or air), foreign bodies in the ear (particularly Q-tips), lightning strikes, otitis media, associated temporal bone fractures.

○ **What is the most common organism which causes pediatric acute otitis media?**

*Streptococcus pneumoniae*, followed by *Haemophilus influenzae* and *Moraxella catarrhalis*.

○ **What is a Bezold abscess?**

A complication of acute mastoiditis where infection spreads to the soft tissues below the ear and sternocleidomastoid muscle.

○ **What is the most common cause of sialoadenitis?**

Mumps.

○ **A patient presents with trismus, fever, and an erythematous, tender parotid gland. Pus is expressed from Stensen's duct. What conditions may predispose a person to bacterial parotitis?**

Any situation which decreases salivary flow. Irradiation, phenothiazine, antihistamines, parasympathetic inhibitors, dehydration or debilitation. Up to 30% of cases occur postoperatively.

○ **In which salivary gland do stones most likely occur?**

80% are submandibular.

○ **What does grunting versus inspiratory stridor indicate?**

Grunting is specific for lower respiratory tract disease, such as pneumonia, asthma, or bronchiolitis. Stridor localizes respiratory obstruction to the level at or above the larynx.

○ **What is the most common cause of epiglottitis?**

*Hemophilus influenzae* (as of the latest literature, though, incidence has dropped dramatically and *Streptococcus* is becoming the more common pathogen since the Hib vaccine).

○ **A lower airway foreign body is suspected. What will plain films show?**

Plain films may show air trapping on the affected side. Inspiration and expiration views demonstrate mediastinal shift away from the affected side.

○ **A patient presents with an itching, tearing, right eye. On exam huge cobblestone papillae are found under the upper lid. What is the diagnosis?**

Allergic conjunctivitis.

○ **A patient is seen with herpetic lesions on the tip of the nose. Why is this a problem?**

The tip of the nose and the cornea are both supplied by the nasociliary nerve. Thus, the cornea may also be involved.

○ **A patient presents with inflammation of the conjunctiva and lid margins. Slit lamp exam reveals a "greasy" appearance of the lid margins with scaling, especially around the base of the lashes. What is the diagnosis?**

Blepharitis. Often caused by staphylococcal infection of the oil glands and skin next to the lash follicles. Treatment consists of scrubbing with baby shampoo, and, in consultation with an ophthalmologist, sulfacetamide drops and steroids.

○ **A patient presents with a pustular vesicle at the lid margin. What is the diagnosis and treatment?**

Hordeolum (stye). An acute inflammation of the meibomian gland most commonly of the upper lid. Treat with topical antibiotics and warm compresses. Surgical drainage may be necessary.

○ **A patient presents with a chronic non-tender, uninflamed nodule of the upper lid. What is the diagnosis?**

Chalazion.

○   **A patient presents with the sensation of a foreign body in the eye. Slit-lamp reveals a dendritic figure which has a Christmas tree pattern. What is the appropriate treatment?**

Antiviral agents and cycloplegics are used to treat herpes simplex keratitis. Steroids spell disaster!

○   **What are complications of a hyphema?**

The 4 S's.

1) Secondary rebleeds, which usually occur between the second and fifth days post injury since this is the time of clot retraction. Rebleeds tend to be worse than the initial bleed.

2) Significantly increased intraocular pressure which can lead to acute glaucoma, chronic late glaucoma, and optic atrophy.

3) Staining of the cornea due to hemosiderin deposits.

4) Synechiae which interfere with iris function.

○   **Why do patients with sickle cell anemia and a hyphema require special consideration when presenting with ophthalmologic concerns?**

Increased intraocular pressure can occur if the cells sickle in the trabecular network, preventing aqueous humor from leaving the anterior chamber. Medication, such as hyperosmotics and Diamox, which increase the likelihood of sickling, must be avoided.

○   **A patient presents with a history of trauma to the orbit with dull ocular pain, decreased visual acuity, and photophobia. Exam reveals a constricted pupil and ciliary flush. What will be found on a slit-lamp exam?**

Flare and cells in the anterior chamber are present with traumatic iritis.

○   **What are causes of a subluxed or dislocated lens?**

Trauma, Marfan's syndrome, homocystinuria, Weill-Marchesani syndrome.

○   **Physiologically, what causes flare?**

Flare is caused by inflammatory proteins resulting in the "dust in the movie projector lights" or "fog in the headlights" phenomena in slit-lamp examination.

○   **Why shouldn't topical ophthalmologic anesthetics be prescribed?**

The anesthetics inhibit healing and decrease the patient's ability to protect his eye due to the lack of sensation.

○   **What is the most common organism in contact lens associated corneal ulcers?**

Pseudomonas.

○   **How can Krazy-Glue (cyanoacrylate) be removed if a patient has stuck their eyelids together?**

Copious irrigation immediately, and then mineral oil. Acetone and ethanol are unacceptable in the eyes. Surgical separation must be done with extreme care to prevent laceration of the lids or globe. Often the patient will have a corneal abrasion, which should be treated in the usual manner.

○   **What test can a physician use to determine if blindness is of a hysterical origin?**

An optokinetic drum can be used. If nystagmus eye movements occur, the patient is seeing the stripes. Prisms may also be used.

○   **A patient presents with traumatic pain behind the left eye, a left pupil afferent defect, central visual loss, and a left swollen disc. What is the diagnosis and potential causes?**

Optic neuritis. This may be idiopathic or may be associated with multiple sclerosis, Lyme disease, neurosyphilis, lupus, sarcoid, alcoholism, toxins, or drug abuse.

○   **In what age group is retropharyngeal abscess most common?**

Children less than four years of age. Symptoms may include difficulty breathing, fever, enlarged cervical nodes, difficulty swallowing, and a stiff neck.

○   **In what age group are peritonsillar abscesses most common?**

Adolescents and young adults. Symptoms may include ear pain, trismus, drooling, and alteration of voice.

○   **What is the most common sight-threatening ocular infection in AIDS patients?**

Cytomegalovirus (CMV) retinitis occurs in 15-40% of AIDS patients.

○   **What are the ocular manifestations of Lyme disease?**

Uveitis, keratitis, and optic neuritis.

○   **Extended wear contact lenses worn overnight increase the risk of infectious keratitis by how much compared to daily wear?**

Approximately 10-fold.

○   **What type of conjunctivitis is caused by adenovirus?**

Acute follicular conjunctivitis.

○   **What is the most common cause of ophthalmia neonatorum in the U.S.?**

*Chlamydia trachomatis.*

○   **What diagnosis is most probable in a newborn who develops "hyperacute" conjunctivitis with copious mucopurulent discharge?**

*Neisseria gonorrhea.*

○   **A patient with chronic follicular conjunctivitis is found to have several smooth, centrally umbilicated papules on the eyelids. What is the most likely diagnosis?**

Molluscum contagiosum.

○   **What two organisms are most likely to cause endogenous bacterial endophthalmitis in a host not otherwise predisposed to infection?**

*Neisseria meningitidis* and *Haemophilus influenzae*

○ **What is the most frequent condition associated with orbital cellulitis?**

Sinusitis.

○ **How common is strabismus during the first few months of life?**

Strabismus during infancy occurs in approximately one-third of infants during the first six months of life.

# PSYCHOSOCIAL AND CHILD ABUSE

○ **From 1970 to 1990, have suicide rates among adolescents aged 15-19 in the United States increased, decreased, or stayed the same?**

Increased. From 5.9 to 11.1 per 100,000.

○ **What is the ratio of attempted suicides to completed suicides?**

10:1.

○ **Is violence more likely between family members or non-family members?**

Between family members. 20–50% of murders in the US are committed by members of the victims' families. Spouse abuse is as high as 16% in the US.

○ **In what percentage of cases of child sexual abuse is the abuser known by the child?**

90%.

○ **In what percentage of cases of child abuse is the mother also abused?**

50%.

○ **What are the most common ages for child physical abuse?**

Two-thirds of physically abused children are under the age of 3, and one-third are under the age of 6 months.

○ **In addition to an evaluation for child abuse, what laboratory studies should be done in the child with multiple bruises?**

CBC with differential, platelet count, PT, and UA.

○ **What is the most common cause of referral to a child psychiatrists?**

Attention Deficit Hyperactivity Disorder.

○ **What are the side-effects of Ritalin?**

Ritalin (Methylphenidate) is a psychostimulant used to treat ADHD. Side-effects include depression, headache, hypertension, insomnia, and abdominal pain.

○ **What is the most frequent first episode of bipolar disease, mania or depression?**

Mania. Depression is rarely the first symptom. In fact, only 5–10% of patients that develop depression first go on to have manic episodes. 1/3 of manic patients never have a depressive episode.

○ **Other than the classic mania, what can lithium be used to treat?**

Bulimia, anorexia nervosa, alcoholism in patients with mood disorders, leucocytosis in patients on antineoplastic medication, cluster headaches, and migraine headaches.

○ **Postural tremor is a major side-effect of lithium. How is this side-effect controlled?**

Minimize the dose during the work day and give small doses of beta blockers.

○ **Should people who are physically active and taking lithium have their lithium dosage increased or decreased?**

Increased. Lithium, a salt, is excreted more than sodium during sweating.

○ **T/F: A patient starting lithium will be expected to gain weight.**

True. All psychotropic medications cause weight gain, hence lithium's usefulness in treating anorexia nervosa.

○ **Lithium toxicity begins at what level?**

14 mg/L. Above this level nausea, diarrhea, vomiting, rigidity, tremor, ataxia, seizures, delirium, coma, and death can all occur.

○ **Why might a patient taking lithium experience polyuria?**

Long term lithium ingestion can cause nephrogenic diabetes.

○ **What is the most common clinical symptom of a patient with a borderline personality disorder?**

Chronic boredom. Other symptoms include severe mood swings, volatile relationships, continuous and uncontrollable anger, and impulsiveness.

○ **A patient presents to your office with parotid gland swelling and erosion of the enamel on her teeth. What findings might you expect to find in this patient?**

The patient described most likely has bulimia. Elevated serum amylase and hypokalemia are associated with bulimia.

○ **List some common laboratory findings associated with eating disorders?**

Hyponatremia, hypokalemia, hypocalcemia, hypophosphatemia, anemia, hypoglycemia, starvation ketoacidosis, abnormal glucose tolerance, hypothyroidism due to low T3 levels, persistently elevated cortisol due to starvation, low FSH, LH and estrogens, and elevated growth hormone.

○ **What is the prevalence of conduct disorder?**

10%. It is much more common in boys and is familial.

○ **Children with conduct disorder are most likely to develop what adult disorder?**

About 40% will have some pathology as adults. The most common disorder is antisocial personality disorder.

○ **What is conversion disorder?**

Internal psychological conflict that manifests itself as somatic symptoms. Voluntary motor or sensory function is affected. Examples include weakness, imbalance, dysphagia, and changes in vision, hearing, or sensation. These symptoms are not feigned or intentionally produced. They are also not fully explained by medical conditions.

○ **Delirium is most likely to occur in what kinds of patients?**

Those with multiple medical problems, decreased renal function, high WBC count, anticholinergic, propranolol, scopolamine, or flurazepam drug use.

○ **Describe delirium.**

"Clouding of consciousness" resulting in disorientation, decreased alertness, and impaired cognitive function. Acute onset, visual hallucinosis, and fluctuating psychomotor activity are all commonly seen. All symptoms are variable and may change over hours.

○ **Name some over-the-counter and "street" drugs that may produce delirium or acute psychosis.**

Salicylates, antihistamines, anticholinergics, alcohols, phencyclidine, LSD, mescaline, cocaine, and amphetamines.

○ **Name some symptoms of major depression.**

IN SAD CAGES:

Interest

Sleep
Appetite
Depressed mood

Concentration
Activity
Guilt
Energy
Suicide

○ **What is dysthymia?**

Dysthymia is a chronic disorder lasting more than 2 years. The severe symptoms of depression, such as delusions and hallucinations are absent. Patients with dysthymia have some good days, they react to their environment, and they have no vegetative signs. 10% of patients with dysthymia develop major depression.

○ **Wild and abundant dreams may result from withdrawal of what drug?**

Antidepressants. Other side-effects of withdrawal are anxiety, akathisia, bradykinesia, mania, and malaise.

○ **What is a dystonic reaction?**

It is a very common side-effect of neuroleptics. Muscle spasm of tongue, face, neck, and back are seen. Severe laryngospasm and extraocular muscle spasm may occur also.

○ **Define the following dyspraxias: ideomotor, kinesthetic, and constructional.**

Ideomotor: The patient is unable to perform simple motor tasks despite adequate understanding, sensory and motor strength.
Kinesthetic: The patient is unable to position his extremities on command despite adequate understanding, sensory and motor strength.
Constructional: The patient cannot copy simple shapes despite adequate understanding, sensory and motor strength.

○ **A 16-year-old male presents to the ED complaining of pleuritic pain, palpitations, dyspnea, dizziness and tingling in his arms and legs. What is the diagnosis?**

Hyperventilation syndrome. This is frequently associated with anxiety. The tingling is due to decreased carbonate in the blood.

○ **In olfactory hallucinations, is the olfactory sensation still intact?**

Yes. Patients remain responsive to normal odors. Hallucinations of foul odors are superfluous to normal smells.

○ **A 17-year-old male arrives somnolent with vitals of P: 130, R: 26, BP: 170/80, and T: 105°F. You note diffuse muscular rigidity and intermittent focal muscle twitching/jerking lasting 1–2 seconds. As you "work him up," your nurse returns from the waiting area with news from the family that the patient has had a progressive decline of mental status for 2 days after seeing his psychiatrist. The patient has had a history of 'psychosis' for almost one year. What process should be included in your differential diagnosis at this time?**

Neuroleptic malignant syndrome.

○ **What labs would you expect to be elevated in this patient?**

CPK is usually elevated and correlates with increasing risk of fatality due to myoglobinuria. Serum alkaline phosphatase, serum aminotransferases and the white cell count are elevated. Hyponatremia, and hypokalemia are also present.

○ **How is lethal catatonia differentiated from neuroleptic malignant syndrome (NMS)?**

They are differentiated by the timing of the hyperthermia. In lethal catatonia, severe hyperthermia occurs during the excitement phase before catatonic features develop. In neuroleptic malignant syndrome, hyperthermia develops later in the course of the disease with the onset of stupor.

○ **What is the difference between the effects of low potency and high potency neuroleptics?**

Low potency neuroleptics have greater sedative, postural hypotensive, and anticholinergic effects. High potency neuroleptics have greater extra-pyramidal side-effects.

○ **Why is Haloperidol one of the preferred neuroleptics?**

It can be used IM in emergencies, and it has few side-effects. It does, however, have a high frequency of extra-pyramidal effects.

○ **What is the treatment for a "bad trip" on LSD?**

Chlorpromazine can be used IM for severe or uncontrollable anxiety. Remind the patient of reality by constantly reminding him that his perceptions are only distortions due to the drug.

○ **What is the difference between malingering and factitious disorder?**

The goal of a malingerer is an external incentive such as workman's comp. The goal of a someone with factitious disorder is to enter into the sick role. Both involve voluntary faking of an illness.

○ **What is an extreme case of factitious disorder?**

Munchausen's syndrome. These patients may actually try to cause harm to themselves (i.e., by injecting feces into their veins) and are very accepting/seeking of invasive procedures. Munchausen by proxy is another example. In this disease the patient seeks medical care for another, usually a child.

○ **A patient has ingested a phenothiazine and arrives hypotensive. What intervention(s) may be considered?**

IV crystalloid boluses usually suffice. Severe cases are best managed with norepinephrine (Levophed), or metaraminol (Aramine). These pressors stimulate $\alpha$-adrenergic receptors preferentially. $\beta$-agonists, such as isoproterenol (Isuprel), are contraindicated due to the risks of $\beta$-receptor stimulated vasodilation.

○ **What are extrapyramidal reactions?**

Dopamine receptor blockade within the nigrostriatal system results in involuntary and spontaneous motor responses including dystonia, akathisia, and Parkinson-like syndrome.

○ **A 14-year-old female comes to your office complaining of sudden episodes of palpitations, diaphoresis, lightheadedness, a fear of losing control, a sense of being choked, tremors, and paresthesias. What is the diagnosis?**

Panic disorder. Panic disorders need not be linked to any events. Though they are commonly associated with agoraphobia, social phobia, mitral prolapse, and late non-melancholic depression.

○ **What percentage of patients with panic disorder also suffer from major depression?**

50%.

○ **What is the most common specific phobia exhibited during childhood?**

Animal phobia.

○ **A 16-year-old female was raped 6 months ago. She has now suddenly developed recurrent, distressing flashbacks of the event; she is having nightmares and intense fear, is avoiding all males. She has a diminished memory of the rape, and an exaggerated startle response. Is this woman experiencing PTSD?**

Yes. This is delayed onset PTSD. The onset of symptoms can occur at least 6 months after the provoking event.

○ **What are the signs and symptoms suggestive of an organic source of psychosis?**

Acute onset, disorientation, visual or tactile hallucinations, age less than 10, and evidence suggesting overdose or acute ingestion, such as abnormal vital signs, pupil size and reactivity, or nystagmus.

○ **What is the difference between schizophrenia and schizophreniform disorder?**

Schizophreniform disorder implies the same signs and symptoms as schizophrenia, yet these symptoms have been present for less than 6 months. The impaired functioning in schizophreniform disorder is not consistent. Schizophreniform disorder is generally a provisional diagnosis with schizophrenia following.

○   **What are the 5 criteria for a diagnosis of Schizophrenia?**

1) Psychosis.
2) Emotional blunting.
3) No affective features or episodes.
4) Clear consciousness.
5) The absence of coarse brain disease, systemic illness, and drug abuse.

○   **Separation anxiety has an average onset of what age?**

Age 9. These children fear leaving home, sleep, being alone, going to school and losing their parents. 75% develop somatic complaints in order to avoid attending school.

○   **A 15-year-old female complains of pain in her calf, headache, shooting pain when flexing her right wrist, random epigastric pain, bloating, and irregular menses, all of which cannot be explained following medical workup. What is the diagnosis?**

Somatization Disorder—multiple, unexplained medical symptoms involving multiple systems. In order to diagnose a patient with somatization disorder, one must have 4 or more unexplained pain symptoms. Symptoms generally begin in childhood and are full blown by the age of 30. This is more common in females than males.

○   **What are some important clinical considerations when handling intoxicated, violent, psychotic, or threatening patients?**

These patients require a careful history and physical with attention to the mental status exam. Look for evidence of trauma, toxic ingestion, or metabolic derangement. Historical sources, such as family, paramedics, mental health workers, police, or medical records may need to be accessed. The patient may need to be physically or chemically restrained to obtain an adequate examination and for the safety of the patient and hospital staff.

○   **What psychiatric problems are associated with violence?**

Acute schizophrenia, paranoid ideation, catatonic excitation, mania, borderline and antisocial personality disorders, delusional depression, posttraumatic stress disorder, and decompensating obsessive/compulsive disorder.

○   **What are the prodromes of violent behavior?**

Anxiety, defensiveness, volatility, and physical aggression.

○   **Define the following:**

Akathisia: Internal restlessness. The patient feels as if he is "jumping out of his skin."

Echolalia: Meaningless automatic repetition of someone else's words. This may occur immediately or even months after hearing the words.

Catalepsy: The patient maintains the same posture over a long period of time.

Waxy flexibility: The patient offers resistance to anyone trying to change his position, then gradually allows himself to be moved to a new posture, much like a clay figure.

○   **What percentage of teenage girls have eating disorders?**

20%.

○ **What are the two subclassifications of anorexia nervosa?**

Restricts (limit intake) and Bulimia (binge eating followed by countermeasures).

○ **How do you diagnose bulimia nervosa?**

A history of overeating followed by forged purging is all that is needed. Erosion of the tooth enamel and back of second and third fingers in the dominant hand should lead you to suspect the diagnosis.

○ **What electrolyte abnormalities are commonly seen in bulimia nervosa?**

Hypokalemia, hypochloremia and metabolic alkalosis.

○ **What are the main causes of death in patients with anorexia nervosa?**

About 10% of these patients end up dying from complications (i.e. electrolyte imbalances, arrhythmias, or congestive heart failure).

○ **How long after intake can marijuana still be detected in the urine?**

From 3 days after one episode to 28 days in a frequent user.

○ **The anesthetic drug Ketamine is related chemically to what illicit drug?**

Phencyclidine (PCP, Angel Dust).

○ **In addition to the history, physical, laboratory tests, and collection of physical evidence, what else needs to be done in a case of sexual abuse of a child?**

File a report with child protective services and law enforcement agencies. Provide emotional support to the child and family. Give a return appointment for follow-up of STD cultures and testing for pregnancy, HIV, or syphilis, as indicated. Assure follow-up for psychological counseling by connecting the child/family to the appropriate services in your area.

# OBSTETRICS AND GYNECOLOGY

○ **What is the <u>most</u> <u>common</u> non-gynecologic condition that presents with lower abdominal pain?**

Appendicitis.

○ **What is secondary amenorrhea?**

No menstruation for 6 months or more in a women who previously had regular menses.

○ **What is the <u>most</u> <u>common</u> cause of secondary amenorrhea?**

Pregnancy. The second most common cause is hypothalamic hypogonadism which can be due to weight loss, anorexia nervosa, stress, excessive exercise, or hypothalamic disease.

○ **What is the <u>most</u> <u>common</u> cause of dysfunctional uterine bleeding in a child?**

Infection. For teenagers, it is most commonly due to anovulation.

○ **Virtually all severe cases of dysfunctional uterine bleeding occur in what age group?**

Adolescent females shortly after the onset of menstruation.

○ **What is the treatment of choice for a Bartholin gland abscess?**

Marsupialization. This prevents recurrences.

○ **B-hCG is secreted by what and for what reason?**

B-hCG is secreted by placental trophoblasts; its purpose is to maintain the corpus luteum, which in turn maintains the uterine lining. The corpus luteum is maintained through the sixth to eighth week of pregnancy, by which time the placenta begins to produce its own progesterone for maintenance of the endometrium.

○ **What are the rates of pregnancy with the following forms of birth control: (1) surgical sterilization, IUDs, or oral contraceptives; (2) coitus interruptus and rhythm method; (3) condoms; and (4) foams, jellies, sponges, or diaphragms?**

1) 0.2–2%, 2) 10%, 3) 12%, and 4), 18–20%.

○ **Failure of the hCG to increase by 66% over 48 hours in a pregnant females is indicative of what?**

An ectopic pregnancy or an intrauterine pregnancy that is about to abort.

○ **What is the <u>most</u> <u>common</u> site of implantation in an ectopic pregnancy?**

The ampulla of the fallopian tube (95%).

○ **What are the risk factors for ectopic pregnancy?**

Prior scarring of the fallopian tubes from infection (i.e., PID or salpingitis), IUDs, previous ectopic pregnancy, tubal ligation, and STDs.

○ **When does an ectopic pregnancy most commonly present?**

6–8 weeks. Patients usually present with amenorrhea and sharp abdominal or pelvic pain. A mass can be felt in 1/2 of the patients. B-hCG confirms pregnancy; ultrasound generally confirms an ectopic pregnancy.

○ **What percentage of pregnancies are ectopic?**

1.5%. Ectopic pregnancies are the leading cause of death in the first trimester.

○ **What is the most common finding on pelvic exam in a patient with an ectopic pregnancy?**

Unilateral adnexal tenderness.

○ **Who is eligible for methotrexate treatment of an ectopic pregnancy?**

Patients who are hemodynamically stable with unruptured gestations of < 4 cm in diameter by ultrasound.

○ **Transient pelvic pain frequently occurs 3–7 days after methotrexate therapy for ectopic pregnancy. What is your concern?**

Pain from rupture may be difficult to differentiate from pain presumed to be due to tubal abortion, which typically lasts 4–12 hours.

○ **For a gestational sac to be visible on ultrasound, what must the B-hCG be?**

At least 6,500 mIU/ml for a transabdominal ultrasound and 2,000 mIU/ml for a transvaginal ultrasound.

○ **When can an abdominal ultrasound find an intrauterine gestational sac?**

In the fifth week. Fetal pole, sixth week. Embryonic mass with cardiac motion, seventh week.

○ **Matching—time to keep those "M"s straight:**

1. Menorrhagia.
2. Metrorrhagia (hypermenorrhea).
3. Menometrorrhagia.

a. Bleeding between menstrual periods.
b. Excessive amount of blood or duration.
c. Excessive amount of blood at irregular frequencies.

Answers: (1) b, (2) a, and (3) c.

○ **Matching—more ways to describe menstrual bleeding:**

1. Hypermenorrhea.
2. Oligomenorrhea.
3. Polymenorrhea.

a. Menstrual periods > 35 days apart.
b. Menstrual periods < 21 days apart.
c. Menorrhagia.

Answers: (1) c, (2) a, and (3) b.

○   **What is the most common complication of ovarian cysts?**

Torsion of the ovary. Torsion is more common with small to medium sized tumors. Emergency surgery is required.

○   **Most cases of PID are caused by what 2 organisms?**

*Neisseria gonorrhoeae* and *Chlamydia trachomatis*.

○   **Which patients with PID should be admitted?**

Admit patients who are pregnant, have a temperature > 38°C (100.4°F), are nauseous or vomiting (which prohibits po antibiotics), have pyosalpinx or tubo-ovarian abscess peritoneal signs, have IUCD, show no response to oral antibiotics, or for whom diagnosis is uncertain.

○   **What are the criteria for diagnosis of PID?**

All of the following must be present: (1) adnexal tenderness, (2) cervical and uterine tenderness, and (3) abdominal tenderness. In addition, one of the following must be present: (1) temperature > 38°C, (2) endocervix Gram's stain positive for Gram-negative intracellular diplococci, (3) leukocytosis > 10,000 /mm$^3$, (4) inflammatory mass on US or pelvic, or (5) WBCs and bacteria in the peritoneal fluid.

○   **Teenage pregnancies are associated with increased risks of what disorders?**

Maternal complications, such as gonorrhea, syphilis, toxemia, anemia, malnutrition, low birth weight babies, and perinatal mortality.

○   **Why is Rh status important in a pregnant patient?**

If the mother is Rh negative and the fetus is Rh positive, fetal anemia, hydrops, and fetal loss can result. Rh immunoglobulin should be given to all Rh negative patients.

○   **What predisposes a female to yeast infections?**

Diabetes, oral contraceptives, and antibiotics.

○   **What organism is the most common cause of vaginitis?**

Candida albicans.

○   **A patient presents with a 2 day history of vaginal itching and burning. On exam, you note a thin yellowish–green bubbly discharge and petechiae on the cervix (also known as "strawberry cervix"). What test do you perform, and what results do you expect to find?**

Look at the discharge mixed with saline under a microscope. If you see a mobile and pear-shaped protozoa (*Trichomonas vaginalis*) with flagella, then the patient should be treated with Metronidazole (Flagyl).

○   **A 16-year-old sexually active female is complaining of a heavy but thin discharge with an unpleasant odor. When you add 10% KOH to the discharge, the combination emits a fishy odor. What would you expect to see on microscopic examination?**

"Clue cells"—epithelial cells with bacilli attached to their surfaces. This patient has *Gardnerella* vaginitis. The patient and her partner should both be treated with Metronidazole (Flagyl).

○   **When should you avoid using Flagyl to treat a female?**

If she is the first trimester of pregnancy. Metronidazole may have teratogenic effects. Clotrimazole (Gyne-Lotrimin) may be used instead. Flagyl has side-effects including nausea, vomiting, and metallic tastes. Most importantly, it acts similarly to disulfiram (Antabuse) and should, therefore, not be taken with alcohol.

○   **A 15-year-old female presents to the ED complaining of a painful sore on her vulva that looks like a pimple at first. On exam, you find an ulcer with vague borders and a gray base. What is the most likely diagnosis?**

Gram's stain, culture, and biopsy (used in combination because of the high false negative rates) should show that this woman has Haemophilus ducreyi, causing chancroid. Treatment is erythromycin or ceftriaxone.

○   **Condylomata acuminata frequently occur in combination with what other STD?**

*Trichomonas* vaginitis.

○   **What is the most common cause of septic arthritis in young adults?**

Disseminated gonococcal infection.

○   **What is the treatment for gonorrhea?**

Ceftriaxone and doxycycline. The latter is given because half of the patients infected with gonorrhea are simultaneously infected with chlamydia.

○   **What is the predominant organism in a healthy female's vaginal discharge?**

Lactobacilli (95%).

○   **What causes toxic shock syndrome (TSS)?**

An exotoxin elaborated by certain strains of *Staphylococcus aureus*. Other organisms causing toxic shock syndrome are group A Streptococcus, *Pseudomonas aeruginosa*, and *Streptococcus pneumoniae*. Tampons, IUDs, septic abortions, sponges, soft tissue abscesses, osteomyelitis, nasal packing, and post partum infections can all house these organisms.

○   **What dermatological changes occur with TSS?**

Initially, the patient will have a blanching erythematous rash that lasts for 3 days. 10 days after the start of the infection there will be a desquamation of the palms and soles.

○   **What criteria are necessary for the diagnosis of TSS?**

All of the following must be present: T > 38.9°C (102°F), rash, systolic BP < 90, and orthostasis, involvement of 3 organ systems (GI, renal, musculoskeletal, mucosal, hepatic, hematologic, or CNS), and negative serologic tests for diseases such as RMSF, hepatitis B, measles, leptospirosis, VDRL, etc.

○   **What is the treatment for TSS?**

Fluids, pressure support, FFP or transfusions, vaginal irrigation with iodine or saline (if the TSS was related to tampon use), and antistaphylococcal penicillin (nafcillin or oxacillin), or cephalosporin.

○   **What is the number one cause of UTIs?**

*E. coli.*

○   **A 16-year-old female presents to the ED complaining of fever, aches and pains, and painful genital sores that looked like blisters 2 days ago until they popped and started hurting. What would you expect to find on culture of the vesicular fluid?**

This patient most likely has the herpes simplex virus, type 2. Tzanck smear or a culture will show multinucleated giant cells by Giemsa stain.

○   **Is appendicitis more common during pregnancy?**

No (1/850). However, the outcome is worse. The WBC count usually does not increase beyond the normal value of 12,000–15,000. In a pregnant patient, pyuria with no bacteria suggest appendicitis. Pregnant patients may lack GI distress, and fever may be absent or low grade.

○   **How is the appendix displaced in pregnancy?**

Superiorly and laterally. Diagnosis of appendicitis in pregnant patients may be further complicated by the fact that normal pregnancy can itself cause an increased WBC. Prompt diagnosis is important because incidence of perforation increases from 10% in the first trimester to 40% in the third.

○   **A 15-year-old, Tanner 5 girl presents with abdominal pain and dysuria; she has not yet started menses. Examination of the genitalia shows a mass at the introitus. What is the most likely diagnosis and cause?**

The most likely diagnosis is hematocolpos, which is due to either a transverse vaginal membrane or an imperforate hymen.

○   **A 3-year-old girl presents with painless vaginal bleeding; there is no history of trauma. Examination of the genitalia reveals a donut shaped, erythematous mass above the introitus. What is the diagnosis?**

Urethral prolapse.

○   **What is the treatment of urethral prolapse?**

If there is no tissue necrosis, management consists of topical estrogen cream for 4-6 weeks. If there is tissue necrosis, excision under general anesthesia is necessary, which can be done as an outpatient.

○   **A mother presents to the ED because she fears her 7 month old daughter's vagina is "closing up". Examination reveals midline fusion of the labia minora, obscuring the view of the introitus. What is the diagnosis?**

Labial adhesions or acquired attachment of the labia minora. This is thought to occur because of low levels of endogenous estrogen in preadolescent girls, resulting in a thin epithelial surface of the labia minora. This thin epithelial surface is prone to maceration and inflammation, leading to fusion of the edges.

○   **What is the treatment for labial adhesions?**

Topical estrogen cream for 4-6 weeks, followed by application of an inert cream, such as zinc oxide, for an additional 2 weeks, to keep the healing surfaces apart.

○ **What is primary dysmenorrhea?**

Painful menses that is not attributable to any other cause, such as endometriosis, PID or structural pelvic disorders.

○ **What are the treatment options for primary dysmenorrhea?**

First line therapy consists of prostaglandin inhibitors such as NSAIDS. For the sexually active teen, oral contraceptives, which will inhibit ovulation, are another alternative, especially if NSAIDS fail to work.

○ **What is the pathophysiology behind dysfunctional uterine bleeding (DUB)?**

DUB is due to anovulatory bleeding, caused by estrogen that is unopposed by progesterone. This causes the endometrium to undergo sporadic growth and sloughing without cyclic coordination. The amount of estrogen secreted by the ovaries varies and bleeding can occur because of a fall in estrogen (withdrawal bleeding) or when the endometrium outgrows its blood supply (breakthrough bleeding).

○ **What is the most common cause of vaginitis in girls who are pubertal but not sexually active?**

*C. albicans.*

○ **Among teenagers who are sexually active, what are the 3 most common causes of vaginitis?**

*Gardnerella vaginalis* (bacterial vaginosis), *C. albicans*, *Trichomonas vaginalis*.

○ **How is the diagnosis of vaginitis by *Trichomonas vaginalis* made?**

Examination of a wet mount preparation of the vaginal discharge showing flagellated protozoa.

○ **How does an adolescent female acquire vaginitis due to *Trichomonas vaginalis*?**

Sexual contact.

○ **When treating vaginitis due to *Trichomonas vaginalis*, what condition must be excluded before metronidazole is prescribed?**

Pregnancy, as metronidazole is teratogenic.

○ **With what drugs does metronidazole interact?**

Ethanol, phenytoin, phenobarbital, warfarin and disulfiram.

○ **A nine-week-old female infant has had a white, malodorous discharge for over seven weeks. Her physical examination is normal except for the aforementioned discharge. A wet prep of the discharge shows motile trichomonads. How did the infant acquire this infection?**

A small number of vaginally delivered female infants may acquire vaginitis due to *Trichomonas vaginalis* from their untreated mothers during delivery. This vaginal discharge may persist for several months if left untreated.

○    **A 10-year-old girl presents with vaginal pain, pruritus and a yellow vaginal discharge. She also has a high fever and a sore throat. A gram stain of the vaginal discharge shows gram positive cocci in pairs. What is the most likely diagnosis, and what is the treatment?**

Group A beta hemolytic streptococcus (GABHS). Vaginitis can appear with or following acute GABHS pharyngitis. Penicillin therapy is curative.

○    **What historical, clinical and laboratory findings are necessary to make the diagnosis of bacterial vaginosis (vaginitis due to *Gardnerella vaginalis*)?**

A whitish, adherent vaginal discharge; vaginal pH > 4.5; amine-like (fishy) odor generated after adding 10% KOH to a sample of the vaginal discharge; when examining the vaginal discharge under the microscope, > 20% of vaginal epithelial cells are studded with gram negative coccobacilli.

○    **What are two treatment options for teenage girls with bacterial vaginosis?**

Oral metronidazole twice daily for 7 days. Topical clindamycin is an alternative for patients who are pregnant.

○    **What is the most common bacteria isolated from a Bartholin's gland abscess?**

*N. gonorrhoeae* is isolated in up to 50% of cultures from Bartholin's gland abscesses. The remaining cases contain mixed growths of aerobic and anaerobic organisms, such as *Bacteroides*, and a smaller number will grow *C. trachomatis*. Up to 30% of cultures will be sterile.

○    **What is Fitz-Hugh Curtis syndrome?**

Fitz-Hugh Curtis syndrome is a peri-hepatitis, or inflammation of the liver capsule, in association with pelvic inflammatory disease (PID). In addition to the signs/symptoms of PID, patients will also complain of right upper quadrant pain and tenderness to palpation.

○    **What other complications are seen in patients with PID and Fitz-Hugh Curtis syndrome?**

20% of patients will have tubo-ovarian abscesses.

○    **What does "RPR" stand for and what does it detect in serum?**

RPR stands for "rapid plasma regain" and detects antibodies against a cardiolipin-cholesterol-lecithin complex. It is a "nonspecific" test for syphilis, as it does not directly detect *Treponema pallidum*.

○    **What is the most likely causes of vaginal discharge in a neonate?**

Physiologic leukorrhea, which is due to the influence of maternal hormones during gestation. The vaginal discharge is clear, white and sticky. A gram stain will show white blood cells but no organisms; cultures will be sterile.

○    **What pathogen is most often responsible for vaginal discharge immediately beyond the neonatal period?**

Trichomonas vaginalis, which is acquired during vaginal delivery of infants born to infected mothers.

○  **A 10-year-old girl presents with chronic vaginal itching; there is no vaginal discharge. On examination her perineum has a hypopigmented, macular rash with telangiectasias in a "figure of 8" pattern. What is the diagnosis?**

Lichen sclerosus, which is a chronic idiopathic dermatitis characterized by atrophy, telangiectasias and hypopigmentation of the perineum, often in a "figure of 8" pattern.

○  **What is the cause of condyloma acuminata (genital warts)?**

Human papilloma virus.

○  **What is the most common etiology of genital ulcers in the United States?**

Herpes simplex, type 2.

○  **How can one make the diagnosis of primary syphilis?**

1) Dark field microscopy of suspicious lesions, which will show the spirochete, 2) RPR, which is a good but nonspecific test, as it does not directly detect *Treponema pallidum*, or 3) fluorescent antibody testing (MHA-TP, FTA), which directly detect antibody response to *T. pallidum*.

○  **A teenage girl presents with milky, non-bloody discharge from her nipples. She is not pregnant. What is the diagnosis and etiology of the discharge?**

This patient has galactorrhea, which is most often caused by a pituitary adenoma that secretes prolactin. Galactorrhea can also be caused by certain drugs, such as phenothiazine, antihistamines, diazepam, cimetidine, metoclopramide, opiates (codeine, morphine), antihypertensive agents (verapamil) and tricyclic antidepressants. If amenorrhea is also present, thyroid disease should be suspected.

○  **What is oligomenorrhea?**

Oligomenorrhea is defined as an interval of more than 6 weeks between menses.

○  **At what point does oligomenorrhea require evaluation?**

Adolescents with a pattern of oligomenorrhea that has continued more than 2 years after menarche or that began after the establishment of a regular menstrual cycle need evaluation.

○  **What are the clinical manifestations of secondary syphilis?**

Maculopapular rash of the trunk, soles, palms, that can resemble pityriasis rosea; mucous patches (white patches on the mucous membranes); condyloma lata, which are flat topped warts present in moist areas of the body, such as the perineum.

○  **What is the treatment for sexually acquired syphilis?**

For primary and early (< 1 year duration of symptoms) syphilis, a single dose of IM benzathine penicillin is sufficient; for late (>1 year duration of symptoms) syphilis, 3 IM doses of benzathine penicillin separated by a weekly interval is required.

○  **What is the most common cause of urethritis among sexually active adolescents in the United States?**

*Chlamydia trachomatis*.

○ **A sexually active 16-year-old male complains of dysuria and a penile discharge. You suspect urethritis. What is the appropriate management of this patient?**

The two most common causes of urethritis in a sexually active male are *C. trachomatis* and *N. gonorrhoeae*: therefore, give a third-generation cephalosporin (ceftriaxone) and an oral course of doxycycline.

○ **What are the clinical manifestations of primary syphilis?**

A painless genital ulcer (chancre), which is the site of inoculation of the spirochete.

○ **Is *Candida albicans* a common cause of vulvovaginitis in pre-pubescent females?**

No, because estrogen promotes fungal growth by stimulating vaginal glycogen stores and acidity.

○ **What are some of the risk factors for developing vulvovaginitis from *C. albicans*?**

Estrogen, which increases vaginal stores of glycogen and increases vaginal acidity; impaired host immunity, due to systemic corticosteroids, diabetes mellitus; and broad spectrum antibiotics.

○ **What are the signs and symptoms of pelvic inflammatory disease (PID)?**

Fever, lower abdominal pain and marked bilateral adnexal tenderness.

○ **What method of contraception is associated with a higher incidence of pelvic inflammatory disease (PID)?**

The risk of PID is twice as high in women who use intrauterine devices (IUD) when compared with women who use no contraceptive method.

○ **Which micro-organisms are responsible for pelvic inflammatory disease (PID)?**

*N. gonorrhoeae, C. trachomatis, Mycoplasma hominis*, and enteric anaerobes as *Bacteroides*.

○ **What is the appropriate antibiotic therapy for the treatment of an adolescent who has cervicitis?**

This patient may have cervicitis from *N. gonorrhoeae* and/or *C. trachomatis*. One strategy would be to give a single intramuscular dose of ceftriaxone and a 7-day course of oral doxycycline (provided the patient is not pregnant). To enhance compliance, a single oral dose of azithromycin may be substituted for the doxycycline. To avoid an intramuscular shot, a single oral dose of cefixime may be substituted for ceftriaxone.

○ **Would the treatment options change if the patient in the previous question were pregnant?**

Yes. If the patient is pregnant, a 7-day course of erythromycin should be substituted for doxycycline.

○ **A ten-year-old girl presents with a unilateral hematoma of the labia majora after a straddle injury. What is the appropriate treatment for this patient?**

Vulvar hematomas usually respond to ice-packs and bed rest.

○ **A teenage girl is treated for secondary syphilis with a single intramuscular dose of benzathine penicillin. Several days later, she develops fever and the maculopapular rash on her trunk becomes much more prominent. What is the cause of her symptoms?**

This patient has an acute systemic febrile reaction, the Jarisch-Herxheimer reaction, which can be seen in up to 20% of patients with acquired or congenital syphilis that are treated with penicillin. This reaction is self-limited and is not a reason to discontinue future therapy with penicillin.

○ **A sexually active teenage girl presents with fever, rash and pain of her knees and elbows. She just completed her menses. Examination reveals fever, a swollen, red, hot knee and erythematous macules of her hands and soles of her feet. What is the most likely diagnosis?**

Disseminated gonococcal infection.

○ **What are the clinical manifestations of disseminated gonococcal infection?**

Arthritis, polyarthralgia, tenosynovitis and a papular rash. Most patients do not have genitourinary symptoms; however.

○ **What is pseudocyesis?**

A rare cause of amenorrhea in women who believe they are pregnant, when they are not. These patients exhibit many symptoms of pregnancy, such as nausea, vomiting, galactorrhea and abdominal distention. The diagnosis is made when the patient insists she is pregnant, despite the absence of fetal heart tones, fetal movement, uterine enlargement and a negative pregnancy test. All patients require psychiatric evaluation.

○ **What is the classic triad of symptoms seen in patients with ectopic pregnancies?**

Lower abdominal pain, vaginal bleeding and an abnormal menstrual history.

○ **What is lymphogranuloma venereum (LGV)?**

An invasive lymphatic infection caused by *C. trachomatis*.

○ **What is the most common presentation of lymphogranuloma venereum (LGV)?**

The initial presentation is that of a local lesion on the genitalia accompanied by regional lymphadenitis.

○ **What is the treatment for lymphogranuloma venereum?**

Tetracycline (patients > 9 years of age), erythromycin, azithromycin or a sulfonamide for 3 to 6 weeks.

○ **How is the diagnosis of infection with *N. gonorrhoeae* made?**

By incubating infected secretions on selective media, such as chocolate agar impregnated with antibiotics, in a 5-10% CO2 environment; this is the gold standard for diagnosing gonococcal infection.

○ **How soon, after conception, do serum pregnancy tests become positive?**

Within 7 days of conception, which is approximately 1 week before the first missed menstrual period.

○ **What is the recommended treatment for the first episode of genital herpes?**

If oral acyclovir is started within 6 days of the onset of lesions, the duration of the lesions may be shortened by 3-5 days.

○   **What is the recommended treatment for recurrent genital herpes?**

Oral acyclovir has minimal effect on the duration of recurrent episodes of genital herpes. If oral acyclovir is started within 48 hours of the onset of symptoms, the duration of the lesions may be shortened only by 1 day.

○   **A 13-year-old girl, Tanner stage 4, presents with yellow vaginal discharge. She has not started menstruating, and is not sexually active. There is no vaginal itching, pain or dysuria. What is the most likely diagnosis?**

Physiologic vaginal discharge, which is usually scant, yellow and without odor; there are no other associated symptoms. This occurs about 6 months prior to menarche.

○   **What are the typical symptoms of "mittelschmerz" (ovulatory pain)?**

1. Sudden onset of right or left lower quadrant pain that occurs 2 weeks after the last menses (mid-cycle).
2. No evidence of intrauterine pregnancy.
3. A pelvic examination that reveals unilateral adnexal tenderness with no mass, no cervical motion tenderness, and no vaginal bleeding.
4. Pain that lasts only 24-36 hours.

○   **In an adolescent female without a history of PID, what is the most common cause of chronic pelvic discomfort?**

Endometriosis.

○   **When is the pain of endometriosis most severe?**

Right before menses.

○   **How soon after conception is the average home pregnancy kit able to detect the HCG and register as positive?**

Depending on sensitivity, anywhere from 1 to 3 weeks.

○   **In a normal uterine pregnancy, what is the doubling time of the HCG levels?**

48 hours. This can be used as one of several screening measures to rule out a hydatidiform mole.

# IMAGING PEARLS

○ **What is a sentinel loop?**

A distended loop of bowel seen on x-ray that lies near a localized inflammatory process. This is a clue to an underlying inflammatory process adjacent to the distended bowel. It can often be seen in pancreatitis or appendicitis.

○ **What is the incidence of allergic reaction to IV contrast materials?**

Severe allergic reactions occur in approximately 1/14,000 patients, whereas fatal reactions occur in about 1/40,000 cases.

○ **What is the prevalence of adverse reactions to ionic and nonionic contrast materials?**

Ionic: 12.7%. Nonionic: 3.1%. Nonionic contrast causes hypotension, bronchospasm, arrhythmia, angioneurotic edema, urticaria, flushing, nausea, and vomiting less often than ionic contrast materials. Whether or not nonionic materials are less nephrotoxic is still controversial.

○ **T/F: Oral contrast should be avoided in patients with marginal renal function.**

False. Little nephrotoxic iodine is absorbed with oral contrast administration. When barium is used, it is inert and not absorbed.

○ **What are the contraindications to administration of oral iodine or barium contrast?**

Barium cannot be given when complete colon obstruction exists or intestinal perforation is suspected. Severe allergy to iodine is the only contraindication to oral iodine-containing preparations.

○ **T/F: IV contrast material is contraindicated in chronic renal failure.**

False. The contrast material can be dialyzed, and the kidney is already maximally impaired.

○ **The magnetic fields of a MRI can be detrimental to patients with what?**

Ferrous metal in their body or electrical equipment whose function can be disrupted by strong magnetic fields. Examples include pacemakers, metal foreign bodies in the eye (welders, sheet metal workers, artists who work with metal, etc.), ferromagnetic cerebral aneurysm clips (unless they are made of nonmagnetic steel), and cochlear implants. Relative contraindications for a MRI include: certain prosthetic heart valves, implantable defibrillators, bone growth, and neurostimulators. One might also include patients who are claustrophobic.

○ **What is the order of ossification centers in the elbow?**

Remember the acronym CRITOE. Capitellum, Radial Head, Internal (medial) epicondyle, Trochlea, Olecranon, External (lateral) epicondyle. These ossify ad 3-5-7-9-11-13 years, in that order. Considerable variation to these ages range, but the order of ossification is usually consistent.

○ **What are the radiographic clues to necrotizing enterocolitis (NEC)?**

Abdominal distention, pneumatosis intestinalis and hepatic portal venous gas. The latter two are felt to be pathognomonic for this entity.

○ **A 5-week-old boy presents with non-bilious projectile vomiting. Initial abdominal x-ray is normal. Most likely diagnosis?**

Hypertrophic pyloric stenosis, also consider milk allergy, eosinophilic enteritis, gastroesophageal reflux, pylorospasm, and midgut volvulus.

○ **What is the recommended initial examination?**

US because it does not involve ionizing radiation.

○ **What are the US criteria for diagnosing HPS?**

- Exaggerated peristaltic waves.
- Delayed gastric emptying of fluid into the duodenum.
- Pyloric muscle wall thickness greater than 3 mm.
- Pyloric canal elongation greater than 14 mm.

○ **What are the signs of HPS that can be demonstrated by an upper GI examination.**

Shoulder sign.
Mushroom sign.
Double- or triple-tract sign.
Beak sign.
Diamond sign.
Teat sign.
Caterpillar sign.

○ **A 1-day-old with choking has an orogastric tube placed. X-ray reveals the tube is coiled in the proximal esophagus. Air is present in the stomach and proximal small bowel. There is situs solitus with a left-sided aortic arch. Most likely diagnosis?**

Tracheoesophageal fistula and Vater syndrome.

○ **If the patient has EA, how did air reach the stomach and proximal small bowel?**

A distal TEF or an H-type fistula allows air to move into the stomach. With an H-type fistula, the tube should not have coiled in the proximal esophagus. Thus, the child probably has EA with a distal TEF.

○ **A newborn has bilious vomiting and abdominal distention. X-rays reveal two large air-filled structures in the mid- and left upper abdomen. Most likely diagnosis?**

Malrotation or midgut volvulus. Other causes of the double-bubble sign: Ladd bands, annular pancreas, preduodenal portal vein duodenal atresia, duodenal stenosis, and duodenal web.

○ **UGI examination demonstrates the duodenojejunal junction to be lower than the duodenal bulb and to the right of the midline. The midgut loops have a spiral course. Diagnosis?**

Malrotation and midgut volvulus.

○ **What is the treatment for midgut volvulus?**

Surgery. If not treated, the volvulus can obstruct blood flow in the distribution of the SMA, leading to intestinal ischemia and necrosis (bloody diarrhea, ileus, abdominal distention).

O    **What signs should raise concern for midgut volvulus?**

Bilious vomiting in an otherwise healthy neonate.

O    **A 3-year-old male presents with a palpable right abdominal mass. CT reveals the mass to be located in the region of the right adrenal gland. The mass does not cross the midline but does invade the IVC. There are no calcifications. The child is noted to have aniridia. Differential diagnosis?**

Wilms tumor versus neuroblastoma.

O    **Which diagnosis is more likely?**

Wilm's tumor is the most common malignant abdominal neoplasm in children 1 to 8 years old. It may cross the midline, invade the IVC, occasionally have curvilinear calcifications, and be associated with aniridia. Neuroblastoma crosses the midline more than half of the time but does not invade the IVC, it usually has stippled course calcifications, and is not associated with aniridia.

O    **What is the leading cause of end-stage renal disease among boys?**

Posterior urethral valves. This condition is the most common cause of urinary tract obstruction among boys.

O    **What complications may occur with posterior urethral valves?**

Neonatal urine leak, urothorax, urinoma, pneumothorax, pneumomediastinum, Prune-belly syndrome and renal dysplasia.

O    **What is the most common cause of adrenal calcification in neonates?**

Adrenal hemorrhage.

O    **What causes adrenal hemorrhage in neonates?**

Birth trauma, hypoxia, septicemia, and hemorrhagic disorders.

O    **Testicular US in a 15-year-old with a low-grade fever, leukocytosis, and acute onset of testicular pain shows testicular and epididymal enlargement with decreased echogenicity, scrotal skin thickening, and a hydrocele. Most likely diagnosis?**

Acute testicular torsion, also consider epididymoorchitis and tumor.

O    **What diagnostic test should be ordered?**

Doppler US. In acute torsion, there is asymmetric or absent blood flow in the affected testicle. In epididymoorchitis, there is increased flow to the affected testicle. Flow to neoplasms is variable. Testicular torsion is the most common scrotal disorder in children. Acute epididymitis is the most common acute process in the postpubertal age group.

O    **What age groups are at highest risk of acute testicular torsion?**

Newborn and puberty (13-16 years)

O   **Doppler US reveals absent arterial flow in the affected testicle. How does the salvage rate depend on the onset of pain and the time of surgery?**

The salvage rate in relation to onset of pain is as follows:

| | |
|---|---|
| 80% to 100% | < 6 hours |
| 76% | 6 -12 hours |
| 20% | 12 - 24 hours |
| Near 0% | < 24 hours |

The test is viable for 3 to 6 hours and spontaneous detorsion occurs in less than 10% of cases.

O   **What age groups are at highest risk of acute testicular torsion?**

Newborn and puberty (13-16 years).

O   **Which organisms are responsible for epididymoorchitis in patients younger than 35 years versus those older than 35 years?**

*Escherichia coli* and *S. aureus*. In patients younger than 35 years, *Chlamydia trachomatis* and *Neisseria gonorrhoeae* should also be considered. In older patients, *E. coli* and *Proteus mirabilis* should be suspected. Orchitis will develop in 20% of patients with mumps.

O   **X-ray of the right femur shows a large, dense diaphyseal/metaphyseal lesion with a sun-burst periosteal reaction. The patient's mother reports painful swelling for 3 months with frequent fevers. Probable diagnosis?**

Central osteosarcoma, also consider osteoid osteoma, sclerosing osteomyelitis, and Charcot's joint. Spontaneous pneumothorax in central osteosarcoma is usually due to subpleural metastasis.

O   **Which paraneoplastic syndrome is present in 25% of patients with central osteosarcoma?**

Diabetes mellitus.

O   **What is the most common malignant bone tumor in children?**

Ewing sarcoma.

O   **A 10-year-old boy presents with left hip pain. X-ray shows widening of the epiphyseal plate.**

Slipped capital femoral epiphysis.

O   **Describe the nature of the injury in slipped capital femoral epiphysis.**

Salter I fracture of the proximal femoral growth plate.

O   **Who are more likely to be affected?**

Overweight adolescent males. It associated with hypothyroidism, renal osteodystrophy, trauma and growth hormone therapy.

O   **What findings can be seen on X-rays?**

Blurring of the junction of the metaphysis and epiphysis and widening of the growth plate.

○ A 9-year-old boy presents with fever, leukocytosis and right ankle pain. X-rays reveal a central area of lucency surrounded by a rim of reactive sclerosis in the distal tibia and a lucent channel-like configuration extending toward the growth plate. Most common diagnosis?

Brodie's abscess caused by *S. Aureus*.

○ If this child had sickle cell disease and osteomyelitis, which organism would you suspect?

*Salmonella* osteomyelitis. In newborns, acquired osteomyelitis is usually caused by group B streptococcus, *S. aureus* or *E. coli*.

○ What are the most common causes of osteomyelitis?

Genitourinary tract infections (#1), lung infections, and dermal infections.

○ What is the most common location of osteomyelitis in children?

The metaphyses of long bones due to the blood supply.

○ X-ray of a 6-month-old mentally retarded boy shows multiple fractures of varying age and location. Diagnosis?

Child abuse.

○ What long bone fractures may be seen in abused children?

- Multiple fractures of varying age and location.
- Avulsion fractures of ligamentous insertions.
- Corner fractures.
- Isolated spiral fractures.
- Common locations include multiple ribs, sternum, vertebral compressions, tibia costochondral or costovertebral separation, clavicles, scapula, skull, and metacarpus.

○ What is the most common cause of death in abused children?

Head trauma.

○ What are the neuroradiologic findings in child abuse?

- Subdural hematoma is the most common finding.
- Contusions.
- Cerebral edema.
- Subarachnoid hemorrhage.
- White matter shear injuries at the corticomedullary junction, centrum semiovale, and corpus callosum.
- Epidural hemorrhage.

○ What are some typical findings of visceral trauma in child abuse?

Duodenal hematoma, organ contusion, bowel or gastric rupture, and traumatic pancreatic pseudocysts. Visceral trauma is the second most common cause of death in child abuse.

○ X-rays of a 2-year-old demonstrate poorly mineralized epiphyses, widening of the growth plates, fraying and cupping of the metaphyses, and bowing of the long bones. The family are strict vegetarians. Diagnosis?

Rickets.

❍   **What is the most common cause of rickets in children?**

Renal disease.

❍   **What causes scurvy?**

Vitamin C deficiency with defective osteogenesis from abnormal osteoblast function.

❍   **What are the four most common posterior fossa masses in children?**

Medulloblastoma and astrocytoma (most common), Brainstem glioma, and Ependymoma.

❍   **CT of a newborn with hepatosplenomegaly and a petechial rash reveals periventricular foci of high attenuation, moderate dilatation of the ventricles, and microcephaly. Probable diagnosis?**

Cytomegalovirus encephalitis, also consider toxoplasmosis and TS.

❍   **Where are intracranial calcifications found in congenital toxoplasmosis and CMV encephalitis?**

*Toxoplasmosis:* intraparenchymal.
*CMV encephalitis:* circumventricular.

❍   **What is the most common congenital solid tumor in the newborn?**

Sacrococcygeal teratoma.

❍   **A newborn infant presents in acute respiratory distress. Chest x-ray shows hypoventilation, a diffuse reticulogranular infiltrate, and prominent air bronchograms. Diagnosis?**

Respiratory distress syndrome (RDS). Also consider pneumonia, pulmonary hemorrhage, pulmonary edema, and sepsis.

❍   **If a pleural effusion is present as well as the above findings, what is your diagnosis?**

Pleural effusion is not a feature of RDS. It is seen in two-thirds of patients with pneumonia.

❍   **What is the pathophysiology of RDS?**

Inadequate surfactant production. It is most commonly seen in low-birthweight infants born before 36 weeks.

❍   **At the end of the first week of life, a child presents to the ED and a repeat x-ray demonstrates diffuse bilateral hazy infiltrates and cardiomegaly. Diagnosis?**

Patent ductus arteriosus. Left-to-right shunt causes pulmonary edema.

❍   **A 4-year-old boy presents with acute respiratory distress, dysphagia, and inspiratory stridor. A lateral x-ray reveals an enlarged epiglottis with thick aryepiglottic folds. DDX?**

Epiglottitis, hemophilia, foreign body, angioneurotic edema, and caustic ingestion.

❍   **What should be the first x-ray examination?**

Upright lateral and anteroposterior (AP) soft tissue x-rays of the upper airway. Acute airway obstruction is more likely if the patient is supine.

○ **What part of the airway is involved in epiglottitis?**

The supraglottic region. In 25% of patients, there is subglottic edema. In croup, the epiglottis and aryepiglottic folds are normal.

○ **What is the most common cause of acute epiglottitis?**

*Haemophilus influenzae* type B.

○ **What is the most common age group to aspirate a foreign body?**

Less than 3 years.

○ **What is the most common object aspirated?**

Peanuts. Few foreign bodies are radiopaque.

○ **Which side is most commonly affected?**

Right.

○ **A nine month old child presents with cyanosis. A chest x-ray reveals decreased pulmonary vascularity and a normal heart size. Diagnosis?**

Tetralogy of Fallott (TOF). Other causes of DDx of right-sided obstruction include pulmonary stenosis with atrial septal defect, transposition of great vessels with pulmonic stenosis, tricuspid atresia with pulmonic stenosis, pulmonary atresia, and Ebstein malformation.

○ **How does heart size help diagnose TOF?**

In TOF, the heart is normal-sized or minimally enlarged. Significant cardiomegaly occurs in tricuspid atresia, pulmonary stenosis/atresia, and Ebstein malformation.

○ **The patient has a normal-sized heart and TOF. What other findings may be present on the chest x-ray?**

Reticular pattern, right sided aorta, asymmetric pulmonary vascularity, concavity in the region of the pulmonary artery trunk (due to a small or absent pulmonary artery), and enlarged right ventricle giving a boot-shaped heart appearance.

○ **An eight-year old boy presents to the ED with a fever, chronic cough and recurrent pneumonia. Chest x-ray findings include reticulonodular infiltrates in the upper lobes, hilar adenopathy, perihilar linear densities, and finger-like opacities in the upper lung fields. Diagnosis?**

Cystic fibrosis (CF).

○ **What CT findings would you expect in a patient with CF?**

Bronchiectasis, bronchial wall thickening, bullae, consolidation, emphysema, interstitial cyst, mucous plugs, and subsegmental or segmental collapse.

○ **What pulmonary complications are expected with CF?**

Mucus plugging (cause of death in 95%), pneumothorax, cor pulmonale, hypertropic pulmonary osteoarthropathy, hemoptysis.

O   **Which organism is most commonly responsible for recurrent pneumonias in CF patients?**

*Pseudomonas aeruginosa.* Less commonly, *Staphylococcus aureus.*

O   **A 14 year-old patient with known CF presents to the ED with abdominal pain and a palpable mass in the right lower quadrant. Abdominal x-ray reveals a granular bubbly mass and a partial small-bowel obstruction. Diagnosis?**

Meconium ileus. Meconium ileus can be complicated by volvulus or intussusception.

O   **X-rays of a newborn shows numerous dilated small-bowel loops and air-fluid levels. The intestinal contents appear bubbly. Diagnosis?**

Meconium ileus associated with CF. Other causes may include Hirschsprung's disease, meconium ileus, ileal stenosis, meconium plug syndrome, small left colon syndrome, and ileal atresia.

O   **A 2-year-old presents with acute violent abdominal pain and vomiting. X-ray of the abdomen reveals a small-bowel obstruction. Diagnosis?**

Intussusception. Other possible causes include appendicitis, adhesions, malrotation, Meckel diverticulum, and incarcerated hernia.

O   **What is the most common cause of acquired small-bowel obstruction?**

Intussusception is the leading cause of small-bowel obstruction between 6 months and 2 years.

O   **What is the initial study of choice?**

Usually ultrasound. If a high level suspicion, consider a water-soluble contrast or air enema. Avoid barium because of the risk of peritonitis if perforation occurs. A retrograde contrast study can diagnose and treat intussusception. The only contraindications to an enema are shock, peritonitis, and pneumoperitoneum. If ultrasound does not demonstrate intussusception, no further study is needed.

O   **What ultrasound findings are expected in intussusception?**

Transverse scans will demonstrate a target, bull's-eye or doughnut signs. On longitudinal scans, pseudokidney, sandwich, or hayfork signs will be seen.

O   **What is the peak incidence of intussusception?**

6 months to 2 years.

O   **What is the most common cause of intussusception?**

95% are idiopathic, usually from mucosal edema and lymphoid hyperplasia following gastroenteritis. The rest are a result of a lead point, most commonly a Meckel diverticulum.

O   **A 7-day-old premature infant presents with blood-streaked stools and diarrhea. X-rays demonstrate tubular-appearing bowel loops with minimal separation. A small triangle of lucency between bowel loops is noted in the right upper quadrant. Diagnosis?**

NEC. Other causes of pneumoperitoneum in a newborn include distal obstruction, idiopathic gastric perforation, and iatrogenic causes. Further inspection may reveal subtle curvilinear lucency around loops of bowel. This suggests pneumatosis intestinalis which is present in 80% of patients with NEC. Pneumoperitoneum indicates perforation. With pneumoperitoneum, air outlines the falciform ligament (football sign).

○ **What is the prognosis if air is discovered in the portal venous system?**

Portal venous air is associated with bowel necrosis and impending perforation.
While portal venous air suggests a poor prognosis, with aggressive treatment, air may be transient and does not imply a hopeless outcome.

○ **What causes NEC?**

NEC is the most common GI emergency in newborns. It develops more than 48 to 72 hours after birth and within the first 10 days of the life in 90% of patients. Risk factors include prematurity, Hirschsprung's disease, and bowel obstruction.

○ **What are the two most common complications of NEC?**

Inflammatory strictures and bowel perforation.

# STATISTICS AND PREVENTIVE

○ **At what point should AZT treatment begin in an asymptomatic patient with HIV?**

When the CD-4+ count reaches 300 cells/mm$^3$ and 500 cells/mm$^3$, respectively.

○ **What is the prophylactic regime of choice for PCP in patients with AIDS?**

Trimethoprim-sulfamethoxazole DS should be started when the CD-4+ count reaches 200 cells/mm$^3$.

○ **At what point should prophylaxis treatment against Mycobacterium acium-intracellulare and toxoplasmosis be started in patients with AIDS?**

When the CD-4+ count reaches 100 cells/mm$^3$.

○ **What percentage of untreated group A *β-hemolytic streptococcal* infections will progress to rheumatic fever?**

3%. Increased incidence of the disease is noted in lower socioeconomic areas.

○ **In what age group is post streptococcal glomerulonephritis <u>most common</u>?**

Peak incidence is between ages 3 and 7.

○ **What is used to control outbreaks of meningococcal meningitis?**

Rifampin and ciprofloxacin are used as chemoprophylaxis for contacts.

○ **Which has a longer incubation period in food poisoning, Staphylococcus or Salmonella?**

Salmonella. It is generally ingested in small doses, then it multiplies in the GI tract. Symptoms occur 6–48 hours after ingestion. With Staphylococcus, the disease process is dependent not on the reproduction of the organism within the host, but rather on the enterotoxin it has already produced on the contaminated food.

○ **How many millimeters indicate a positive reaction to the Mantoux skin test in a person with HIV?**

$\geq 5$ mm. In individuals with risk factors for TB, induration must be $\geq 10$ mm. For those with no risk factors, induration must be $\geq 15$ mm to be positive.

○ **What is the principal vector for Lyme disease in the northeastern United States?**

The black-legged tick, also known as the "deer tick", *Ixodes scapularis*.

○ **An 8 year-old boy has recently acquired a pet iguana. This may place the household at increased risk of what disease?**

Salmonellosis.

○  **What is the most important factor for reducing infectious disease transmission in day care centers?**

Hand-washing.

○  **You have diagnosed an *E. coli* O157:H7 infection in an 18 month old child who attends day care. When should you allow the child to return to day care?**

After diarrhea resolves and two stool cultures are negative.

○  **A 4-year-old child who attends day care has impetigo. When should the child be allowed to return to day care?**

24 hours after treatment has been initiated.

○  **A 4-year-old child who attends day care has streptococcal pharyngitis. When should this child be allowed to return to day care?**

24 hours after treatment has been initiated and after the child has been afebrile for 24 hours.

○  **A three-year-old girl has varicella. When should she be allowed to return to day care?**

6 days after the onset of the rash or sooner if all lesions have dried and crusted.

○  **A 15-month-old boy has a mild case of hepatitis A. When should he be allowed to return to day care?**

1 week after onset of illness or jaundice.

○  **A friend of yours tells you his wife has caught "a bad case of the flu", with all the typical signs and symptoms. He is concerned that he and their children will catch it, and they want to avoid that. What can they do to prevent catching it?**

Wash your hands frequently, avoid touching your face, and maintain a healthy diet.

# LEGAL PEARLS

○ **In general, do minors have the right to give consent for their own treatment?**

No--this right belongs to their parents or guardians.

○ **In an emergency, is it necessary to obtain consent in order to treat a child?**

No.

○ **May a child who lives away from home, is no longer subject to parental control, is economically self-supporting, is married, or is a member of the armed forces give or refuse consent to treatment?**

In general, yes. Such children are considered *emancipated minors*.

○ **May a child who is sufficiently mature to understand the nature of his/her illness and the potential risks and benefits of proposed therapy give or refuse consent to treatment?**

In general, yes. Such children are considered *mature minors*.

○ **Are there other circumstances in which a child has the right to give informed consent to treatment?**

Yes--many states have laws giving children such rights for treatment of sexually transmitted or other communicable diseases, crisis counseling, or substance abuse.

○ **What are the physician's legal obligations where a minor child requests that information obtained in the course of treatment not be communicated to the child's parents?**

In the absence of circumstances such as those outlined in the preceding questions, the physician may not legally honor such a request.

○ **May Jehovah's Witness parents refuse blood transfusions for their minor children?**

No.

○ **May parents be criminally prosecuted if their child dies because they treated the child with prayer rather than with medicine?**

Yes, in some jurisdictions.

○ **May parents authorize removal of life support for a minor child in a persistent vegetative state?**

Yes.

○ **Is it legally required for a physician who suspects child abuse or neglect to report it?**

Yes.

❍ **Is reporting required only for suspected physical abuse?**

No--emotional abuse, sexual abuse, and other forms of abuse are covered by reporting statutes.

❍ **May a parent's refusal to authorize indicated medical treatment be considered child neglect for purposes of the reporting statute?**

Yes.

❍ **May a physician suffer a penalty for failure to report suspected abuse, neglect, or endangerment?**

Yes.

❍ **May a physician be sued by a child or family for failing to report suspected abuse, neglect, or endangerment?**

Yes.

❍ **What would it take for the child or family to win such a suit?**

They must show that the failure to report contributed significantly to a subsequent injury that might have been averted.

❍ **May a physician be sued for defamation based on her/his report of suspected abuse, neglect, or endangerment?**

No, if the report was made in good faith.

❍ **May mothers who engage in substance abuse while pregnant be the subject of criminal prosecution?**

No--such prosecutions have been brought but not upheld.

❍ **In order for a physician to be guilty of malpractice, must the existence of a physician-patient relationship be proven?**

Yes.

❍ **What is medical negligence?**

Acting below the accepted standard of care.

❍ **Is an emergency physician legally required to do what the best specialist in the field would do?**

No--only what a typical reasonable competent physician would do under the circumstances.

❍ **In order for a physician to be found guilty of malpractice, must it be shown that the patient was injured?**

Yes.

❍ **How are practitioners and hospitals that provide care for children legally judged?**

By widely accepted pediatric standards of care.

○ **In order for a physician to be found guilty of malpractice, must it be shown that the patient's injury was caused by the physician's act or omission?**

Yes.

○ **Are there any exceptions to the "informed consent" doctrine?**

Yes, consent may be implied if needed treatment is emergent or the patient's ability to make a decision is lost.

○ **Do all states follow the same common-law definition of "informed consent"?**

No, you must strictly adhere to your state's regulations.

○ **Does the law protect the parents in fully determining the care of their child?**

Yes, if the parents act in the best interest of the child.

○ **T/F: "Baby Doe" cases involve ethical decisions by providers refusing to treat a child with an infectious disease.**

False. "Baby Doe" cases include decision making in cases with severely handicapped or critically ill newborns. Decisions are made by the parents and physicians involved in the child's care.

○ **Identify one resource the provider can utilize in dealing with complex decisions surrounding the care of neonates?**

The hospital ethics committee is a valuable resource for the healthcare providers.

○ **How can a child acquire status of an "emancipated minor"?**

Marriage, judicial decree, military service, parental consent, failure of parents to meet legal responsibilities, living apart from and being financially independent of parents, motherhood.

○ **T/F: Under the term "vicarious liability," the team leader is responsible for the actions of others.**

False. Each team member is held responsible for his or her actions. Each team member is held to the standard of care for his or her level of training.

○ **What specific criteria for brain death in children have been established and validated?**

None. There are a number of definitions used to define brain death in children. Circumstances such as hypothermia, drug use, or idiopathic causes of brain injury or insult may alter neurologic criteria determining the diagnosis of death.

○ **T/F: If the healthcare provider can safely care for the adult patient, he or she can safely care for a child.**

False. Children are different from adults. The provider must have a sound knowledge base with pediatric standards of care.

○ **Is organ donation a consideration when a child is the victim?**

Yes. If approached with respect and sensitivity, organ donation may ultimately benefit the child's family.

○ **When does the legal duty to meet a "reasonable standard" of care commence for the healthcare provider?**

Once he or she performs an act that may be construed as rendering care.

○ **What form of consent traditionally applies to the emergency situation?**

Implied consent.

○ **If a healthcare provider treats a patient without first being granted permission, what may that provider be guilty of committing?**

Assault.

○ **What are the three essential operational elements of informed consent?**

1) A careful assessment of the patient's decision-making capacity.
2) A judgment as to the "voluntariness" of the decisions.
3) A determination of the nature and extent of the information to be disclosed.

○ **In what three ways is patient decision-making capacity reflected?**

In his or her ability to comprehend, communicate, and appreciate the consequences of available choices.

○ **To what does "voluntariness" refer?**

The absence of internal or extrinsic pressures that may coercively restrict patient options.

○ **What does the "reasonable person" standard require physicians to disclose when obtaining informed consent from a patient?**

Those material facts concerning treatment alternatives and risks that a reasonable person would need to make an informed decision.

○ **What is "therapeutic privilege?"**

If there is strong reason to believe that the disclosure involved in obtaining informed consent may cause serious psychological harm, physicians may be excused for failing to obtain it.

○ **T/F: States vary considerably with respect to their statutory or common-law definition of informed consent.**

True.

○ **When may parents make medical decisions on behalf of their children contrary to physician advice?**

On condition they fulfill the duty to provide necessary care for minor children.

○ **When may the state assert its interests in protecting the welfare of children by invoking child protection statutes to override parental wishes?**

If parents fail to provide their children with at least a minimum standard of medical care.

○ **If a parent makes a decision on behalf of his or her child motivated by strong family convictions, can the courts interfere?**

Courts regularly uphold such interventions when parent refusals may be life threatening.

○ **What if the consequences are grave, but not life threatening?**

States have varied in their willingness to intervene in such cases, reflecting the continuing struggle to balance the rights of individual children and family privacy.

○ **Are there exemptions to child protection statutes for parents who seek non-traditional forms of treatment based on religious convictions?**

Many state child-protection statutes have included such exemptions, although the American Academy of Pediatrics has urged states to repeal such provisions.

○ **According to Congressional guidelines, under what three conditions may treatment be withheld from neonates?**

1) The infant is chronically and irreversibly comatose.
2) Treatment would merely prolong dying or would not be effective in ameliorating or correcting all of the infant's life-threatening conditions.
3) Treatment would be virtually futile in terms of survival and therefore inhumane.

○ **How is a "minor" defined?**

Historically, the right of self-determination is recognized at the legal age of maturity, 18 years. Below this age a patient is considered a minor.

○ **Do minors have the right to consent to medical treatment?**

Many state legislatures and courts have expanded minors' rights to consent to medical treatment, although great variability in this approach exists from state to state.

○ **What are "mature minor" rules?**

Statutory rules that uphold the validity of consent given by minors if the treatment is appropriate and the minor is considered capable of comprehending the clinical circumstances and therapeutic options.

○ **What are two conditions that some states allow minors to consent to treat?**

Venereal disease and substance abuse.

○ **What is a "variable competence approach" to minors' consent?**

One that considers developmental aspects of cognitive and psychosocial maturation.

○ **In order to prevail in a malpractice suit, what must the patient prove?**

That the healthcare provider failed in his or her *duty* to provide the patient with the degree of knowledge, skill, and care usually exercised by a reasonable and prudent provider under similar circumstances, given the prevailing state of medical knowledge and available resources, and that the *specific injury* was *caused* by that failure.

○ **Are errors in judgment evidence of malpractice?**

Not by themselves.

○ **When does a provider's legal duty toward a patient begin?**

With a mutual agreement to provide care for compensation or with any act that may represent an undertaking to provide care.

○ **Must a patient have suffered an injury in order to prevail in a malpractice suit?**

Yes. Even if evidence demonstrates that the care provided was substandard, a claim of medical malpractice will fail if the patient escaped injury.

○ **What is "standard of care"?**

The degree of care and skill expected of a reasonably competent practitioner of the same class, acting in the same or similar circumstances.

○ **T/F: Failure to obtain consent can be considered malpractice.**

True. Proof of negligence in malpractice cases may be based on failure to obtain informed consent.

○ **What three things must be proven in order to prove malpractice based on lack of consent?**

1. That the provider failed to disclose all the material facts that a reasonable person would require to make an informed decision.
2. That the patient's injury was caused by the provider's act, for which the patient granted uninformed permission.
3. That a reasonable person would have withheld consent had the material facts been disclosed.

○ **Since consent in CPR may be implied in cardiac arrest cases, when may problems arise?**

In emergency situations when documents on the victim's person or statements made by family members purport to represent the victim's intended refusal of CPR.

○ **What is the generally recognized practice in such situations?**

To initiate resuscitative efforts, with the understanding that CPR may be discontinued based on subsequent authentication of the patient's previously expressed wishes.

○ **What is the "captain-of-the-ship" doctrine?**

That a leader be held vicariously liable for the conduct of others in the group, depending on his or her level of control or right of control of the group members.

○ **Once you have initiated CPR, do you incur a legal liability to continue?**

Once steps are initiated and termination would place the victim in a worse position or compromise the likelihood of assistance from others, the potential rescuer incurs a legal duty to perform appropriately.

○ **How are conflicts between legitimate parental rights of family privacy and the state's interest in protecting the welfare of children decided?**

On whether life-sustaining treatment serves the best interest of an individual child.

○ **What two important elements should hospital policies governing orders not to resuscitate contain?**

1) Requirements that do-not-resuscitate orders be written on the order sheet, accompanied by progress notes that explain the rationale for the decision and identify the participants in the decision-making process.
2) Guidelines for prior judicial review in specifically enumerated circumstances.

○ **What one of two conditions must be met to conform to the Model Uniform Determination of Death Act?**

1) Irreversible cessation of circulation and respiratory function OR
2) Irreversible cessation of all functions of the entire brain including the brain stem

○ **T/F: Criteria developed for brain death in adults and children are the same.**

False. Specific criteria for brain death developed for adults have not been validated for children.

○ **T/F: Cardiopulmonary support systems may be withdrawn from brain-dead patients without judicial review or fear of legal repercussions.**

True.

# RANDOM PEARLS

○   **What signs should be charted when performing a neurological exam on a patient with a suspected anterior dislocation of the shoulder?**

Sensation over the lateral deltoid. In anterior dislocations of the shoulder, the radial nerve may be easily torn. Intact sensation to the lateral deltoid will indicate an intact radial nerve.

○   **A patient recently hit in the eye during a brawl has diplopia when looking up. The injured eye does not appear able to look up. What is the diagnosis?**

Orbital blowout fracture with entrapment of inferior rectus or inferior oblique.

○   **When estimating vaginal blood loss in the gynecological patient, sanitary pads are often used as a means of measurement. How much blood loss can be estimated per pad?**

20-30 ml.

○   **Which organism is typically responsible for causing bacterial conjunctivitis?**

*Staphylococcus*. The second most common organism is *Streptococcus*.

○   **Which virus causes herpangina?**

*Coxsackievirus Group A*. A sore throat, fever, malaise, and vesicular lesions on the posterior pharynx or the soft palate are often seen with this disease.

○   **Which organisms most often induce lymphedema?**

*Staphylococcus* or β-hemolytic *Streptococcus*.

○   **Name two causes of toxic epidermal necrolysis.**

1) Drug or chemical. The onset of this condition by drug and chemical-related causes typically occurs in adults and is characterized by cleavage at the derma-epidermal junction.
2) Staphylococcal. Bacterial-related SSSS is usually contracted by children < 5 years and results in the an intraepidermal cleavage beneath the stratum granulosum.

○   **Describe the presentation of SSSS.**

This disease begins after URI or purulent conjunctivitis. Initially, the lesions are tender, erythematous, and scarlatiniform and they are usually found on the face, neck, axillae, and groin. Later, the skin peels off in sheets with lateral pressure, and a + Nikolsky's sign is displayed.

○   **Which nerve is usually injured in glenohumeral dislocation?**

Axillary nerve (numb area over lateral deltoid).

○   **What is the most common form of anorectal abscess?**

Perianal abscess.

○ **Describe the mechanism and cause of a boutonniere deformity.**

A Boutonniere deformity is secondary to rupture of the extensor apparatus of the PIP joint. The cause of the injury is a PIP joint which is flexed and a DIP joint which is hyperextended. Treat by splinting the PIP joint in full extension.

○ **What are the 4 causes of central cyanosis with decreased $SaO_2$?**

1. Decreased $PaO_2$ or decreased $O_2$ diffusion.
2. Hypoventilation.
3. V-Q mismatch, pulmonary shunting.
4. Dysfunctional hemoglobin, which includes sickle cell crisis and drug-induced hemoglobinopathies.

N.B. Hb-CO does not cause cyanosis, although the cherry red appearance of skin and mucous membranes can suggest cyanosis.

○ **What is a positive Chvostek's sign?**

Chvostek's sign is characterized by a twitch in the corner of the mouth that occurs when the examiner taps the facial nerve located in front of the ear. It is present in approximately 10–30% of normal individuals. Eyelid muscle contraction resulting from the Chvostek's maneuver is generally indicative of hypocalcemia.

○ **What is Trousseau's sign and when is it exhibited?**

Trousseau's sign is a carpal spasm that is induced when a blood pressure cuff on the upper arm maintains a pressure above systolic for approximately 3 minutes. Fingers become spastically extended at the interphalangeal joints and flexed at the metacarpophalangeal joints. Trousseau's is generally a more reliable indicator of hypocalcemia than the Chvostek's sign.

○ **What are the two most common causes of fatal anaphylaxis?**

1) Drug reactions (95% of which are due to penicillin). Parenteral administration results in the deaths of approximately 300 people/year.
2) Hymenopteran stings cause fatal anaphylaxis in 100 people/year.

○ **Which type of hypersensitivity reaction is responsible for anaphylaxis?**

Type I (IgE mediated) hypersensitivity reaction. Immediate IgE binds allergen, and stimulate mast cells and basophils. Examples include food allergy and asthma.

○ **What is the single most common cause of upper GI tract hemorrhage?**

Duodenal ulcers.

○ **What are Kanavel's four cardinal signs of infectious digital flexor tenosynovitis?**

1. Tenderness along the tendon sheath.
2. Finger held in flexion.
3. Pain on passive extension of the finger.
4. Finger swelling.

○ **Which organism most commonly causes acute infectious endocarditis?**

*Staphylococcus aureus.*

○ **Describe the skin lesions found in a patient with disseminated gonococcemia.**

Umbilicated pustule with a red halo.

○ **Describe the skin lesions associated with a *Pseudomonas aeruginosa* infection.**

*Pseudomonas aeruginosa* typically produces pale, erythematous skin lesions that are approximately 1 cm in size with an ulcerated necrotic center (ecthyma gangrenosum).

○ **Describe the signs and symptoms of spinal shock.**

Spinal shock represents complete loss of spinal cord function below the level of injury. Patients have flaccid paralysis, complete sensory loss, areflexia, and loss of autonomic function. Such patients are usually bradycardic, hypotensive, hypothermic, and vasodilated.

○ **Active adduction of the thumb tests which nerve?**

Ulnar nerve.

○ **Describe the rash that is present with exanthem subitum (roseola).**

The rash is usually found on the trunk and the neck and is maculopapular.

○ **What is the most common site of Crohn's disease?**

The ileum.

○ **What are the signs and symptoms of Crohn's disease?**

Fever, diarrhea, right lower quadrant pain with mass possible, fistulas, rectal prolapse, perianal fissures, and abscesses. Arthritis, uveitis, and liver disease are also associated with this condition.

○ **What systemic diseases are associated with Crohn's disease?**

Pyoderma gangrenosum, uveitis, episclerosis, scleritis, arthritis, erythema nodosum, and nephrolithiasis.

○ **What contrast x-ray findings are associated with Crohn's disease?**

The segmental involvement in the colon with an abnormal mucosal pattern and fistulas, often without involvement of the rectum. A narrowing of the small intestine may also be displayed.

○ **What are the principal signs and symptoms of ulcerative colitis?**

Fever, weight loss, tachycardia, panniculitis, and six bloody bowel movements per day.

○ **Does toxic megacolon commonly occur with ulcerative colitis or with Crohn's disease?**

Toxic megacolon is a very common, serious complication of ulcerative colitis.

○ **What are the two most common causes of acute diarrhea?**

Rotavirus and Norwalk agent.

O   **What is the most common cause of diarrhea in a child less than one year old?**

Rotavirus.

O   **Which cause of diarrhea is most commonly associated with seizures?**

*Shigella.*

O   **What induces rose spots and watery diarrhea, as well as high fever and relative bradycardia?**

*Salmonella.*

O   **What is the treatment for individuals infected with *Salmonella*?**

Supportive care without antibiotics. However, if a severe fever is exhibited, antibiotic therapy may be warranted.

O   **Which microbial agents are associated with mesenteric adenitis and pseudoappendicitis?**

*Yersinia.*

O   **What is the most common food–borne pathogen?**

Staphylococcus. This pathogen produces diarrhea and vomiting within 6–12 hours after ingestion.

O   **Which type of infectious gastroenteritis is associated with the consumption of seafood?**

Vibrio parahaemolyticus.

O   **Which type of diarrhea is perfuse and bloody, but does not involve vomiting?**

*Entamoeba histolytica.* Diarrhea that is not necessarily bloody and that is associated with contaminated meat may be due to *Clostridium perfringens*.

O   **What type of defect produces diminished pulses in the lower extremities of a pediatric patient?**

Coarctation of the aorta.

O   **What are the signs and symptoms of aortic stenosis in a child?**

Exercise intolerance, chest pain, and a systolic ejection click with a crescendo, decrescendo murmur radiating to the neck with a suprasternal thrill. No cyanosis!

O   **What are the signs of left-sided heart failure in an infant?**

Increased respiratory rate, shortness of breath, and sweating during feeding.

O   **What is the single most common cause of CHF in the second week of life?**

Coarctation of the aorta.

O   **What is the most common cause of impetigo?**

Group A *ß-hemolytic Streptococcus*.

○ **What is the most common cause of bullous impetigo?**

*Staphylococcus aureus.*

○ **What is the most common cause of orbital infections?**

*Staphylococcus aureus.* Periorbital infections are usually caused by *H. influenzae.*

○ **What is the most common cause of pediatric bacteremia?**

*Streptococcus pneumonia.*

○ **A patient presents with a staccato cough and a history of conjunctivitis in the first few weeks after birth. What causes this type of pneumonia?**

*Chlamydia trachomatis.*

○ **What is the most common cause of viral pneumonia in the pediatric patient?**

RSV.

○ **How do steroids function in the treatment of asthma?**

Steroids increase cAMP, decrease inflammation, and aid in restoring the function of ß-adrenergic responsiveness to adrenergic drugs.

○ **Which two viral illnesses are prodromes for Reye syndrome?**

Varicella (chicken pox) and influenzae B.

○ **What are the signs and symptoms of Reye syndrome.**

Irritability, combativeness, and lethargy, right upper quadrant tenderness, history of influenzae B or recent chicken pox, papilledema, hypoglycemia, and seizures. Lab results reveal hypoglycemia, an ammonia level greater than 20 times normal, and a bilirubin level that is normal.

○ **Describe the five stages of Reye syndrome.**

Stage I: Vomiting, lethargy, and liver dysfunction.
Stage II: Disorientation, combativeness, delirium, hyperventilation, increased deep tendon reflexes, liver dysfunction, hyperexcitable, tachypnea, fever, tachycardia, sweating, and pupillary dilatation.
Stage III: Coma, decorticate rigidity, increased respiratory rate, and a mortality rate of 50%.
Stage IV: Coma, decerebrate posturing, no ocular reflexes, loss of corneal reflexes, and liver damage.
Stage V: Loss of deep tendon reflexes, seizures, flaccidity, respiratory arrest, and 95% mortality.

○ **In the pediatric esophagus, where is a foreign body most commonly lodged.**

The cricopharyngeal narrowing.

○ **What is the most common cause of cardiac arrest in an uremic patient?**

Hyperkalemia.

○ **What is the most common cause of right sided endocarditis in IV drug addicts?**

*Staphylococcus aureus.*

○ **Which valve is the usually affected in IV drug addicts?**

The tricuspid.

○ **What is the most common cause of osteomyelitis or septic arthritis in an IV drug addict?**

*Serratia marcescens.*

○ **A baby boy is brought to the emergency department with vomiting and persistent crying for two hours. On exam, a testicle is tender and enlarged. What is the most common cause?**

A testicular torsion.

○ **What is the most common cause of hyponatremia?**

Dilution.

○ **A fracture of the acetabulum may be associated with damage to what nerve?**

The sciatic nerve.

○ **What are the causes of normal anion gap metabolic acidosis?**

Diarrhea, ammonium chloride, renal tubular acidosis, renal interstitial disease, hypoadrenalism, ureterosigmoidostomy, and acetazolamide.

○ **What are some common causes of respiratory alkalosis?**

Hyperventilation, such as shock, sepsis, trauma, asthma, PE, anemia, hepatic failure, heat stroke, and exhaustion, emotion, salicylate poisoning, hypoxemia, pregnancy, and inappropriate mechanical ventilation.

○ **How should neurogenic shock be managed?**

With the replacement of volume deficit followed by vasopressors.

○ **What is the order of appearance of a CHF on a chest x-ray?**

Initially cephalization and the redistribution of blood flow is observed, with the subsequent appearance interstitial edema with evident Kerley B lines, as well as a perihilar haze. These findings are followed by alveolar infiltrates in the typical butterfly appearance. Finally, flagrant pulmonary edema and effusions become evident.

○ **What is the classic EKG for Wolff-Parkinson-White syndrome?**

A change in the upstroke of QRS, the delta wave.

○ **What are the most common dysrhythmias associated with digitalis?**

PVC's.

○ **How many days after a measles vaccine could a fever and a rash be expected to develop?**

7–10 days.

○ **What is the most common complication of acute otitis media?**

Tympanic membrane perforation. Other complications include mastoiditis, cholesteatoma, and intracranial infections.

○ **Describe a mallet finger deformity.**

A mallet finger deformity is produced by forced flexion of the DIP joint when the finger is in full extension. The deformity is a result of either a rupture of the distal extensor tendon, or an avulsion fraction of the tendon insertion on the distal phalanx with a dorsal plate avulsion.

○ **What agents commonly induce the onset of laryngotracheitis?**

*Parainfluenza virus* type I.

○ **What electrolyte abnormality is commonly associated with the transfusion of packed red blood cells?**

Hypocalcemia secondary to citrate toxicity. Citrate, when rapidly infused, binds ionized calcium and therefore decreases the calcium level. Hyperkalemia may also develop with rapidly packed red blood cell transfusion, especially if the patient is in renal failure or if the blood products are old.

○ **Describe a typical patient with intussusception.**

Intussusception usually occurs in children between the ages of 3 months to 2 years. The majority are 5-10 months old, and it is more common in boys. The area of the ileocecal valve is typically the source of the problem.

○ **A patient suffers a rotational knee injury and hears a pop. Within 90 minutes a hemarthrosis develops. Where is the suspected location of the injury?**

The anterior cruciate.

○ **What are the signs and symptoms of acute pericardial tamponade?**

Triad of hypotension, elevated CVP, and tachycardia are usually indicative of either acute pericardial tamponade or a tension pneumothorax in a traumatized patient. Muffled heart tones may be auscultated.

○ **What EKG result is pathognomonic of pericardial tamponade?**

Total electrical alternans. Pulsus paradoxus is nonspecific. Muffled heart tones are subjective findings and are difficult to appreciate.

○ **What cause of death is secondary to an untreated tension pneumothorax?**

Decreased cardiac output. The vena cava is compressed, which lowers the right heart blood return and severely compromises stroke volume, blood pressure and cardiac output.

Ed. Note: 2° arrhythmias can also occur. V-tach in a young, apparently healthy person is 2° to a tension pneumothorax until proven otherwise. (JNA)

○ **Describe the symptoms and signs of varicella (chicken pox).**

The onset of varicella rash is 1–2 days after prodromal symptoms of slight malaise, anorexia, and fever. The rash begins on the trunk and scalp, appearing as faint macules and later becoming vesicles.

○ **Describe the signs of roseola infantum.**

Roseola infantum usually affects children ages 6 months to 3 years. It is characterized by a high fever that begins abruptly and lasts 3–5 days, possibly precipitating febrile seizures. A rash appears as the temperature drops to normal.

○ **How does a patient older than 12 months present with sickle cell disease?**

Initial symptoms are often pain in the joints, bones, and abdomen. The child may have abdominal tenderness and even rigidity. Mild icterus and anemia may be present.

○ **How does a child present with erythema infectiosum (fifth disease or slapcheek syndrome)?**

Fifth disease typically does not infect infants or adults. There are no prodromal symptoms. The illness usually begins with the sudden appearance of erythema of the cheeks, followed by a maculopapular rash on the trunk and extremities that evolve into a lacy pattern.

○ **Which organism typically causes paronychia?**

*Staphylococcus.*

○ **Describe the signs and symptoms of neuroleptic malignant syndrome.**

Muscle rigidity, autonomic disturbances, and acute organic brain syndrome. Blood pressure and pulse fluctuate wildly, and a fever as high as 42°C (108°F) may be evident. Muscle necrosis may occur with resultant myoglobinuria.

○ **Which organism commonly induces a septic joint in a child?**

*Staphylococcus aureus.*

○ **What organism commonly causes a septic joint in an adolescent?**

*Neisseria gonorrhoeae.*

○ **What are the signs of tension pneumothorax on a physical exam?**

Tachypnea, unilateral absent breath sounds, tachycardia, pallor, diaphoresis, cyanosis, tracheal deviation, hypotension, and neck vein distention.

○ **Which organism most commonly causes bacterial pneumonia, except for in the first week of life?**

*Streptococcus pneumoniae.*

○ **What is the most common cause of abdominal pain in children?**

Constipation.

○ **What is the most common cause of an intestinal obstruction in children under 2 years of age?**

Intussusception.

○ **What is the most common cause of pulsus paradoxus in a child?**

Asthma.

○ **What is the most common dysrhythmia associated with Wolff-Parkinson-White syndrome?**

A paroxysmal atrial tachycardia.

○ **What drug should be used to treat a patient in cardiac arrest secondary to hyperkalemia?**

Calcium chloride—IV acts fastest. Also provide $NaHCO_3$.

○ **What is an anaphylactoid reaction?**

An anaphylactoid reaction is very similar to anaphylaxis; however, it does not require prior exposure to the reaction product. Cases may occur from a radiopaque contrast media or from medications, such as NSAIDs.

○ **What are the common presentations of a transfusion reaction?**

Myalgia, dyspnea, fever associated with hypocalcemia, hemolysis, allergic reactions, hyperkalemia, citrate toxicity, hypothermia, coagulopathies, and altered hemoglobin function.

○ **What are the signs of the Cushing reflex?**

Increased systolic blood pressure and bradycardia, as a result of cerebral edema.

○ **When evaluating a pediatric cervical spine film, what are the normal values?**

The predental space in a child is < 5 mm; in an adult, it is < 3 mm. The posterior cervical line attaching the base of the spinous process of C1 to C3 should be considered. If the base of C2 spinous process lies > 2 mm behind the posterior cervical line, a hangman's fracture should be suspected. The anterior border of C2 to the posterior wall of the fornix distance is < 7 mm. Finally, the anterior border of C6 to the posterior wall of the trachea distance is 14 mm in children younger than 15 years of age; it is < 22 mm in an adult.

○ **What is the most serious complication associated with dental infections, besides possible respiratory compromise from Ludwig's angina?**

Septic cavernous sinus thrombosis.

○ **What are the complications of impetigo?**

Post streptococcal glomerulonephritis.

○ **Describe the key features of the Rocky Mountain Spotted Fever (RMSF) rash.**

Around the fourth day of fever, a rash begins on the wrists and ankles and spreads centripetally.

○ **What is the most serious transfusion reaction?**

Hemolytic. Treat with aggressive fluid replacement and Lasix.

○ **What is the most common transfusion reaction?**

Febrile.

○ **Describe the scarlet fever rash.**

The rash has a sandpaper type texture and begins on the face, neck, chest, and abdomen. It then spreads to extremities. Patients may also have strawberry tongue.

○ **Describe a patient with Chlamydial pneumonia.**

Chlamydial pneumonia is usually seen in children 2–6 weeks of age. The patient is afebrile and does not appear toxic.

○ **A patient has had 3 days of diarrhea which was abrupt in onset. The patient reports slimy green, malodorous stools that contain blood. In addition, the patient is febrile. What is the most likely cause?**

Salmonella.

○ **What is the ferric chloride test and what toxic ingestion does it detect?**

Add a few drops of 10% ferric chloride solution to a few drops of urine. A purple color indicates presence of salicylic acid. Ketones or phenothiazine can lead to falsely positive results.

○ **In what type of patients is Staphylococcal pneumonia likely?**

Patients that are in hospital, debilitated, or abusing drugs.

○ **What effect will heparin or warfarin overdose have on the prothrombin time (PT) the partial thromboplastin time (PTT)?**

When administered in excessive doses, both cause increases in PT and PTT.

○ **What are the classic findings of shaken baby syndrome?**

1. Failure to thrive.
2. Lethargy.
3. Seizures.
4. Retinal hemorrhages.
5. CT may show subarachnoid hemorrhage or subdural hematoma from torn bridging veins.

○ **Conjunctivitis is an associated finding in about what percentage of neonates with chlamydia pneumonia?**

About 50%.

○ **Neonates with chlamydia pneumonia are usually tachypneic with a bad cough. Are they febrile?**

Usually not.

○ **What is the most common bacterium causing septic arthritis of the hip?**

*Staphylococcus aureus*.

○ **Newborns should stop losing weight how many days after birth?**

About 6 days.

○ **What are some entities in the differential diagnosis of bloody diarrhea in the neonate?**

Necrotizing enterocolitis, bacterial enteritis, allergic reactions to milk, and iatrogenic causes secondary to antibiotics.

○ **Neonates with necrotizing enterocolitis are sick; what are some of the signs of sepsis to look for?**

Poor feeding, lethargy, fever, jaundice, abdominal distention, and poor color.

○ **What should be considered in the case of a neonate who has never passed stool?**

Meconium ileus or plug, Hirschsprung's disease, intestinal stenosis, or atresia.

○ **Anal stenosis, hypothyroidism, and Hirschsprung's disease can all present with what clinical sign?**

Constipation that was not present at birth but which began before the infant was 1 month old.

○ **Describe the signs and symptoms of a slipped capital femoral epiphysis. What x-ray tests are necessary for its diagnosis?**

Gradual onset of hip pain and stiffness with restriction of internal rotation; patient may walk with a limp. X-ray analysis should include both the anterior-posterior and lateral views of both hips. The slip of the epiphyseal plate posteriorly is best seen on the lateral view.

○ **Describe the signs and symptoms of a patient with chondromalacia patellae.**

Chondromalacia patellae typically occurs in young, active females. The pain is localized to the knee. There is no effusion and no history of trauma. Patella compression tests are usually positive.

○ **Describe the presentation of a patient with post extraction alveolitis.**

"Dry socket" pain occurs on the second or third day after extraction.

○ **Ludwig's angina typically involves what spaces in the head?**

The submental, sublingual, and submandibular spaces.

○ **What are the signs and symptoms of a peritonsillar abscess?**

Sore throat, dysarthria (hot potato voice), odynophagia, ipsilateral otalgia, low grade fever, trismus, and uvular displacement.

○ **What is the presentation of a patient with diphtheria?**

Sore throat, dysphagia, fever, and tachycardia. A dirty, tough gray fibrinous membrane so firmly adherent that removal causes bleeding may be present in the oropharynx. *Corynebacterium diphtheriae* exotoxin acts directly on cardiac, renal, and nervous systems. It can cause ocular bulbar paralysis that may suggest botulism or myasthenia gravis. The exotoxin may also cause flaccid limb weakness.

○ **What is the most common cause of acute food-borne disease?**

*Staphylococcus aureus* and the enterotoxins it produces.

○ **What are the common features of *Vibrio parahaemolyticus*?**

This condition is caused by organisms associated with oysters, clams, and crabs. Symptoms include cramps, vomiting, dysentery, and explosive diarrhea. Severe infections are treated with tetracycline and Chloramphenicol.

○ **Painful, bright red rectal bleeding is most often due to:**

Anal fissure. External hemorrhoids present with acute painful thrombosis and are not typically associated with constant, bright red bleeding. Internal hemorrhoids present with painless bright red bleeding, usually with defecation.

○ **How much protamine is required to neutralize 100 units of heparin?**

1 mg of protamine will neutralize ≈ 100 units of heparin. The maximum dose of protamine is 100 mg.

○ **What patient position will enhance the murmur of mitral stenosis?**

Left lateral decubitus.

○ **What is the optimal patient position and maneuver for auscultation of aortic insufficiency?**

Have the patient sit up and lean forward with his or her hands tightly clasped. During exhalation, listen at the left sternal border.

○ **What murmurs will the Valsalva maneuver increase?**

Only IHSS. All other murmurs are diminished.

○ **What is an interesting diagnostic feature of aortic regurgitation?**

Head bobbing.

○ **What effect does furosemide have on calcium excretion?**

Furosemide causes increased calcium excretion in the urine.

○ **What is the most common arrhythmia in mitral stenosis?**

Atrial fibrillation.

○ **How does dobutamine differ from dopamine?**

Dobutamine decreases afterload with less tendency to cause tachycardia.

○ **Describe Kerley A and B lines.**

Kerley A lines are straight, non-branching lines in the upper lung fields. Kerley B lines are horizontal, non-branching lines at the periphery of the lower lung fields.

○ **How should a patient with neuroleptic malignant syndrome be treated?**

1. Ice packs to the groin and axilla.
2. Cooling blankets.
3. Fan.
4. Water mist evaporation.
5. Dantrolene at an IV rate of 0.8 to 3 mg/kg IV q 6 hours to a total of 10 mg/kg.

○ **What are the effects of using ketamine in a pediatric patient?**

The child's eyes will be wide open with a glassy stare. He or she will have nystagmus, hyperemic flush, and hypersalivation. There will also be a slight rise in the heart rate. A very rare complication of ketamine use is laryngospasm. Hallucinations are a common side-effect in children over the age of 10. Sympathetic stimulation occurs increasing intracranial pressure.

○ **What are the contraindications to TAC?**

Mucus membranes, burns, and large abrasions. TAC used on the tongue and mucus membranes has led to status epilepticus and patient death due to the cocaine content.

○ **Why are quinolones contraindicated in children?**

Quinolones impair cartilage growth.

○ **A patient presents with a symmetric weakness that has progressed over several days and associated paresthesia. Diminished reflexes are noted. What is the diagnosis?**

Guillain-Barré syndrome. Other signs and symptoms are diminished reflexes, minimal loss of sensation, paresthesias, and leg weakness.

○ **What conditions may make the end tidal $CO_2$ monitor inaccurate?**

Monitor may be falsely yellow due to contamination from acid dilutants and drugs, such as lidocaine-HCl and epinephrine-HCl. Contamination with vomit or acid dilutants may also produce false readings.

○ **Under what conditions does neurogenic pulmonary edema occur?**

Associated with increased intracranial pressure from head trauma, subarachnoid hemorrhage, and even with seizures.

○ **What is the most commonly missed fracture in the elbow region?**

A radial head fracture. Like the navicular fracture, radiographic signs of a radial head fracture may not show up for days after the injury. A positive fat pad sign may be the only finding suggestive of this injury.

○ **What is the most common cause of food-borne viral gastroenteritis?**

Norwalk virus commonly found in shell fish.

○ **What signs indicate an HIV positive patient is at increased risk for opportunistic infections like PCP?**

An absolute CD-4 count of less than 200 and a CD-4 lymphocytic percentage of less than 20.

○ **A patient with a temperature of 29°C develops V-fib. Is defibrillation likely to be successful?**

Defibrillation should be attempted but is unlikely to be successful at temperatures less than 29°C.

○ **In the evaluation of retropharyngeal abscess, what is the usual age of the patients, how do they present, what diagnostic tests are used in their evaluation, and what treatment modalities are recommended?**

Retropharyngeal abscess is most commonly seen in children less than 4 years old. Usual presentation is with dysphagia, a muffled voice, stridor, and a sensation of a lump in the throat. Patients usually prefer to lie supine. Diagnosis is made with a soft tissue lateral neck film which may demonstrate edema and air/fluid levels. CT may be useful. Treatment includes airway, IV antibiotics, and admission to the ICU. Intubation may rupture the abscess.

○ **What is the usual cause of facial cellulitis in children less than 3 years of age?**

*H. influenzae*.

○ **What antibiotics should be avoided in myasthenia gravis patients?**

Polymyxin and aminoglycoside have curare-like properties that may cause paralysis in these patients.

○ **What is a chalazion?**

This is a Meibomian gland granuloma, a complication of conjunctivitis. A chalazion can deform the eyelid which can lead to blindness.

○ **How should a chalazion be treated?**

Surgical curettage.

○ **Patient presents with eye pain. She has a constricted pupil, ciliary flush, and red injected sclera at the limbus. What is the diagnosis?**

Acute iritis.

○ **A patient presents with fever, neck pain or neck stiffness, and trismus. Exam reveals pharyngeal edema with tonsil displacement and edema of the parotid area. What is the diagnosis?**

Parapharyngeal abscess.

○ **Describe Stevens-Johnson syndrome?**

It is a bullous form of erythema multiforme that involves mucous membranes. It may cause corneal ulcerations, anterior uveitis, or blindness.

○ **What is the most common site of aseptic necrosis?**

The hip.

○ **Which epicondyle is involved in tennis elbow?**

The lateral epicondyle.

○ **What is the most common site of infectious arthritis?**

The knee, followed by the hip. *Staphylococcus* is the most common cause.

○ **Describe the Gram stain appearance of *Staphylococcus aureus*.**

Gram-positive cocci in grape-like clusters.

○ **What findings mark the presentation of a patient with rapidly progressive glomerulonephritis?**

Hematuria (most common), edema (periorbital), HTN, ascites, pleural effusion, rales, and anuria.

○ **What arrhythmia is frequently encountered during renal dialysis?**

Hypokalemia induced ventricular fibrillation.

○ **A heroin addict presents with pulmonary edema. What is the best treatment?**

Naloxone, $O_2$, and ventilatory support. Don't bother using diuretics.

○ **How much energy should be used to cardiovert an unstable infant with a wide complex tachycardia?**

0.5–1.0 J/kg.

○ **How much energy should be used to cardiovert unstable VF in an infant?**

2 J/kg.

○ **Under what conditions should staphylococcal pneumonia be considered as a possible diagnosis?**

Although it only accounts for 1% of bacterial pneumonias, it should be considered in patients with sudden chills, fever, pleurisy, and cough—especially following a viral illness, such as measles or influenza.

○ **After the first month of life, what is the number # 1 cause of meningitis and the # 1 cause of pneumonia in children?**

Meningitis: *Streptococcus pneumoniae*.
Pneumonia: *Streptococcus pneumoniae*. *H. influenzae* is the second most common cause.

○ **Discuss infantile spasms.**

Onset is by 3–9 months of age. It typically lasts seconds, and may occur in single episodes or bursts. The EEG is often abnormal. 85% of these patients will be mentally handicapped.

○ **What causes Q fever?**

*Coxiella burnetii*, also known as *Rickettsia burnetii*. It is found in *Dermacentor andersoni* tick.

○ **Ludwig's angina pathology:**

Hemolytic streptococci, staphylococcus, mixed aerobes and anaerobes.

❍ **What is the most likely cause of CHF in a premature infant?**

PDA.

❍ **What is the most likely cause of CHF in the first 3 days of life?**

Transposition of the great vessels which leads to cyanosis and failure.

❍ **What is the most likely cause of CHF in the first week of life?**

Hypoplastic left ventricle.

❍ **What is the most likely cause of CHF in the second week of life?**

Coarctation of the aorta.

❍ **What is the most common cause of painless upper GI bleeding in an infant or child?**

Varices from portal hypertension.

❍ **What is the most common cause of major painless lower GI bleeding in an infant or child?**

Meckel's diverticulum.

❍ **Common cause of orbital cellulitis:**

*Staphylococcus aureus*.

❍ **What is the most common symptom in RMSF?**

Headache occurs in 90% of patients.

❍ **What is the causative organism of otitis externa?**

Pseudomonas.

❍ **What are the signs and symptoms of Lyme Disease, stages I–III?**

Stage I:   Erythema Chronicum Migrans, malaise, fatigue, headache, arthralgias, fever, and chills.
Stage II:  Neurologic and cardiac symptoms include headache, meningoencephalitis, facial nerve palsy, radiculoneuropathy, ophthalmitis, and 1°, 2° and 3° AV blocks.
Stage III: Arthritis (knee > shoulder > elbow > TMJ > ankle > wrist > hip > hands > feet).

❍ **With brain stem herniation, is decorticate or decerebrate posturing expected?**

Decerebrate posturing (hyperextension). Decorticate posturing is flexion of the upper extremities and extension of the lower extremities.

❍ **A patient presents after experiencing trauma to the head. He has an elevated systolic blood pressure and bradycardia. What is the diagnosis?**

Cushing reflex.

○ **What are the most common sites of stress fractures in the foot?**

Second and third metatarsals.

○ **What is the most common cause of subarachnoid hemorrhage in teenagers?**

AV malformations.

○ **What is the most common cause of acute aortic regurgitation?**

Infectious endocarditis.

○ **What is the most common congenital valvular disease?**

Bicuspid aortic valve.

○ **What metabolic abnormality is commonly associated with hypercalcemia?**

Hypokalemia.

○ **How may mydriasis caused by mydriatics and anticholinergic drugs be distinguished from mydriasis caused by third cranial nerve compression?**

Pilocarpine will reverse cranial nerve compression, but it won't have any effect on anticholinergic drugs or mydriatics.

○ **What is the chief benefit of dopamine, and what is its chief complication?**

The chief benefit is prompt elevation of blood pressure with ß-adrenergic effects at low doses and α-adrenergic effects at high doses.

○ **What is the chief effect of dobutamine?**

Dobutamine increases the cardiac contractility without increasing blood pressure.

○ **What is the most common cause of post splenectomy (postsplenic) sepsis?**

*Streptococcus* pneumonia.

○ **What is the most common cause of tricuspid regurgitation?**

Right heart failure secondary to left heart failure, typically caused by mitral stenosis.

# BIBLIOGRAPHY

**BOOKS/ARTICLES:**

Aaron CK, Bania TC: Insecticides: Organophosphates and Carbamates. In Goldfranks, LR (ed): Goldfrank's Toxicologic Emergencies. East Norwalk, CT, Appleton and Lange, 1994, pp 1105-1116.

*Acad Emerg Med* 1997; 4:1025

Plantz, S.H. Emergency Medicine Pearls of Wisdom. (6th Ed.). Lincoln, NE: Boston Medical Publishing, 2005.

Advanced Cardiac Life Support. Dallas: American Heart Association, 2001.

Advanced Trauma Life Support. Chicago: American College of Surgeons, 1995.

American Academy of Ophthalmology. Basic and Clinical Science Course. Section 8 (1994-95), Section 9 (1996-97) and Section 12 (1997-98).

Anderson, J.E. Grant's Atlas of Anatomy (10th Ed.). Baltimore: Williams & Wilkins, 1999.

Auerbach, P.S. Management of Wilderness and Environmental Emergencies (4th Ed.). St. Louis: C.V. Mosby Company, 2001.

Bakerman, S. ABCs of Interpretive Laboratory Data (3rd Ed.). Greenville: Interpretive Laboratory Data, Inc., 1994.

Barkin, R.M. Emergency Pediatrics (4th Ed.). St. Louis: C.V. Mosby Company, 2004.

Bartlett, J.G. and Gorbach, S.L., The triple threat of aspiration pneumonia. Chest . 1975. 68: 4.

Berkow, R. The Merck Manual (17th Ed.). Rahway: Merck Sharp & Dohme Research Laboratories, 1999.

Bork, K. Diagnosis and Treatment of Common Skin Diseases (2nd Ed). Philadelphia: W.B. Saunders Company, 1999.

Bryson, P.D. Comprehensive Review in Toxicology (2nd Ed.) Aspen Publishers, Inc., 1989

Cahill, B.C. and Ingbar, D.H., Massive hemoptysis. Clinics in Chest Medicine. 1994. 15: 147.

Cost factors in pediatric trauma: D. Gurses, A. Sarioghu-Buke, M. Baskan, et al. Can J Surg 46:441-445, (December), 2003. J Pediatr Surg. 2004 Jul;39(7):1149.

Cullom, RD Jr. and Chang, B (eds.) The Wills Eye Manual: Office and Emergency Room Diagnosis and Treatment of Eye Disease, Second Edition. JB Lippincott Co., Philadelphia. 1994.

Dambro, M.R. Griffith's 5 Minute Clinical Consult. Lippincott, Williams and Wilkins, 1998.

DeGowin, E.L. Bedside Diagnostic Examination (7th Ed). New York: Macmillan Publishing Co. Inc., 1999.

Diagnostic and Treatment Guidelines on Domestic Violence, AMA Publication.

Diagnostic and Treatment Guidelines on Sexual Assault, AMA Publication.

Ellenhorn M.J., Schonwald S., Ordog G., Wasserberger J., *Ellenhorn's Medical Toxicology* (3$^{rd}$ Edition), Williams & Wilkins, 2003.

Firearm Violence: Community Diagnosis and Treatment, Publication and slide show of Physicians for Social Responsibility

Fitzpatrick, T.B. Color Atlas and Synopsis of Clinical Dermatology (4$^{th}$ Ed). New York: McGraw-Hill Publishing Company, 2000.

General Russ Zajtchuk, M.C., U.S. Army Editor in Chief; Textbook of Military Medicine: *Medical Aspects of Chemical and Biological Warfare,* Published by the Office of the Surgeon General, Department of the Army, USA, 1997.

Goldrank, L.R., Flomenbaum N.E., Lewin N.A., Weisman R.S., Howland M.A., Hoffman R.S., *Goldfrank's Toxicologic Emergencies* (6$^{th}$ Edition), Appleton & Lange 1998, Stamford, CT.

Greenberg M.I., Hamilton R.J., Phillips S., *Occupational, Industrial and Environmental Toxicology* (2$^{nd}$ Edition), Mosby 2003, St Louis, MO.

Guidelines 2000 for Cardiopulmonary Resuscitation and Emergency Cardiac Care: An International Consensus on Science. *Circulation* 2000; 102:8 (suppl I): 1-I-370.

Harris, J.H. The Radiology of Emergency Medicine (4$^{th}$ Ed.). Baltimore: Lippincott, Williams and Wilkins, 2000.

Harrison, T.R. Principles of Internal Medicine (15$^{th}$ Ed.). New York: McGraw-Hill Book Company, 2001.

Harwood-Nuss, A. The Clinical Practice of Emergency Medicine (3$^{rd}$ Ed). Philadelphia: J.B. Lippincott, Williams & Wilkins, 2001.

Haxhija EQ, Nores H, Schober P, Hollwarth ME. Lung contusion-lacerations after blunt thoracic trauma in children. Pediatr Surg Int. 2004 Jun;20(6):412-4.

Hazinski, Mary Fran, et al., eds. *2000 Handbook of Emergency Cardiovascular Care for Healthcare Providers*. Dallas: American Heart Association, 2000.

Hazinski, Mary Fran, et al. eds. *Pediatric Advanced Life Support Provider Manual*. Dallas, American Heart Association, 2002

Hoppenfeld, S. Physical Examination of the Spine and Extremities. Norwalk: Appleton-Century-Crofts, 1976.

Kirk M  Smoke Inhalation. In Goldfranks, LR (7$^{th}$ ed): Goldfrank's Toxicologic Emergencies. East Norwalk, CT, Appleton and Lange, 2002, pp. 1183-1272.

Leaverton, P.E. A Review of Biostatistics (3rd Ed.). Boston: Little Brown and Company, 1986.

Marriott, H.J.L. Practical Electrocardiography (10$^{th}$ Ed.). Baltimore: Lippincott, Williams and Wilkins, 2001.

Moore, K.L. Clinically Oriented Anatomy. Baltimore: Williams & Wilkins, 1982.

Nelson, Waldo E. Textbook of Pediatrics. Philadelphia: W.B. Saunders Comany, 2004.

Pediatric Advanced Life Support (Part 10)," *Circulation* 2000; 102 (suppl. I): I-291—I234.

Pepose, JS, Holland, GN, and Wilhelmus, KR. Ocular Infection and Immunity. Mosby, St. Louis. 1995.

Perkins, E.S. An Atlas of Diseases of the Eye (4th Ed.). London: Churchill Livingstone, 1993.

Physicians' Desk Reference (58th Ed.). Oradell: Medical Economics Company Inc., 2004.

Plantz, SH. Emergency Medicine PreTest, Self-Assessment and Review, McGraw-Hill, 1990.

Rivers, C.S. Preparing for the Written Board Exam in Emergency Medicine. Milford: Emergency Medicine Educational Enterprises, Inc. 1992.

Roberts J, Tafuri J: Organophosphate and Carbamate Poisonings. In Tintinalli, JE (ed) Emergency Medicine: A Comprehensive Study Guide. New York, NY, McGraw-Hill, 1996, pp 822-827.

Robbins, S.L. Pathologic Basis of Disease (6th Ed.). Philadelphia: W.B. Saunders Company, 1999.

Rosen, P. Emergency Medicine Concepts and Clinical Practice (5th Ed.). St. Louis: Mosby Year Book, 2000.

Rowe, R.C. The Harriet Lane Handbook (16th Ed.). Chicago: Year Book Medical Publishers, Inc., 2002.

Simon, R.R. Emergency Orthopedics The Extremities (3rd Ed.). Norwalk: Appleton & Lange, 1995.

Simon, R.R. Emergency Procedures and Techniques (3rd Ed.). Baltimore: Lippincott, Williams and Wilkins, 2001.

Slaby, F. Radiographic Anatomy. New York: John Wiley & Sons, 1990.

Squire, L.F. Fundamentals of Radiology (5th Ed.). Cambridge: Harvard University Press, 1997.

Stedman, T.L. Illustrated Stedman's Medical Dictionary (27th Ed.). Baltimore: Lippincott, Williams & Wilkins, 2000.

Stewart, C.E. Environmental Emergencies. Baltimore: Lippincott, Williams and Wilkins, 1990.

The Hand Examination and Diagnosis (2nd Ed.). London: Churchill Livingstone, 1983.

The Hand Primary Care of Common Problems (2nd Ed.). London: Churchill Livingstone, 1990.

The Physician's Guide to Domestic Violence, Salber and Taliaferro, Volcano Press, 1995

Tietjen, P., Kaner, R.J. and Quinn, C.E., Aspiration Emergencies. Clinics in Chest Medicine. 1994. 15: 117.

Tintinalli, J.E. Emergency Medicine A Comprehensive Study Guide (5th Ed.). New York: McGraw-Hill, Inc., 1999.

Tomaszewski C: Carbon Monoxide. In Goldfranks, LR (ed): Goldfrank's Toxicologic Emergencies. East Norwalk, CT, Appleton and Lange, 1994, pp 1199-1210.

Tsang T, Demby AM. Penile fracture with urethral injury. The Journal of Urology, 1992;147:466-468.

Weinberg, S. Color Atlas of Pediatric Dermatology (4th Ed.). New York: McGraw-Hill, 2001.

Weiner, H.L. Neurology for the House Officer (6th Ed.). Baltimore: Lippincott,Williams & Wilkins, 2004.

Wilkins, E. W. Emergency Medicine (3rd Ed.). Baltimore: Lippincott, Williams & Wilkins, 1989.

# NOTES

# NOTES

# NOTES

# NOTES

# NOTES

UMDNJ-SMITH LIBRARY
30 12TH AVENUE
NEWARK, N.J. 07103

DEMCO